Instructor's Manual
to accompany

CRITICAL THINKING IN MEDICAL-SURGICAL SETTINGS
A Case Study Approach

Maryl L. Winningham, APRN, PhD, FACSM
Assistant Professor
and
Barbara A. Preusser, APRN, PhD, CCRN
Assistant Professor

University of Utah College of Nursing
Salt Lake City, Utah 84112

Mosby

St. Louis Baltimore Boston Carlsbad Chicago Naples New York Philadelphia Portland
London Madrid Mexico City Singapore Sydney Tokyo Toronto Wiesbaden

Mosby
Dedicated to Publishing Excellence

A Times Mirror Company

Publisher: Nancy L. Coon
Editor: Michael S. Ledbetter
Senior Developmental Editor: Teri Merchant
Project Supervisor: Gayle Morris
Cover Design: David Zielinski

Printed in the United States of America

Mosby-Year Book, Inc.
11830 Westline Industrial Drive, St. Louis, Missouri 63146

International Standard Book Number 0-8151-9419-6

96 97 98 99 90 00 / 9 8 7 6 5 4 3 2 1

CONTRIBUTORS

Kathleen Baldwin, RN, PhD, CEN, CCRN
Assistant Professor
College of Nursing
University of Utah
Salt Lake City, Utah
(Multiple system disorders)

Julie Balk, MS, ANP
Advanced Nurse Practitioner
The Heart Center of Salt Lake
Salt Lake City, Utah
(Genitourinary, cardiovascular disorders)

Nancy Brazelton, RN, MS
Clinical Instructor
College of Nursing
University of Utah
Salt Lake City, Utah
(Neurologic disorders)

Sheryl Davey, RN, MS
Assistant Professor (Clinical)
College of Nursing
University of Utah
Salt Lake City, Utah
(Cardiovascular disorders)

Cynthia Godsey, FNP, MS
Health Care Consultant
Salt Lake City, Utah
(Respiratory disorders)

Carol Green-Nigro, RN, PhD
Nursing Instructor
Johnson County Community College
Overland Park, Kansas
(Immunologic disorders)

Lynn Hollister, RN,C, MS
Nursing Practice Coordinator
HCA St. Marks Hospital
Salt Lake City, Utah
(Introduction to *Instructor's Manual*; Genitourinary disorders)

Kathleen Kaufman, RN, MS
Assistant Professor (Clinical)
College of Nursing
University of Utah
Salt Lake City, Utah
(Gastrointestinal disorders)

Penny Marshall, RN, PhD
Nursing Instructor
Johnson County Community College
Overland Park, Kansas
(Endocrine disorders)

Shirley Otto, RN, MSN, AOCN, CRNI
Clinical Nurse Specialist
St. Francis Regional Medical Center
Wichita, Kansas
(Hematologic, oncologic disorders)

Barbara A. Preusser, APRN, PhD, CCRN
Assistant Professor
College of Nursing
University of Utah
Salt Lake City, Utah
(Pulmonary, gastrointestinal, endocrine, and neurological disorders; emergency situations)

Janet Reilly, RN, MS, CCRN
Assistant Professor (Clinical)
College of Nursing
University of Utah
Salt Lake City, Utah
(Pulmonary disorders)

Janyce Streeter, RN, MS, CCRN
Instructor
College of Nursing
Brigham Young University
Provo, Utah
(Musculoskeletal disorders)

Mary Jo Westin, RN, MS
Instructor
College of Nursing
Brigham Young University
Provo, Utah
(Musculoskeletal disorders)

Russ Wilshaw, RN, MS, CEA
Instructor
College of Nursing
Brigham Young University
Provo, Utah
(Musculoskeletal disorders)

Maryl L. Winningham, APRN, PhD, FACSM
Assistant Professor
College of Nursing
University of Utah
Salt Lake City, Utah
(Instructor's manual; Cardiovascular, endocrine, hematologic, musculoskeletal, and oncologic disorders)

Barbara J. Wirick, RN, MS, CEN
Assistant Professor
Weber State University
Ogden, Utah
(Emergency situations, endocrine disorders)

CONSULTANTS

Kathleen Baldwin, RN, PhD, CEN, CCRN
Assistant Professor
College of Nursing
University of Utah
Salt Lake City, Utah

Brian Barker, RPh
Clinical Pharmacist
Health Science Center
University of Utah
Salt Lake City, Utah
(Pharmacological science)

Sheila A. Dunn, RN, MSN, ANP
Clinical Instructor
St. Louis University
St. Louis, Missouri
Adult Nurse Practitioner
Southern Illiois Healthcare Foundation
Centerville, Illinois

Renata J. M. Engler, MD, COL, MC, USA
Allergy-Immunology Service
Walter Reed Army Medical Center
Washington, DC

L. Joan Goe, RN, EdD
Associate Professor
College of Nursing
University of Utah
Salt Lake City, Utah

Kim Litwack, RN, PhD, CPAN
Associate Professor
College of Nursing
University of New Mexico
Albuquerque, New Mexico

Judith L. Myers, RN, MSN
Assistant Professor
St. Louis University
St. Louis, Missouri

Linda K. Olinger, BS, BSMT, ASCP
Medical Technologist
Summa Health Systems
Akron, Ohio
(Laboratory Science)

Nimmi Welikala-Rasiah, RN, MSN, CCRN
Instructor
University of Nevada-Las Vegas
Las Vegas, Nevada

Linda J. Winningham, RD, MS
Ray, Michigan
(Nutritional Science)

Barbara J. Wirick, RN, MS, CEN
Assistant Professor
Weber State University
Ogden, Utah

To our students,
"who taught us everything we thought we knew!"

M.L.W. & B.A.P

ACKNOWLEDGMENTS

We would like to thank:

- Our patients who let us learn nursing by practicing on them.
- Those nurses we saw in action and told ourselves, "Now *that's* a *great nurse*!"
- The teachers who encouraged us to follow our convictions.

To them we humbly acknowledge our gratitude and indebtedness.

This book would never have become a reality if it weren't for the forbearance and help of the following individuals:

- Sue Meeks, whose job (and talent) it was to organize the raw material and make everything look good.
- Teri Merchant, Senior Development Editor, who tried to keep us on the straight and narrow, patiently listened to us complain, coordinated the review process, and edited this work.
- Michael Ledbetter, Editor, who made this book a reality, and Julie Council, Editorial Assistant, for their support.
- Our consultants and contributors, for the creative work they shared with us.
- Our colleagues and friends who put up with us during the months of heavy writing.
- Our dogs, who felt neglected over the past few months, and who will probably take a copy of this book and bury it deeply in the back yard.

M.L.W. & B.A.P.

INTRODUCTION

To the Instructors

Warning: Sacred cows sacrificed here.

It takes courage to lead into the future. We need new ways of thinking, functioning, and interacting as we enter the coming millennium. Nursing must either march into the future with bold and creative initiatives that address the health-care needs of our society, or it will mourn over the ashes of lost dignity and a dying profession. This book represents but one small step in our participation in that process. It started with our search for ways to encourage critical thinking in undergraduate students and anchor it to clinical realities. Although there were many detailed case studies in print, no books could be found that provided many different cases in a flexible context that could be a "prn" resource for faculty and students. Whenever we asked publisher's representatives if they knew of a large case studies book, they would ask if we wanted to write one. No, we didn't. But we were desperate; we wanted material to prepare our students for the type of clinical challenges and decisions they soon would be facing in the workplace. It didn't take long to discover the difficulty of developing a large repertoire of good cases. Over the last year, we have invited others to help us. Together, we offer this book in the hope that it will make teaching a little easier for you and learning more relevant to the students. As students study these cases, we also hope they will practice and apply critical thinking in developing answers.

The need for nurses with well-practiced, critical thinking skills is urgent; new graduates are being expected to make decisions and take actions of increasing sophistication. The need to consider the complexity of problems, along with a wide variety of variables (e.g., social, emotional, physical, financial, spiritual), in decision-making is unprecedented. Further, these decisions must be made in a fluid clinical arena with little guidance and limited resources. The problem of how we best prepare graduates to function in this constantly changing environment can be viewed either as a threat or a challenge. Bold experiments in educational processes are needed. Meanwhile, there can be no compromise in our social contract to produce graduates who consistently provide from the beginning, safe, effective, and efficient nursing care. Since magic is not available, we are left with the need to use critical thinking techniques to meet these challenges ourselves.

Historical Background to Critical Thinking in Nursing

The identified desire and need for critical thinking has a long and honorable history. The process of critical thinking has been practiced and taught, in some form or another, since the time of Socrates. In this century, Wallis (1926) identified a model of "creative thinking" with preparation, incubation, illumination, and verification stages. Einstein also expressed his interest in this process and suggested, "the formulation of a problem is often more essential than its solutions" (Einstein & Infield, 1938, p. 83). The post-World War II resurgence in faculty scholarship focused on defining critical thinking in the educational arena. In 1954, Dressel and Mayhew proposed components of critical thinking as consisting of (1) defining a problem, (2) selecting pertinent information to solve that problem, (3) recognizing stated and unstated assumptions, (4) formulating and selecting relevant and/or promising hypotheses, (5) drawing valid conclusions, and (6) judging the validity of inferences.

The competency-based education movement in nursing led to the acknowledgment that mere measurement of the ability to perform tasks was insufficient for practice. It was recognized that higher-level cognitive skills were required and used by professional nurses. This lead to a shift in emphasis to the process by which nursing professionals learned and practiced their art (Benner, 1984; del Bueno, 1990). The focus on critical thinking outcomes in the curriculum was inspired by the National League for Nursing (NLN) in 1991, when it was established as a criterion for nursing programs seeking NLN-accreditation. Since then, the struggle to integrate process, as well as outcome, in critical thinking has become a major obsession for nursing faculty everywhere. Despite decades of discussion, a universally acceptable definition of critical thinking in nursing remains elusive. This is probably less related to professional insight and confidence than to our unwillingness to appear authoritarian (a definite "no, no" in the critical thinking arena)!

Barriers to Critical Thinking

Barriers to critical thinking also have existed since the time of Socrates. Although the context specific to nursing may vary, barriers include:

1. *Social resistance:* including the contemporary world view of authority figures. (Fortunately, we know a few nursing faculty who have been ordered to drink poison, as Socrates was.) Individuals in authoritative roles, whether emperors, bureaucrats, deans, directors of nursing, or parents, often do not appreciate a challenge to established norms. Hence, society frequently presents conflicting demands such as, "think critically but don't ask questions or challenge authority." This barrier affects both faculty and students in nursing.
2. *Emotional resistance:* nurses frequently experience an inner reluctance (i.e., guilt or fear) to "stand out" or "make trouble," a consequence of our personal as well as cultural heritage.
3. *Intellectual resistance:* the educational system frequently "punishes" individuals who challenge or question, labeling them as aberrant or "trouble makers."
4. *Spiritual resistance:* the spirit of excitement and inquiry with which children are endowed is often squelched by authoritative practices in education or at home. Excitement and inquiry soon are replaced by boredom, discouragement, and dullness. Moreover, students may initially view attempts to make education "relevant" with some suspicion.
5. *Professional resistance:* professional rigidity ("We've always done it that way... or "We've never done it that way before") is a primary barrier to professional creativity and critical thinking in both faculty and students. We speak of empowering patients. How can patients be empowered when students do not feel empowered? How can students feel empowered when faculty do not feel empowered? How can unempowered students acquire critical thinking skills when unempowered faculty have been stifled from exhibiting and promoting critical thinking?

How Is This Case Study Book Different?

The use of case studies to stimulate critical thinking in "real life" problem solving is common to every practice discipline. The practice in nursing of using a few complex case studies is excellent to study pathophysiologic mechanisms and detailed processes, but it limits flexibility. In addition, students do not have the opportunity to repeatedly practice the fundamental steps of solid, clinical decision making. We have assembled a large collection of case studies entirely composed of real life based scenarios that faculty can use to illustrate theoretical presentations, whether in textbooks or didactic interactions. To keep information as current as possible, we worked with Mosby to produce this book in nine months, incorporating computerized on-line services and current journal articles for state-of-the-knowledge information from all the health care sciences. This should help faculty who are asked to teach in clinical areas that are not specific to their area of expertise to identify current clinical practices in those areas.

Guaranteeing Success or Failure?

One of the most effective ways to stifle student attempts at critical thinking and curiosity, is by using unnecessarily rigid grading criteria. It is true, that in some situations, there are absolute answers (particularly at the knowledge and comprehension level). As the cognitive challenges increase (as with application and analysis questions) and good judgment becomes more critical to outcomes, students need the opportunity to "experiment" without being punished. From a student's perspective, "punishment" usually consists of (1) having points taken off for "wrongthink" behaviors, and (2) embarrassing them in front of others for a particular response. This sends a clear message; students who take chances, think creatively, or don't toe the line, are punished. Students become confident, empowered, and courageous nurses when they are encouraged in the professional and therapeutic steps they take, and when taking intellectual chances is fostered and rewarded. This is surely the measure of success for nursing faculty. *The answers in this book are only suggestions.* Getting a response partially correct is an opportunity to reinforce the "good judgment" response, while discovering the source of incorrect perceptions. There is no question that teaching critical thinking in nursing requires intelligent, experienced, and creative faculty!

What if you have never taught case studies or used this style before? We suggest you announce an optional study session (maybe a brown bag lunch or something similar) and try one of the easier, system-related cases to illustrate one or more points made in class. Students who attend extra study sessions tend to be more motivated, and this may provide a good audience on which to practice. When you finish, get feedback from the students about what they did or did not find helpful. It will also help you feel more confident in incorporating clinical exemplars in didactic classes.

Instructor's Manual versus Student Workbook

The *Instructor's Manual* contains everything in the student's workbook, with the addition of the answers and several other items. While both books contain Notes, Instructor Notes are specific to this manual. This manual also contains a section on clinical tips for students. The title of each case and a box containing information on difficulty, setting, and index words are only in this manual. Eliminating this information from the workbook is necessary because this information may tip students off to the answers. Enough space has been left between questions for students to provide a concise response but not enough room for "multiple guess" responses (printing should be encouraged to facilitate faculty review). The types of questions asked vary widely and depend on the difficulty of the case, the clinical context, and the cognitive level of the case.

Provided answers are suggestions, not written in stone. Faculty should feel free to supplement or replace printed questions with questions of their choosing. This works particularly well in the context of small group and discussion groups, where additional questions may be posed by students. In our experience, discussion of a particular case often leads to students sharing clinical experiences of a similar or contrasting nature. Change anything you like.

To facilitate preparation for beginning students, a "Case Study Prepsheet" is located in the Appendix. This form can be photocopied and used by students to look up definitions, diagnoses, abbreviations, laboratory tests, medications, and other related material before class discussions. The "Prepsheet" also offers evidence of out-of-class preparation by students.

What Are Those Mysterious Codes?

At the beginning of each case in the *Instructor's Manual,* is a box with three headings: *Difficulty* (cognitive level) of the case, *Setting* (where the case took place), and *Index Words* (key terms listed in the index).

Difficulty of each case was evaluated according to the cognitive demands required of students in thinking through and responding to each of the questions; the overall difficulty of the questions determined the difficulty of the case. Because high acuity is the rule rather than the exception in hospital settings, even first-year students are exposed to patients with complex emotional, social, and medical problems. For that reason, cases are organized within each chapter according to cognitive level rather than clinical difficulty.

Symbol	Difficulty	Cognitive Level of Questions
*	Beginning	Knowledge, comprehension, rare application and analysis
**	Intermediate	Few knowledge, some comprehension and application, few analysis
***	Advanced	Rare knowledge, few comprehension, more application and analysis

Setting ranges from home care and outpatient clinics to intensive care units. In many instances, the case involves more than one setting. This is to help students learn to recognize issues related to case management and continuity of care. Although the majority of cases take place in the hospital, outpatient, extended care, and home care settings are increasingly featured in student placement.

Index words are major diagnostic and problem terms referenced in the index. For instance, type I diabetes mellitus may be in other chapters as a preexisting condition or complicating factor in addition to the endocrine chapter.

Strategic Focus of Questions

This book is designed for use with any textbook and is organized according to organ system. As explained above, cases in each chapter are evaluated according to cognitive demands and ranked from easier to more difficult independent of the condition of the patient. Relevant educational and psychosocial needs of the patients and their families were included in many of the cases, reflecting reality. *All of the cases are based on genuine clinical events. Select changes were made to protect the anonymity of the individual or to streamline the case presentation.*

Questions were analyzed according to nursing process, cognitive level, client needs, and NLN criteria. At the end of each question is a bolded, bracketed phrase with letters inside. These letters, alternating upper- and lower-case letters, are to be interpreted as follows:

[NURSING PROCESS/cognitive level/CLIENT NEEDS/nln criteria]

NURSING PROCESS:

- A = Assessment
- PD = Problem, Analysis, or Diagnosis
- P = Plan
- I = Implementation
- E = Evaluation

cognitive level:

- k = Knowledge
- c = Comprehension
- ap = Application
- an = Analysis

CLIENT NEEDS:

- S = Safety
- PI = Physiologic Integrity
- PSI = Psychosocial Integrity
- HP = Health Promotion

nln criteria:

- ct = Critical thinking
- ni = Therapeutic nursing intervention(s)
- tc = Therapeutic communication

Standard definitions of the above terms for nursing process, cognitive level, and client needs, as presented in the NCLEX literature, are used. In addition, the following definitions for the NLN criteria of critical thinking, nursing interventions, and therapeutic communication were used:

Critical Thinking: "Critical thinking is the disciplined process of actively and skillfully conceptualizing, applying, analyzing, synthesizing, and evaluating information gathered from, or generated by, observation, experience, reflection, reasoning, or communication as a guide to belief and action. In its exemplary form, critical thinking is based on universal intellectual values that transcend subject matter divisions: clarity, accuracy, precision, consistency, relevance, sound evidence, good reason, depth, breadth, and fairness. Critical thinking entails proficiency in the examination of those structures or elements of thought implicit in all reasoning: purpose, problem/question-at-issue, assumptions, concepts, empirical grounding, reasoning leading to conclusions, implications/consequences, objections from alternative viewpoints, and frame of reference" (Paul, 1993). It is important to note that when students hear the term *critical thinking*, they think they are supposed to criticize something or someone (in a negative sense). It is important to clarify what critical thinking is and why it is important to the education of professionals.

Therapeutic Nursing Intervention: "Therapeutic nursing interventions are acts (behaviors) carried out by nurses or their representatives to foster and enhance the physical, emotional, social, spiritual, and cultural well being of individuals, families, groups, or communities. These nursing behaviors/acts are conducted in an environment of compassion, trust, empathy, ethical caring, and respect. Therapeutic nursing interventions are based in nursing knowledge, skills, and problem solving abilities that guide a holistic approach to health care. Holistic nursing interventions are inclusive of a consideration of the physical, emotional, social, spiritual, and cultural dimensions of an individual, group, or situation" (University of Utah College of Nursing, 1993). The only addition we would like to make is that therapeutic nursing interventions also should be based on relevant scientific findings, regardless of the disciplinary source.

Therapeutic Communication: "Communication is the exchange of information, thoughts, feelings, and behaviors. Communication in nursing is further defined as the effective utilization of a variety of methodologies that maintain and promote safe, competent, and humanistic practice" (University of Utah College of Nursing, 1993).

Nursing Diagnosis

We were amazed at the emotional extremes generated by the question of including nursing diagnosis. On the one hand, some well-intended nursing leaders advised us, "It's on the NCLEX. Every book has it. It's wonderful because it defines what nurses truly do. You should include nursing diagnoses with every case." Other equally well-meaning leaders confided, "Nursing diagnosis is on the way out...thank goodness. My publisher made me include it, but I resented it. We should be focusing on diagnostic and reimbursement codes and how nurses can gain access to some financial control in the health care system." So we made the following decision: when nursing diagnosis questions are asked, responses are given in terms of NANDA-approved nursing diagnosis as a matter of quality control. They are not included in every case; but then, no other question appears with every case either. We would like to leave it up to you; you are intelligent professionals, add nursing diagnosis wherever you like. Some cases, involving long-term follow-up, may involve significant changes in nursing diagnoses over time for a single patient. If you don't like nursing diagnoses, have your students ignore the related questions and substitute some other form of problem statements or analyses. *Most important is that the students learn to systematically gather data and information, analyze it, learn what it means, and know what to do with it.* And, please, when we discuss controversial issues, such as nursing diagnosis, let us do it in an open environment of critical thinking, respect, and collegial kindness!

Consistency of Process and Outcome

There is a rule in exercise science about "specificity of training." It means, if you want to become a better speed skater, practice speed skating! We need to apply this concept to nursing education. If we want students to become better nurses, have them practice good nursing. There is much discussion today about matching process with outcomes; yet many of the outcome instruments are incongruent with the process and the true desired outcome! It is our belief that, by practicing making sound decisions in simulated settings, students find it easier to make sound decisions in the chaos and confusion of clinical settings. It is essential to practice basic steps of decision making again and again, until students feel confident in what they are seeing and doing. We need to listen to the echoes of the past revolution in education, "Back to basics!" We assume and presume far too much of our beginning students. The more we worked on these cases, the more we realized how much we assumed students knew or didn't know, and the more we realized we had been barriers to learning rather than facilitators.

Many of the case-related questions in this book reflect a mixture of processes as well as recognition of desired outcomes. In some cases, you may disagree with the strategic focus of our question analysis (i.e., you may think a question requires application rather than comprehension), and you may be right. In reviewing the questions, we realized that some questions required different levels of response; indeed, depending on point of view, several different categories could be appropriate. The bracketed codes are included to help faculty identify characteristics of the process involved in the outcome. Feel free to disagree. After all, isn't that part of what critical thinking is about?

Focusing on Student Strengths and Weaknesses

Dealing with process (cognitive limitations), not just outcomes (right answers), can lead to discoveries about a student's cognitive level of problem solving. Watch for consistencies in error or inability to understand a next step. Identifying whether these problems happen at a particular cognitive level (for instance, the student has no problem with knowledge and comprehension questions, but doesn't seem to "get the hang" of application questions) can help the instructor analyze where the student needs help. By working through the book and focusing on such questions (or by making your own exercises), the student can gain confidence through tiny, step-by-step success experiences.

Uses for the Case Studies Approach

There are many ways these case studies can be applied. It is our belief that many beginning students are not capable of using case studies alone as a means of learning. (Case studies alone are more appropriate for practicing professionals who have clinical experience on which to build.) The cases in this book should be used to illustrate theory and can help build bridges between didactic and clinical classes. It is difficult for students to "pin the tail on the donkey" if there is no donkey! Having said that, these are some of the ways in which these case studies can be used:

1. *Small group discussion:* assign a case for take-home work and allow them to work in groups to find the answer; some groups like to split up with every person taking a different question or using a different reference.

2. *Homework assignments:* assign a case for a take-home quiz or to prepare to turn-in or to present in class.

3. *Class presentations:* individuals or small groups can prepare a case to present in class before their peers; this is also an excellent way to prepare them for professional presentation after graduation. Encourage students to develop their own case studies from patients they have worked with.

4. *Diagnostics:* it can be very humbling, as well as revealing, to have students work on the cases individually. It is a fast way to see if they really understand what you thought was "crystal clear;" especially note what kind of questions were troublesome to individuals or groups, and if there is a pattern to their responses.

5. *Classroom illustration:* cases can be used for an in-class, change-of-pace after teaching a heavy portion of theory.

6. *Assignment or quiz:* cases can be used as unannounced, in-class assignments or quizzes to reward students who come to class prepared, and to generate enthusiasm for preparation in those who don't.

7. *Promoting interaction:* case studies can help in small group discussions to elicit student responses; discussions also can give you an idea of how articulate and able a particular student is in verbal communication among peers.

8. *Buying you some respite:* every instructor has bad days when there has been, for whatever reason, inadequate preparation time. Because these cases come loaded with answers, you can use them to help in "quick fix" lectures and presentations, and go to bed early for a change!

9. *Success imaging:* competitive athletes use imaging to visualize themselves doing something well. Work through cases with students having them, step-by-step, visualize themselves going through the motions of working with patients and performing certain assessments, skills, or interventions; have them picture themselves as competent and confident professionals.

10. *Identifying creative and exceptional students:* watch for the student who has different answers than many of the others; not wrong, just different or unusual. Students sometimes show surprisingly creative responses. This is an opportunity to identify potential candidates for your graduate program several years from now!

11. *Inservices:* since we started developing this idea, institutional nursing educators have asked if they could use these cases for staff development and inservices. Absolutely! Presenting one or two of these cases on a unit where you teach may be good "PR" and a positive payback to the nursing staff for their help with your students. The "Emergency Situations" chapter may be especially useful because many nurses don't feel comfortable about their decision-making abilities in critical situations. These inservices can be kept to 15 to 20 minutes, which may fit in well with high acuity and large patient work loads.

Strange Abbreviations, Bad Habits, and Regional Differences

When we first planned this book, we wanted to use more abbreviations to help students acquire the language and culture of nursing. Alas, one cannot expect beginning students to understand that MAEW, MOEx4, and MAEx4 all mean the same thing (maybe), depending on your background. The order of written vital signs were just as bad (P,BP,R,T; T,P,R,BP; BP,P,R,T). We decided to use the same order for the entire book: BP,P,R,T. (When taking vital signs, the most important thing is to look at the patient's face at least once!) We compromised by spelling out more terms, and focusing on the most common and consistent abbreviations and symbols. We used temperature values in F or C, depending on the case, so students can have practice converting the numbers. Laboratory values presented another problem. Emphasize to students that each institution or laboratory has its own system and "normal" range, and they cannot use the same numbers universally. Until everyone gets on the SI (international system) bandwagon, this will continue to be a particularly significant problem. We encourage students to read laboratory values carefully and get an "official" list of abbreviations for medical records in their institution and avoid creativity in this area.

A Personal Comment: Some faculty may be offended because we used the term "patient" rather than "client." Both authors have been patients in the hospital and are firmly convinced that "patient" and "prisoner" must be related concepts. We were not in the hospital by choice, and it is not a place you would choose for a vacation. We are convinced that no change in terminology can lend dignity to hospital gowns, lack of privacy, and loss of choice and control. On the other hand, one of us calls the people we see in our faculty practice "clients," and the other calls them "her folks." Call us politically incorrect if you will.

Please Give Us Feedback!

There is an "Evaluation/Problem Report" form in the Appendix. Please share with us what is helpful to you, as well as what is not. Did you find a mistake? Please let us know. It is customary for someone at Mosby to contact anyone who sends in corrections or comments. We appreciate your comments and will consider them in planning future editions of this book. Thanks!

References:

Benner, P. (1984). *From novice to expert*. Menlo Park, CA: Addison Wesley.
del Bueno, D. J. (1990). Experience, education, and nurses' ability to make clinical judgments. *Nursing and Health Care, 11*(6), 290-294.
Dressel, P. L., & Mayhew, L. B. (1954). *Critical thinking in social science: A handbook for evaluation and teaching.* Debuque, IA: William C. Brown, Co.
Easton, G. (1992). *Learning from case studies* (2nd ed.). London: Prentice Hall.
Einstein, A., & Infeld, L. (1938). *The evoution of physics*. New York: Simon & Schuster.
Paul, R. (1993). *Paper prepared for the National Council for Excellence in Critical Thinking.* Rohnert Park, CA: Sonoma State University.
National League for Nursing (NLN). (1991). *National League for Nursing education plan.* New York: Author.
University of Utah College of Nursing. (1993). *Self-study report.* Submitted to the Council of Baccalaureate and Higher Degree Programs, National League for Nursing. Salt Lake City, UT: Author.
Wallis, G. (1926). *The art of thought.* New York: Harcourt Brace.

Pointers for Students:
How To Look Like You Know What You Are Doing

Clinical experiences can be overwhelming and confusing; the environment is filled with distractions. It doesn't look at all like the book! The following are "tips and tricks" contributed by the writers of these cases. They have been included in the hope that there might be some points you will find useful. Don't read them all at once; read a few here and a few there, and apply them as you get the opportunity.

General Suggestions

- There are five instruments every nursing student should carry at all times. Never lend these items to anyone unless you can afford to replace one or more without complaint. They are a good black ink, ballpoint pen; a good stethoscope; a pocket penlight—preferably with pupil sizes or centimeter ruler on the side; a medium-sized hemostat (straight Kelley); and bandage scissors. Purchase a good quality stethoscope. Try listening with several different types, and choose the one that is best for you—engrave your name on it. The stethoscope is your most important tool.
- Staying hydrated will help you stay more alert. Drink plenty of fluids (besides, it gives you an excuse to go to the bathroom for a 30-second break).
- Keep a quick snack handy. Sometimes you need a pick-me-up and don't have time to leave the unit to get something.
- Plan something special you can do to help alleviate stress, and stick to your plan on a regular basis.
- Use of slang or words that could offend the patients should be avoided. Be aware of your patient's comfort level.
- Assume nothing and take nothing for granted.
- Listen and observe carefully. Be aware of changes and try to anticipate their significance.
- Watch how nurses do things, and pick out things that work best for you.
- Projecting confidence and a "matter of fact" manner will usually put the patient, and yourself, at ease.
- Care should always be taken to respect each patient's privacy; conduct interviews and examinations in a professional manner.
- Be sensitive to hesitation and nonverbal cues when gathering information. What is left unsaid may be extremely important. Use phrases such as "could you tell me more," or "couldyou help me understand.to"elicit more information.
- Watch for physical or emotional scars. Individuals—both men and women—who have been subjected to the degradation of sexual abuse and molestation may be especially prone to shame, aversion, or aggressive reactions.
- Don't be surprised to find that many adults may not be knowledgeable about the basics of elimination and sexual functioning. This often is covered up by humor.
- Documentation is critical, tools should be simple to use and developed for use at a 6th grade reading level. If you have a limited budget and a clinical setting of patients who speak more than one language, ask for volunteers to help translate educational material.
- As the patient's resting respiratory rate doubles from baseline, s/he will need to be intubated and placed on mechanical ventilation.
- Never trust equipment. Double check to make sure all equipment is functional.
- Treat the patient, not the monitoring devices or numbers.
- Not every patient with hepatitis or cirrhosis is an alcoholic.
- Not every alcoholic will go into DT.

- Do not assume the patient is anorexic if s/he looks malnourished.
- Do not assume a patient is well-nourished just because s/he is obese.

Assessment

Learn to assess pain without leaving out important data. Suggestion: use the COLDERRA method where C = characteristics, O = onset, L = location, D = duration, E = exacerbation, R = relief, R = radiation, and A = associated signs and symptoms.

- Begin with the basics and keep reviewing them: Airway, Breathing, Circulation (ABC).
- Become a keen observer; use all your senses.
- Don't be distracted by the obvious. Keep looking!
- Formulate a systematic way of assessing patients and make it a habit. You will be less likely to overlook or omit something.
- You can't find something if you don't look for it.
- Don't trust (1) machines, (2) numbers, (3) what you can't see.
- With the first assessment of your shift, check the patient's ID bracelet and the rate and type of every fluid infusing—*you* are responsible for fluids under your control from the moment of shift change until your shift is over.
- Remember to auscultate before palpating: Watch! Listen! *Then* Touch!
- Testing pH of NGT drainage is easier if you slip the litmus paper into the end of the NGT and reconnect the tube to suction. Drainage will be pulled over the paper which can then be removed. (Of course, antacids in the tube will negate this.)
- Any abrupt change in color or amount of drainage from drains or wounds needs to be explored and reported.
- Do not suggest words to describe feelings or events to your patients. You may miss subtle nuances if you jump to conclusions; listen to what your patients have to say and how they say it.
- Perform a thorough psychosocial assessment that includes the values of patients and their significant others.
- Include the significant other when you assess sleep patterns. They may be able to tell you more about snoring and other sleep disturbances than the patient can.
- Accurate records of data, such as intake and output, is a must. Lawsuits have been won—and lost—over one single I/O sheet. Involve the patient and family in helping keep records.
- Always double check calculations; use a calculator, if necessary.
- Acute cardiovascular and musculoskeletal injuries require frequent evaluation and documentation of the 5 Ps: Pulse, Pallor, Pain, Paresthesia, and Paralysis. Deterioration of status in any of these variables may indicate a medical emergency.
- Be alert for substance abuse as an underlying diagnosis in individuals whose hospitalization is sudden and unanticipated. Many nurses have been injured by patients in undiagnosed withdrawal. This may be a particular risk in motor vehicle accidents (MVAs) or medical crises, where alcohol or drug use may be contributing factors.

Problem/Diagnoses

- You have gathered your data, now look at it. Do you see any patterns? Do the data fit the history?
- Ask the following questions:
  - Do the data make sense in the context of this patient?
  - Do the data create a complete picture?
  - Do you need additional data?
- Use the data to formulate your list of patient problems.

- Prioritize specific problem statements, and guard yourself against distractions.
- Never be too smart to look something up.

Planning

- Plan and coordinate care with your patient. By discussing interventions and priorities, you will learn to understand more about your patient's value system.
- Noncompliance is rare when there is true teamwork.
- Educate the patient as you carry out this process; process and outcome can and should be integrated. A better educated patient is more prepared to comply with the medical and nursing care regimen.
- Always include relationships, self-esteem, and emotional issues in planning care.
- Prevent infection. Teach your patients and their families to wash their hands properly. Take them to the sink in the room and demonstrate hand washing techniques that you were taught in Nursing 101. Show them how to use a paper towel to turn off the faucet. Have them practice.
- Check equipment; double check if you have any doubt. You are responsible for reporting equipment that is not in working order.
- Substance abuse is not uncommon in the recovery of trauma patients. Consider a psychiatric nurse practitioner or social services consultation if you suspect this is a problem.

Implementation

- Frequently check your patient's charts for STAT orders.
- Document everything you do; if it isn't charted, you didn't do it.
- Document the patient's response to treatments, medications, and activities.
- Let the patient's values and preferences be the guide.
- Get the family and significant others to help, if appropriate.

Evaluation

- Monitor carefully for changes, whether dramatic and sudden, or subtle and gradual.
- Include the patient in helping evaluate care. Ask, "Do you feel that what we have done is helping? What do you think?"
- Is the patient getting better? If yes, then continue with the plan. If not, reassess and revise the plan as needed.
- Evaluate patients' and spousal cooperation. Never label patients as "noncompliant." Determine why patients do not take their medication, complete treatments, etc. The side effects of treatment make him/her feel worse than the disease, and s/he is exercising their right of choice. "Noncompliance" on the part of the patient is more often "knowledge deficit" on our part!
- Long-term problems, particularly pain, often contribute to depression. Involve other health care professionals and pain specialists in addressing these complex issues.

CONTENTS

CHAPTER 1. CARDIOVASCULAR DISORDERS

Case Study 1: Hypertension

Difficulty: *	*Setting:* Outpatient office practice
Index Words: Hypertension, coronary artery disease	

You have just accepted a new position as an office RN for a busy internal medicine physician. During your interviews with her, she told you that patient education was very important to her but she has found that she never has enough time to give adequate teaching. Part of your new job is to help her with patient management and education in her already-established hypertension clinic.

On your first day at the hypertension clinic, you meet M.P., a 78 year-old-woman who was told about 6 months ago that her blood pressure was elevated. You take her blood pressure using the 1993 American Heart Association guidelines and get 160/102. She tells you that the physician told her she has hypertension and that she should take a pill everyday. She seems confused and asks you, "What is hypertension, anyway?"

1. How would you explain hypertension to M.P.? **[P,I/c/PI,PSI/ct,ni,tc]**
   - Establish what her educational and cognitive levels are and adjust the information accordingly. Many times, in clinical settings, use terms that are not familiar to the lay public. You should start by explaining to M.P. that hypertension (HTN) is the medical term used for high blood pressure. You should go on to explain that hypertension is very common and affects approximately 20% of white and 30% of black Americans 18 years of age and older. You can also explain that hypertension increases with age and that 50% of all people over the age of 65 are affected.

M.P. goes on to say that she feels just fine and doesn't think she needs this pill anyway. She shows you a prescription for enalapril (Vasotec) 2.5 mg daily and states, "The doctor gave this to me but I don't think I'll get it filled. Right now I feel fine."

2. What is your next nursing intervention? **[P/ap/PI,PSI/ct,ni,tc]**
   - Explain to M.P. that high blood pressure is usually asymptomatic but that treatment is essential. By explaining what hypertension can do if left untreated, you will enhance her understanding of her condition and, ideally, help with medication compliance. Start by explaining that HTN is the most significant risk factor for the development of atherosclerotic coronary artery disease (CAD). You should also explain that HTN, if left untreated, can cause damage to numerous organs but especially her eyes and her kidneys. Worst of all, HTN can lead to a cerebrovascular accident (CVA or stroke) with resulting impairment or death. The possibility of a stroke is for most patients the most dramatic and convincing.

M.P. thanks you for explaining everything to her and reports she will get her prescription filled today on the way home from the doctor's office. She goes on to ask if there is anything else she should do to treat her HTN.

3. What nonpharmacologic measures might help someone like M.P. control her blood pressure? **[P/c/PI,PSI,HP/ct,ni,tc]**
   - If M.P. is more that 15% over her ideal weight, weight loss should be recommended. Considerable drops in blood pressure often occur even before patients reach their ideal weight. Of more importance than weight loss is a decrease in the waist-hip ratio (WHR). Modest improvements in WHR can result in optimal improvements in blood pressure and the lipid profile.
   - Dietary instruction may include limiting the salt in her diet and reducing overall fat intake. There should also be a dietary balance between calcium, potassium, sodium, chloride, and magnesium intake. Although sodium restriction has been controversial, it appears safe and effective in modestly lowering the BP in patients over 40 years of age.
   - Routine aerobic exercise, like walking, is also encouraged. Patients at risk for CAD should begin an exercise program under supervision. It is important to start slowly and build up gradually. Earlier recommendations for exercise to be performed at least 3 times per week for at least 30 minutes at a heart rate of 65% to 70% of the predicted maximal heart rate have changed. It is now recognized that *any* moderate activity is better than none. Studies have shown that long-term exercise compliance is better in individuals engaging in lower-to-moderate intensity exercise than the higher intensity. While some patients may need to start walking as little as 3 to 5 minutes daily and increase by 1 to 2 minutes per week, the eventual goal is to walk briskly (without discomfort or shortness of breath) for 30 minutes 5 to 6 times per week. Patients receiving beta-blockers cannot use normal exercise heart rate recommendations and require special guidelines. Here are some general rules of thumb for exercise: (1) if the individual is stiff, sore, or exhausted as a result of the exercise, he/she has done something wrong or done too much; (2) if he/she is out of breath during exercise, he/she is doing too much. Slow down and enjoy and live!
   - If M.P. drinks alcohol, she should be instructed to limit her intake to 1 drink per day because ethanol has a direct vasopressor effect.

M.P. leaves your office a much more informed health care consumer and says she will see you in a month at her follow-up appointment. M.P. returns to the office 4 weeks later. She sits down to get her blood pressure taken and tells you she has been doing everything you taught her and has no questions about your previous teaching.

4. You are getting ready to take M.P.'s blood pressure. What are important factors to keep in mind to guarantee an accurate reading of M.P.'s blood pressure? **[A/c/S,PI/ct,ni]**
   - Cuff size: you need to verify that the size of the sphygmomanometer cuff is appropriate for the circumference of the arm when you take a blood pressure. If the cuff is too small, a false high reading may be obtained; conversely, if the cuff is too large, you can obtain a false low reading by as much as 10 mm Hg.
   - Position: M.P. should also be sitting with her arm supported at the level of her heart. If the reading seems higher than usual, let her sit for 5 to 10 minutes and retake it. Patients will often rush to their appointment and have a transient elevation in BP that will resolve once they are relaxed.

You escort M.P. to the exam room. While you are walking with her she tells you that she has a cough that has been bothering her for the past 3 weeks. She reports it is so bad that she can't even sleep. She tells you she is going to ask the doctor "for an antibiotic to get rid of this cough."

5. Knowing what you do about M.P.'s treatment plan, what is the most likely cause of her cough? **[PD/c/PI/ct]**
   - Enalapril (Vasotec) was the medication prescribed for her HTN. Enalapril belongs to the drug class of ACE inhibitors, which are commonly used in the treatment of hypertension. ACE inhibitors lower BP by decreasing peripheral vascular resistance. The most common side effect of ACE inhibitors is a chronic, nonproductive cough. Since M.P.'s cough began shortly after initiating enalapril this is the most likely cause.

M.P. sees the physician and tells you that the doctor stopped her medication to see if her cough got better. She has substituted metoprolol (Lopressor) 50 mg bid. M.P. is curious what side effects this new medication will have.

6. List 4 things you would include in teaching M.P. about her new medication. **[P/S,PI,PSI,HP/ct,ni,tc]**
   - Metoprolol belongs to the drug class of beta-adrenergic antagonists, more commonly referred to as beta-blockers. Beta-blockers are widely prescribed as antihypertensives and act by reducing heart rate and cardiac output, as well as reducing plasma renin levels. The major side effects include that her heart won't beat as hard when she gets excited or works hard (negative inotropic) and it won't beat as fast (chronotropic effects). She may experience a narrowing of her airway (bronchospasm), decreased circulation to her fingers and toes (provocation of Raynaud phenomenon), calf pain when walking (claudication), and a masking of low blood sugar in patients with diabetes (masking of hypoglycemia).
   - Because treatment with beta-blockers blunts the heart rate response to exercise, M.P. should be supplied with new heart rate guidelines (often defined in terms in how many beats above resting rather than calculated from a percent). She *will* continue to get benefits from her exercise despite the lower heart rate. She should be warned that she needs to be more careful about exercising in hot weather because she may not have the normal vasodilatory skin response for cooling.
   - Beta-blockers are sometimes associated with depression; changes in mood should be reported.
   - Beta-blockers may inhibit abdominal weight loss because abdominal (gut) fat cells are sensitive to epinephrine stimulation of fat metabolism.
   - It is also important to tell her to not abruptly stop her medication because sudden cessation of therapy can cause bronchospasm and irregular heart beats.

M.P. calls you 3 weeks later and states she is feeling fine and does not have any side effects from her new medication. She has had her blood pressure checked twice at the senior citizens' center, and those readings were 138/78 and 142/82.

7. M.P. asks if these blood pressures readings are OK. What do you tell her? **[P/c/PI,PSI/ct,ni,tc]**
   - Tell her you're proud of her! Therapeutic goals are individualized; however, these BP readings are within normal ranges. Tell M.P. that these readings are normal and that you will pass them onto the doctor.
   - She should continue on with her prescribed medications and not make any alterations without talking to you first. You should then pass on the information to the physician and make sure there are no additional instructions.

M.P. comes in for routine follow-up 1 year later. She continues to do well on her metoprolol 50 mg daily with average BP readings of 132/78. She participates in a routine walking program and eats a low-fat, no added salt diet. She tells you she recently was at a luncheon with her garden club and that most of those ladies take different blood pressure pills than she does. She is curious if she would be better off on a different medication.

8. How can you best respond to M.P.'s statement? **[P/c/PI,PSI/ct,ni,tc]**
   - Start by explaining that there are many different drugs used to treat HTN. The goal of her therapy is to find a medication that adequately controls *her* blood pressure with few or no side effects. Each patient is individual in his/her medical history and tolerance for specific medications so she may find her friends on different medications. Her BP has been well controlled, and she denies any side effects from her metoprolol, so there would be no benefit to changing her medication. You should encourage her to also seek feedback from the doctor during her appointment if she has any further questions or concerns about her treatment.
   - There are generic versions of many drugs and there are different doses and formulations for each. All of these will have different shapes and colors, so the same drug may have several different appearances. This can be confusing, so patients should always double-check with their pharmacist to make sure there has been no mistake if their medication looks different.

Case Study 2: Coronary Artery Disease

Difficulty: *	*Setting:* Outpatient clinic
Index Words: Coronary artery disease, hyperlipidemia	

As an occupational health nurse at a free-standing HMO clinic, one of your primary responsibilities is providing information to all employees on healthy lifestyles. While you are waiting in the supermarket check-out line, your neighbors seek you out for advice. He reports that he recently had a physical and was given a "clean bill of health." He tells you he feels great but confides in you that his family history of premature coronary disease worries him. He said he wants to limit his risk factors but he just doesn't know what to do. You agree to see him later in the week to guide him in identifying lifestyle changes he can make.

During your initial interview you learn that K.N. is 55 years old and has no chronic medical problems. His family history is significant for premature coronary artery disease in both his father and mother. His father experienced his first MI at the age of 49 and his mother died of an MI at the age of 60. He has never smoked and denies any hypertension, diabetes, or other medical problems. He is 5'10" and weighs 200 lb. His VS are 128/70, 72, 16. He has a sedentary job and gets no routine exercise. He gives you a lipid profile laboratory analysis that reveals the following values: total cholesterol 243 mg/dl, LDL 165 mg/dl, HDL 31 mg/dl, triglycerides 240 mg/dl.

1. His waist and hip circumferences are 48.5" and 40.5", respectively. Describe at what location and how these measurements are made. **[A/k/PI,HP/ct,ni]**
   - Measuring waist-hip ratio (WHR): WHR determination requires use of a tape measure to obtain the abdominal (waist) circumference and the hip circumference in inches or centimeters. The abdominal circumference is measured at the level of the umbilicus (or level of greatest anterior extension of the abdomen) with the individual standing. The hip circumference is determined by measuring the greatest circumference at the level of the buttocks. Both measurements should be performed at the end of a normal expiration and without indenting the skin with the tape measure. The formula for calculating WHR is *Abdominal Circumference* divided by *Hip Circumference.* WHR values above 1.0 for men and above 0.8 for women are associated with increased risk of diabetes, hypertension, heart disease, and stroke. *These data should be an essential part of all nursing physical and health-promotion assessments.* (From Office of Disease Prevention and Health Promotion, 1994.)

2. Calculate K.N.'s WHR, and explain the significance of your finding. **[A,PD/c/PI/ct,ni]**
   - 48.5" (waist circumference) divided by 40.5" (hip circumference) yields a WHR of 1.2. This is considerably higher than the 1.0 maximum recommended for men. This indicates that K.N. has a more dangerous, higher cardiac risk body fat pattern than obesity alone would indicate.

3. Identify all the cardiac-related risk factors in K.N.'s previous information. Place a check mark (✓) next to those that are modifiable risk factors **[A,PD/c/PI,HP/ct]**
   - 55-year-old man.
   - Family history of cardiac disease on both sides.
   - ✓ Sedentary life-style.
   - ✓ Overweight with a high WHR.
   - ✓ Hyperlipidemia.

4. Based on the information you received in the initial interview, what lifestyle modifications would you prescribe for K.N.? **[P/ap/PI,HP/ct,ni,tc]**
   - K.N.'s lifestyle modifications should be directed toward weight loss, establishing a routine exercise program, and management of his hyperlipidemia.

You and K.N. decide that his first efforts will be directed toward dietary modification. Successful dietary modification could help his weight loss efforts, as well as his hyperlipidemia.

5. What information would you give to K.N. regarding a healthy diet? **[P/c/PI,HP/ct,ni,tc]**
   - Because of K.N.'s age, he should be instructed that a healthy diet consists of the basic 4 food groups. The use of the more recent food pyramid can make teaching health dietary principles easy and effective. The pyramid's base comprises grains, rice, cereal, and breads, which should account for 6 to 10 servings a day. The next level of the pyramid is divided between fruits and vegetables. Continuing up the pyramid is the meat/protein group and, finally, the top comprises fats and sweets, which should account for a very small portion of daily intake (Office of Disease Prevention and Health Promotion, 1994).

The 1993 National Cholesterol Education Program (NCEP) recommendation for initial diet therapy is called a Step 1 Diet. This involves reduction of dietary fat to less than 30% of total calories and a reduction of saturated fat to less than 10% of total calories. Cholesterol intake is limited to less than 300 mg/day. More recent data suggest that a very low-fat diet (less than 20% fat) may be more effective where CAD already exists.

K.N. already appears overwhelmed and states, "Just tell me how I can do this in my everyday life."

6. How would you explain this to him in plain English? **[P/k/HP/ct,ni,tc]**
   - Unnecessary fat, in general, can be reduced by cutting portion sizes of beef, chicken, pork, or fish to 3 oz per serving for a total of 2 servings per day; 3 oz is approximately the size of the palm of his hand. He should pick fish and poultry over red meat whenever possible and avoid all fried food.
   - Because some vegetable oils, such as coconut and palm oil, are high in saturated fats, encourage him to stick with such vegetable oils as canola or olive oil. Recent data indicate that "margarine" products with "partially hydrogenated" oils may actually be harmful. Dairy products can be high in fat; however, there are excellent and tasty low-fat or no-fat dairy products now available.

K.N. tells you he was not fasting when his lipid profile was drawn. He is curious if this made his cholesterol higher than it really is.

7. How would you answer K.N.'s question? **[P/c/HP/ct,ni,tc]**
   - Cholesterol levels are not affected by fasting; however, triglyceride levels are. Most lipid profiles calculate the LDL cholesterol using the following formula: LDL-cholesterol = Total cholesterol - HDL-cholesterol = VLDL. VLDL = triglycerides/5. In this equation, if the triglycerides are elevated from a recent meal, then the VLDL will be falsely elevated, resulting in an inaccurately low LDL. Since K.N.'s triglycerides were within normal range, this is probably an accurate assessment of his cholesterol status.

You write down the name of two inexpensive books on low-fat, healthy eating that K.N. can get locally. K.N. sets up a follow-up appointment with you in 2 months. When he returns, he has the results of his most recent lipid profile. The results are total cholesterol 220 mg/dl, LDL 143 mg/dl, HDL 32 mg/dl, and triglycerides 165 mg/dl. His vital signs remain within normal limits. He has lost 8 lb since you last saw him; even better, his WHR is 1.12!

8. What diet instruction would you give K.N. now? **[P/c/PSI,HP/ct,ni,tc]**
   - First, congratulate him on how well he has done. Talk with him about how things have gone and any problems he may have run into. Praise his problem-solving behaviors. He is making excellent progress.
   - Although his lipid profile has improved, he still is above the goal of an LDL of 130 mg/dl or less. He should be progressed to the NCEP Step II Diet, which limits the saturated fat to 7% per day and cholesterol to 200 mg/day.

K.N. states he understands the goal for his LDL cholesterol is less than 190 and that LDL is his "bad" cholesterol. He questions what his goal is for his HDL cholesterol and is curious if this is what people mean by "good" cholesterol.

9. What information would you give K.N. about HDL cholesterol? **[P/c/PI,HP/ct,ni,tc]**
   - HDL, or high-density lipoprotein, is considered to be the "good" cholesterol and appears to have a cardioprotective effect. Values less than 35 mg/dl are considered to be a separate risk factor for CAD. HDL values are difficult to modify; however, they can be raised by routine, moderate aerobic exercise.
   - Although some people recommend moderate ETOH intake to raise HDL levels, the value of this intervention is dubious and requires a careful assessment of other factors in an individual's life, including potential for alcoholism and cancer.

K.N. verbalizes understanding of the teaching regarding HDL cholesterol. He feels he adequately understands his diet therapy and would now like to start a routine exercise program.

10. What general information would you give him regarding an exercise program? **[P/c/PI,HP/ct,ni,tc]**
    - Many factors should be included when picking an exercise program. First, inquire what K.N. likes to do. The specific exercise is not as important as that it be something he will keep doing. Some people like to alternate types of exercise so they do not get bored; it also allows for specific muscle groups to recover between workouts and reduce the risk for inflammation. For weight-bearing activities, a good pair of shoes is essential, but they don't have to be expensive. Good quality, well-fitting shoes are significant to preventing injuries. Remind K.N. to start out slowly and increase his workouts gradually. He should obtain clearance from his physician before beginning his exercise program. A good way to start a walking program is to start walking briskly for 20 minutes 3 days a week on alternating days. Shortness of breath or discomfort is a good reason to slow down a little. Every week, he can increase his time by 5 minutes until he reaches 40 minutes. When he reaches this point, he can start working out 4, then 5, then 6 days per week. His goal should be to briskly exercise 5 to 6 days/week at an intensity that will get his heart going but never provoke dyspnea. Men who walk between 15 to 18 miles a week achieve optimal lipid regulating response. For women, 12 to 15 miles per week usually is adequate. Hydration is important! Drink plenty of water before, during, and after exercise to prevent dehydration.

K.N. follows up with you in 2 months. He has lost an additional 10 pounds and feels great. More important, his WHR is 0.93. He denies any problems regarding his dietary or exercise programs and expresses appreciation for your help. His repeat HDL is 50 mg/dl and LDL is 130 mg/dl.

Case Study 3: Coronary Artery Disease Prevention and Rehabilitation

Difficulty: *

Setting: Outpatient rehabilitation center

Index Words: Coronary artery disease, hypertension, angina pectoris, substance abuse, sleep disorders

You are a nurse at a free-standing cardiac prevention and rehabilitation center. Your new client in risk-factor modification is B.J., a 37-year-old traveling salesman, who is married with 3 children. During a recent evaluation for chest pain (including a cardiac catheterization), he was diagnosed with angina pectoris, given a prescription for SL nitroglycerin, told how to use it, and referred to your cardiac rehabilitation program for sessions 3 days a week. B.J.'s wife comes along to help him with healthy lifestyle changes. You take the following nursing history: B.J.'s father died of sudden cardiac death at age 42 and his mother (still living) had a CABG x 4 (quadruple coronary artery bypass graft of 4 vessels) at age 52; his hypertension is controlled with nifedipine (Procardia) 90 mg PO qd, which he has taken regularly; he has a 35 pack/year smoking history; an occasional beer ("a beer every weekend with the football game"); and a dietary history of fried and fast foods. His current weight is 205 at 5'8"; waist/hip ratio of 1.21. His VS are 132/86, 82, 18, 98.4°F.

1. List 3 nonmodifiable risk factors for CAD. **[A/k/S,Pl/ct]**
   - Nonmodifiable (predisposing biologic) risk factors: age, gender, family history/genetics.

2. List 6 modifiable risk factors for CAD. **[A/k/Pl,HP/ct]**
   - Modifiable (predisposing lifestyle) risk factors: cigarette smoking, physical inactivity, obesity (fat distribution pattern), stress, oral contraceptives, hypertension (even if maintained by medication), hyperlipidemia, glucose intolerance.

3. Underline each of the responses in #1 and #2 above that represent B.J.'s CAD risk factors. **[A/c/Pl,HP/ct]**
   - Underline family history, gender, cigarette smoking, physical inactivity, obesity (fat distribution pattern), stress, hypertension (even if maintained by medication), and suspect hyperlipidemia (genetics and high-fat diet).

4. You would like to know more about B.J.'s hyperlipidemia. What 4 common laboratory values do you need to know? **[A/k/Pl/ct]**
   - Triglyceride level, total cholesterol, high density lipoprotein (HDL), low-density lipoprotein (LDL).

B.J. laughingly tells you he believes in the 5 all-American food groups: salt, sugar, fat, chocolate and caffeine.

5. Identify health-related problems in this case description; the problem that is potentially life-threatening should be listed first. **[A/c/PI/ct]**
   - High risk for sudden cardiac death (family history; male over age 35; multiple risk factors); inactivity (sedentary lifestyle); obesity; smoking; stressful lifestyle; hypertension; probable hyperlipidemia; and a high-fat, low-fiber diet.

6. What is the most important priority problem that you need to address with B.J.? Identify the teaching strategy you would use with him. **[PD,P/an/PI,PSI,HP/ct,ni,tc]**
   - The most important problem is the one B.J. and his wife are willing to work on; the one *they* identify as most important. This helps cement their commitment to behavioral change. For example, they decide he needs to exercise. Inform him that cardiac rehabilitation will help him become active and do it safely—he might even enjoy it! You may help him change his outlook because this is something *he* thinks is important.
   - Praise his wife for being supportive in helping both of them live a healthier lifestyle.

   Instructor Note: Research has shown that the spouses of men with CAD tend to have more CAD themselves. She is not only helping him, she is helping herself and serving as a role model for her children who will inherit B.J.'s heart disease risk.

7. What is the second problem you would work with B.J. to change? Identify an appropriate strategy to resolve the problem. **[PD,P/an,PI,PSI,HP/ct,ni,tc]**
   - Once again, negotiate with B.J. and his wife what they would like to work on.
   - Obesity: inform them that eating low-fat meals does not mean that they have to give up tasty foods. Give the wife a few low-fat recipes that taste good, and encourage her to swap recipes with other people in cardiac rehab. Center teaching around the low-fat diet to decrease obesity and hyperlipidemia risks. There are many excellent books as well as magazines available on tasty low-fat, healthy eating.
   - Smoking: give B.J. and his wife a list of smoking cessation classes and explain how stopping smoking will reduce his risk of heart attack. Assure him that although it will not be easy, he can do it.
   - Stress: teach relaxation techniques that B.J. can use when he is on the road.

8. B.J.'s wife takes you aside and tells you, "I'm so worried for B. I grew up in a really dysfunctional family where there was a lot of violence. B. has been so good to the kids and me. I'm so worried I'll lose him that I have nightmares about his heart stopping. I find myself suddenly awakening at night just to see if he's breathing." How are you going to respond? **[A,PD,P/an/PSI/ct,ni,tc]**
   - Thank her for sharing with you. Acknowledge that heart disease in a loved one can be a very frightening thing.
   - Suggest she practice stress-relaxation techniques with him.
   - Ask if she would like to talk to someone about her anxiety.

Note: Nightmares about losing a loved one to heart disease are not rare, especially during the time of diagnosis or disease-related crisis. However, a background of childhood violence can have deep roots and often requires special help. Clearly, this is woman is in distress. Depending on her willingness at this time, it would be good for her to talk with a therapist. If she doesn't think she needs it, try suggesting that it might be good for B. and the kids and that it would help her relax and be more responsive to them. At the appropriate point, it would be important for her to be able to share with B. how she feels. From her description, this sleep disturbance is an unhealthy situation that should be addressed. If she refuses, keep an open relationship; it is important that she keep talking to someone about her fear.

9. Six weeks after you start working with B.J., he admits that he has been under a lot of stress. He rubs his chest and says, "It feels really heavy on my chest right now." You feel his pulse and note that his skin is slightly diaphoretic, he is agitated, and appears to be very anxious. What are you going to do to obtain additional information? **[P,I/c/S,PI,PSI/ct,ni,tc]**
   - Have B.J. stop any activity and lie down because you want to decrease the workload on his heart and decrease his body's need for oxygen.
   - Monitor his vital signs.
   - Give B.J. 1 nitroglycerin and observe for changes; see if the pain subsides. You may repeat the nitroglycerin tablets 5 minutes apart x 2 (total of 3 tablets SL over 15 minutes). The nitroglycerin will dilate the coronary arteries and increase the blood supply and oxygen delivery to his heart muscles.
   - Reassure him that you will stay with him; you just want to be sure everything is OK.

10. B.J. continues to feel symptomatic. Now what are you going to do? **[I/ap/PI/ct,ni,tc]**
    - Dial 911 and request emergency transport to the nearest ED.
    - While you are waiting for the medics, start 2 to 4 L/O_2 per nasal cannula and an IV TKO in case IV medications have to be administered.
    - Run a 12-lead ECG or rhythm strip to look for dysrhythmias. Run a long rhythm strip. If he needs to be transported by the paramedics to the ED, it may be valuable to the medical personnel at the hospital.
    - Continue to observe B.J. carefully and reassure him, making him as comfortable as possible.
    - Notify B.J.'s attending physician and his wife.

    Instructor Note: This may be a good opportunity to discuss the concept of emergency protocols with students. They need to know that different facilities have different protocols and they must be followed. If your students are placed in more than one agency, it may be useful to have them look up the protocols used by each agency or unit and compare them as a postclinical group activity. As students are spread out into more diverse settings, it will be more difficult for faculty to be aware of details and speak to the protocols of each agency. This exercise will not only help you be aware of what is expected in the various settings, it is a first step in management—and leadership—training for nursing students, who will need to learn how to develop such protocols as professional nurses.

Case Study 4: Rule Out Myocardial Infarction

Difficulty: * *Setting:* Hospital ED, hospital

Index Words: Myocardial infarction, substance abuse, coronary artery disease, hypertension, angina

W.R., a 48-year-old construction worker with a 36-pack/year smoking history, is admitted to your floor with a diagnosis of rule out myocardial infarction (R/O MI). He has significant male-pattern obesity ("beer belly," high WHR), a barrel chest, and reports a dietary history of high-fat food. His wife brought him to the ED after he complained of unrelieved "indigestion." His admission VS were 202/124, 96, 18, 36.8°C. W.R. was put on O_2 2 L/nc, an IV of D_5W at KVO was started, and he was given sublingual nifedipine (Procardia) in the ED. He was admitted to Dr. Adam's service. He tells you he's just fine in a loud and angry voice and demands a cigarette.

1. Are these VS reasonable for a man his age? If not, which one(s) concern(s) you. State your reasons why? **[PD/c/S,PI/ct]**
   - His blood pressure is dangerously high and his pulse is rapid for a 48-year-old man who is at rest. Both these can contribute to myocardial ischemia.

2. Identify 5 priority problems associated with the care of a patient like W.R. **[PD/c/S,PI,PSI/ct]**
   - Blood pressure control: monitoring for efficacy of medication and side effects.
   - Myocardial ischemia: (1) increased O_2 demand due to increased cardiac output (high BP and P); (2) probable decreased O_2 availability r/t coronary artery disease (CAD) and/or (chronic obstructive pulmonary disease (COPD); (3) possible decreased diffusion of gases across the alveolar/capillary membrane. (2) and (3) are directly related to his smoking history.
   - Cigarette smoking: he is going to want to smoke; smoking negatively affects the heart because of the increased stress on the lungs and the vascular vasoconstriction that restricts oxygenation; you need to caution him about not smoking during his stay in the hospital and ask his wife to take his cigarettes and lighter or matches home with her.
   - Diet modification: he is used to a high-fat diet and may find hospital food unappetizing; enlist the cooperation of his wife when she comes in, discuss the necessity of modifying their eating habits; reassure her that a low-fat diet can still be very tasty and ask her if she would like to talk to the dietitian.
   - Constipation: his high-fat, low-fiber dietary preferences as well as decreased activity during hospitalization increase his risk for constipation; the pattern of breath-holding during a bowel movement is termed the "Valsalva maneuver." In cardiac patients who are constipated, it can lead to an MI or sudden death.
   - Hostility: his anger is probably masking fear of death and fear of loss of control, which can contribute to more stress on his heart and would be dangerous at this time.
   - Denial: his denial is a coping mechanism related to his fear. Although denial sometimes serves a positive purpose, in this situation it is contributing to behaviors that increase his risk of cardiac damage.

3. List 3 relevant nursing diagnoses for a cardiac patient like W.R. **[PD/c/PI/ct]**
   - Risk for altered cardiopulmonary tissue perfusion r/t increased cardiac output and decreased oxygen availability.
   - Fear r/t threats to health and self-concept.
   - Knowledge deficit of behavioral risk factors (smoking and diet) r/t cardiopulmonary disease.
   - Risk for constipation r/t dietary intake and activity restrictions.

4. Which of the following laboratory tests might be ordered to investigate W.R.'s condition? If the order is appropriate, place an "A" in the space provided. **[A/c/PI/ct]**
   ___ CBC.
   ___ EEG in the AM.
   ___ Chem 7 (electrolytes).
   ___ PT/PTT.
   ___ Bilirubin q AM.
   ___ Urinalysis.
   ___ STAT 12-lead ECG.
   ___ Type and cross (T&C) for 4 units PRCs (packed red cells)
   Answers:
   A The CBC, Chem 7, PT/PTT, and urinalysis are appropriate admitting laboratory tests for all patients with blood pressure disorders.
   A The STAT 12-lead ECG is appropriate for this patient because his heart is involved.
   I The EEG, bilirubin, and T&C are not appropriate for this patient.

5. What significant laboratory tests are missing from the above list? **[A/k/PSI/ct]**
   - Serial cardiac enzymes; the order should read CPK and LDH (with isoenzymes if elevated).

6. How are you going to respond to his angry demands for a cigarette? He also demands something for his "heartburn." How will you respond? **[P,I/an/PI,PSI/ct,ni,tc]**
   - Address his feelings of loss of control by acknowledging his legitimate issues of craving (cigarettes) and pain/discomfort. Assure him you will call the physician and get something to help him feel more comfortable.
   - Explain that smoking could cut off oxygen to his heart and increase his pain/burning/discomfort (use his choice of words).
   - Reassure him that you will be available if he needs help.
   - Offer him a choice by asking him if he would like some Milk of Magnesia (MOM, magnesium hydroxide) for his heartburn while you contact the doctor (you may offer him 30 ml Maalox according to your unit protocol). Ask if there is anything else you can do to make him more comfortable. (And no, he still can't smoke!)
   - Professional confidence and competence communicate themselves to people experiencing fear and help meet their needs for security.

You call Dr. Adam's resident who prescribes 10 mg morphine sulphate IV push q1h prn for pain (burning, pressure, angina).

7. Explain 2 reasons for this order. **[P/c/PI,PSI/ct]**
   - Morphine sulphate, a narcotic analgesic, will address his discomfort and make him more comfortable. This should help reduce his stress. (With narcotics, be sure to institute a bowel care program to prevent constipation.)
   - Morphine sulfate also functions to dilate pulmonary vessels and decrease preload on the heart.

8. What special precautions should you follow when administering morphine sulfate IV push? **[I/c/S,PI/ct,ni]**
   - Ask about prior allergy, hypersensitivity reaction to morphine sulfate, or impaired liver function.
   - Assess VS, type, location, and intensity of pain before and 30 to 60 minutes following administration.
   - Administer IV push over a 4- to 5-minute period.

9. What safety measures/instructions would you give him before you leave his room? **[P/c/S/ct,ni,tc]**
   - He should press the nurses' call light as soon as he starts to experience any uncomfortable feelings (the word pain may be misunderstood), becomes nauseated, or experiences more "indigestion."
   - Inform him of his activity status, such as, "The doctor has placed you on bed rest with bathroom privileges. That means if you need to use the bathroom, you need to turn on your call and someone will assist you. Do not try to get up by yourself."
   - It is against the law for him to smoke in the hospital. Have his wife take his cigarettes and lighter or matches home.

10. One of the housekeeping staff asks you, "If the poor guy can't smoke, why can't you give him a nicotine patch?" How will you respond? **[PD/c/S,PI,PSI/ct,tc]**
    - Explain that use of the nicotine patch can lead to chest pain, hypertension, and tachycardia in patients with heart disease. In W.R.'s current condition, this would be contraindicated.

    Instructor Note: This point is controversial; some physicians will use patches and others will not. If the patch is used, manufacturers recommend starting with a 14 mg patch.

11. Before leaving for the night, Mrs. R. approaches you and asks, "Did W. have a heart attack? I'm really scared. His father died of one when he was 51." How are you going to respond to her question? **[P/ap/PSI/ct,ni,tc]**
    - It is important to recognize and address Mrs. R.'s anxiety. Reassure her that he is getting excellent care and he will be closely monitored.
    - Explain that no one can tell whether he's had a heart attack until the test results come back. Thank her for the additional information and tell her you will pass it along to the physician. Tell her that he is going to need her help when he goes home so that he can begin to live a more healthy lifestyle.

12. When you come into W.R.'s at 2200 to answer his call light, you see he is holding his left arm and complaining of aching in his left shoulder and arm? What information are you going to gather? What questions will you ask him? **[A/an/PI,PSI/ct,ni,tc]**
    - Take his vital signs.
    - Evaluate his level of anxiety.
    - Observe his color.
    - Feel for diaphoresis.
    - Ask about the presence of pain/symptoms: quality, intensity (have the patient rate the pain on a scale of 0 to 10; 0=no pain, 10=the worst it could be), location (where did it start and has it traveled anywhere), duration.
    - Ask about nausea.

13. Based on your assessment findings, you decide to call the physician. What information are you going to report to her? **[A/an/PI/ct,ni]**
    - Identify yourself and give information about the patient: W.R. in room xyz; was admitted to Dr. Adams with a diagnosis of R/O MI; arrived at X PM; report anything unusual that happened on admission.
    - The most recent set of VS and whether or not they have changed since admission.
    - Briefly explain the signs you observed on entering the room and report his symptoms
    - Report the information given by the wife in case the doctor was not informed.
    - Make sure you have the medication sheet and chart with you when you call so you can knowledgeably address questions.

It was determined that W. R. has coronary artery disease (CAD). The physician suggested it would be best to treat him medically for now. He was discharged with a referral for a follow-up visit to the cardiologist in 1 week.

14. Before discharge, what 4 educational issues are you going to discuss with W.R. and his wife? **[P/an/S,PI,PSI,HP/ct,ni,tc]**
    - Medications: review his medications again with him and his wife; give the patient a preprinted medication instruction sheet, and highlight important information; instruct them to call their local pharmacist if they have questions about medications after they get home.
    - Diet: review dietary instructions with both W.R. and his wife; suggest they look in their local bookstore for *Healthy Heart* and tasty, low-fat recipes.
    - Smoking: review availability of smoking cessation programs offered by the American Lung Association/American Heart Association and give him the telephone numbers of the local chapters.
    - Exercise: review the importance of regular, moderate-intensity exercise; instruct him to check with his insurance program about covering the cost of a supervised cardiac rehabilitation program, otherwise ask his physician for exercise heart rate recommendations and safety guidelines. *W.R. should not start an exercise program until cleared to do by by his physician.*
    - Regular BP checks: explain the importance of having his blood pressure checked on a regular basis to make sure his medication is adequate; inform him that local fire departments will check his blood pressure.

Case Study 5: Deep Vein Thrombosis

Difficulty: * *Setting:* Hospital

Index Words: Deep vein thrombosis, coronary artery disease, atrial fibrillation

You are assigned to care for L.J., a 70-year-old retired bus driver who has just been admitted to your medical floor with R leg deep vein thrombosis (DVT). L.J. has a 48 pack/year smoking history, although he states he quit 2 years ago. He has had pneumonia several times, frequent episodes of atrial fibrillation, 2 previous episodes of DVT, and was diagnosed with rheumatoid arthritis 3 years ago. Two months ago he began experiencing shortness of breath on exertion and noticed swelling of his R foreleg that became progressively worse until it also involved his thigh to the groin. His wife brought him to the hospital when he complained of increasingly severe pain in his leg. When a Doppler study indicated a probable thrombus of the external iliac vein extending distally to the lower leg, he was admitted for bed rest and IV heparin therapy. Significant admission lab values are: PT 12.4 sec, PTT 25 sec, Hgb 13.3 g/dl, Hct 38.9%, cholesterol 206 mg/dl. Electrolytes are normal.

1. List 6 risk factors for DVT. **[A/k/Pl/ct]**
   - Most risk factors fall within the 3 categories of Virchow's triad:
     - Venous stasis: lengthy surgery, immobility, over age 40, pregnancy, atrial fibrillation, CHF, obesity, stroke, denervated limb, hip/knee replacement.
     - Venous endothelial injury: previous DVT, IV catheter, fractures, chemical injury (e.g., cigarette-smoke products, elevated glucose), trauma, varicose veins, hypertension.
     - Hypercoagulability: malignant neoplasms, dehydration, oral contraceptives, estrogen therapy, sepsis, blood dyscrasias, burns.

2. Identify the problems from L.J.'s history above that represent his personal risk factors. **[A/c/Pl/ct]**
   - Smoking history.
   - Decrease in mobility related to shortness of breath.
   - Atrial fibrillation.
   - Previous DVTs.
   - 70 years of age.

3. Keeping in mind L.J.'s health history and admitting diagnosis, what are the most important assessments you should make during your physical examination and assessment? **[A/ap/S,Pl/ct,ni]**
   - Baseline VS.
   - Cardiopulmonary: baseline VS, assess heart sounds, compare perfusion of extremities.
   - Venous compromise of affected leg: assess warmth, redness, pain, edema, Homan's sign, distal pulses, capillary refill, baseline calf and thigh girth. Don't forget to compare both legs.
   - Lungs: assess breath sounds and for dyspnea, chest pain.
   - Mental status: assess for confusion, restlessness, lethargy.

4. What is the most serious complication of DVT? **[A/k/S,Pl/ct]**
   - Pulmonary embolism.

Your assessment of L.J. reveals bibasilar crackles with moist cough; normal heart sounds, BP 138/88, P 104, 3+ pitting edema R lower extremity, mild erythema of R foot and calf, and severe R calf pain. He is alert and oriented but a little restless. He denies shortness of breath and chest pain.

5. Which of these assessment findings should you monitor closely for development of the complication identified in #4? **[A/ap/S,Pl/ct,ni]**
   - Crackles.
   - Cough.
   - Tachycardia.
   - Restlessness.

6. List 6 other common signs/symptoms of this complication in order of priority. **[A/k/Pl/ct]**
   - Dyspnea and tachypnea (occur in 85% of cases).
   - Sudden pleuritic chest pain (occurs in 74% of cases).
   - Apprehension.
   - Hemoptysis.
   - Fever.
   - Nausea and vomiting.
   - Cyanosis.

   Note: If a pulmonary embolism is massive, the signs/symptoms are more like those of myocardial infarction: crushing, substernal chest pain, marked respiratory distress, feeling of impending doom, rapid, shallow breathing, dysrhythmias, shock.

You place L.J. on bed rest and give him a bolus of 5000 units of heparin SC, followed by a continuous IV heparin drip. You give him acetaminophen (Tylenol) as ordered, for pain.

7. The heparin comes premixed as heparin 20,000 units in 500 ml D_5W. If the physician prescribed the patient to receive 1240 U/h, how fast would you infuse the drip? What will be the method of infusion? **[A/c/S/ct,ni]**
   - 31 ml/h.
   - Heparin IV should be infused by pump only.

8. What instructions will you give him about his activity? **[P/c/S,Pl/ct,ni,tc]**
   - Maintain bed rest to prevent dislodgment of an embolus from the DVT. Ask him to immediately report to you any signs/symptoms of pulmonary embolism (see above).
   - Frequently change positions in bed; this helps prevent problems of immobility.
   - Perform frequent gentle dorsiflexion and plantarflexion of the feet and ankle circles to promote circulation and facilitate venous return.
   - Do not cross legs; crossing legs can decrease circulation.
   - Do not massage R leg; massage could dislodge a thrombus.
   - Keep R leg elevated without pressure under the knee; promote circulation.
   - Avoid sudden muscle movement of affected limb that could dislodge a thrombus.

   Note: Significant others often want to do something helpful. Having them remind the patient to do their ankle exercises, in particular, can be a valuable adjunct.

9. What pertinent laboratory values/test results would you expect the physician to order (and that you should monitor)? **[A/k/S,PI/ct,ni]**
   - PTT to monitor therapeutic dose of heparin. Normal PTT: 25-38 seconds; therapeutic PTT: 1½ to 2½ times the normal level.
   - PT.
   - Platelet count.
   - Chest x-ray.
   - Ventilation/perfusion (V/Q) scan.
   - CBC.
   - ABGs.
   - Guaiac stool, any emesis.

10. One of your nursing diagnoses/patient problems is pain. List 4 interventions you would choose for L.J. associated with this diagnosis? **[PD/AN/PI/ct,ni]**
    - Get specific information on the symptom; verify with the patient the location, quality, intensity, onset, and expression of pain.
    - Assess and monitor those factors that increase or decrease pain.
    - Assess and monitor emotional responses and coping mechanisms to pain.
    - Eliminate or modify those stimuli that increase pain.
    - Evaluate the effectiveness of his pain medication.
    - Teach him techniques he can use to modify his own pain (e.g., relaxation, imagery, distraction).

    Instructor Note: It is not uncommon for older adults to reject imagery and relaxation techniques. Students should be encouraged to explore the patient's values and preferences.

A week has passed. L.J. responded to heparin therapy, was started on warfarin (Coumadin) therapy, and is being discharged to home for home care follow-up. "Good," he says, "just in time to fly out West for my grandson's wedding." His wife, who has come to pick him up, rolls her eyes and looks at the ceiling. You almost drop the discharge papers in disbelief at what you have just heard (and you thought you did such a good job of discharge teaching!).

11. What are you going to say to him? **[P,I/an/S,PI,PSI/ct,ni,tc]**
    - Wrong! You observe that L.J. doesn't seem to have realistic expectations associated with his recovery, so you explain...
    - He is going to require daily follow-up visits to monitor his status.
    - Sitting on a plane for several hours, along with the vigorous activity required to make plane changes, is not safe for him at this time; he is likely to have another DVT develop from sitting on the plane (not to mention sitting at the wedding dinner, wedding, reception); he is going to continue to receive Coumadin for an extended period of time and will be at risk for bleeding and bruising; in addition, following his hospitalization and bed rest, it will take him weeks or even months to adapt to the vigor of everyday life.
    - Explore with him the possibility of sending an audio- or video-taped message from him to the newlyweds. Ask if anyone can tape the ceremony and parts of the reception for him to view at home so he won't feel so isolated.

L.J. listened to you and Mrs. J. was quite relieved (she has been telling her friends about this "wonderful nurse who talked some sense into my husband"). L.J.'s son arranged to video-tape the entire ceremony and guests at the reception taped special greetings for him. It's been 2 weeks and he seems quite pleased. He watches the tape daily and points out his favorite parts to the home care nurse every time she visits.

Case Study 6: Congestive Heart Failure

Difficulty: ** *Setting:* Hospital ED, hospital, home care

Index Words: Congestive heart failure, coronary artery disease, hip fracture, communication deficit

You are just getting caught up with your work when you receive the following phone call, "Hi, this is Deb in the ED. We're sending you M.M., a 63-year-old Hispanic woman with a PMH of CAD. Her daughter reports that she's become increasingly weaker over the last couple weeks and has been unable to do her housework. Apparently she has been c/o swelling in her ankles and feet by late afternoon, and has nocturnal diuresis x 4. Her daughter brought her in because she has complained of heaviness in her chest off and on over the last few days but denies any discomfort at this time. The daughter, N., took her to see her family physician who immediately sent her here. VS are 146/92, 96, 24, 37.2°C. She has an IV of D_5W at KVO in her right forearm. Her labs are as follows: Na 134 mEq/L, K 3.5 mEq/L, Cl 103 mEq/L, HCO_3 23, BUN 13 mg/dl, creatinine 1.3 mg/dl, glucose 153 mg/dl, WBC 8.3 mm^3, Hct 33.9%, Hgb 11.7 g/dl, platelets 162 mm^3. PT, PTT, and UA are pending. She has had her CXR and ECG and her orders have been written."

1. What additional information do you need from the ED nurse? **[A/an/PI,PSI/ct,tc]**
   - What is her admitting diagnosis?
   - Does she speak English? If not, is her daughter coming up with her?
   - Have any cardiac enzymes been drawn?
   - What did her chest x-ray show?
   - Did her ECG show any changes from the last time?

   Instructor Note: A very astute student also may observe the lack of an order for Mg (see below).

2. How are you going to prepare for this patient? **[P/an/PI,PSI/ct,tc]**
   - If the patient doesn't speak English and the daughter isn't coming to the floor with her, does the hospital have an interpreter or someone who speaks Spanish?
   - Turn the bed down and place an IV pole in her room.
   - Make sure there is a thermometer, BP cuff, and admission pack in the room.

3. M. M. arrives by wheelchair (w/c). As she transfers from the w/c to the bed, what observations should you make? **[A/an/S,PI/ct]**
   - Observe the following before she gets out of the w/c: general skin color, respiratory rate and pattern, texture of the hair.
     Instructor Note: People who have prolonged chronic illnesses tend to have poor nutritional intake. Poor intake leads to course, thin, sparse hair; edema (decreased protein levels); bruising (vitamin K deficiency); poor general hygiene (it takes a lot of energy to complete ADL).
   - Place your hands on the patient's skin to note temperature, turgor, and moisture on the skin; this can be done in the process of obtaining initial VS.
   - Observe the following as she moves from the w/c to the bed: gait, need for assistance, balance, coordination, effort, change in color or respiratory pattern.

4. Given the information above, which of the following orders would be appropriate for this patient? Carefully review each order to determine if it is appropriate or inappropriate as written. If the order is appropriate, place an "A" in the space provided; if the order is inappropriate, place an "I" in the space provided and underline the inappropriate part. **[A/an/S,PI,HP/ct]**

   ___ Routine VS.
   ___ Serum magnesium STAT.
   ___ Up ad lib.
   ___ 10 g sodium, low animal fat diet.
   ___ Change IV to NS at 100 ml/h.
   ___ Cardiac enzymes on admission and q8h x 24 then q AM.
   ___ CBC, Chem 7 and lipid profile in AM.
   ___ Schedule for abdominal CT scan for AM.
   ___ Heparin 10,000 U sq q8h.
   ___ Docusate sodium 100 mg PO, qd.
   ___ Ampicillin 250 mg IVPB q6h.
   ___ Furosemide 200 mg IVP STAT.
   ___ Nitroglycerin 0.4 mg 1 SL q4h prn for chest pain.

   _I_ Routine VS: q4h.
   _A_ Serum magnesium STAT.
   _I_ Up ad lib: chair ad lib/ambulate with assist.
   _I_ 10 g sodium, low animal fat diet: 2 g low-sodium diet:
   _I_ Change IV to NS at 100 ml/h: D_5 NS if on Lasix, Na is borderline.
   _A_ Cardiac enzymes on admission and q8h x 24 then q AM.
   _A_ CBC, Chem 7, and lipid profile in AM.
   _I_ Schedule for abdominal CT scan for AM: not needed at this time.
   _I_ Heparin 10,000 U sq q8h: 5000 U sq.
   _A_ Docusate sodium 100 mg PO, qd.
   _I_ Ampicillin 250 mg IVPB q6h: no current indication for this.
   _I_ Furosemide 200 mg IVP STAT: dose too large, 40 to 80 mg may be more appropriate.
   _I_ Nitroglycerine 0.4 mg SL q5min prn for chest pain: SL prn for chest pain x 3 doses; call the house officer (HO) if no relief.

   Missing orders:

   - K at 3.5 mEq/L; K is borderline, should have 40 mEq/L in maintenance IV or give 20 mEq PO bid plus 40 mEq PO now.
   - Also, based on serum Mg results, magnesium supplementation may be required.

Serum magnesium is rapidly becoming recognized as an essential laboratory test with respect to blood pressure and cardiac functioning in general. Both Mg and K should be evaluated together. Unfortunately, Mg is not on any of the standardized laboratories "batteries" and must be specifically requested.

5. When you respond to M.M.'s call light, you observe she is talking rapidly in Spanish and pointing to the bathroom. Her speech pattern indicates she is SOB. You assist her to the bathroom and note that her skin feels clammy. While sitting on the commode she vomits. On a scale of 1 to 10 (1 = being no problem, 10 = being a CODE-level emergency), how would you rate this situation and why? **[A/an/PI/ct]**

   - 8 to 10: the patient's skin is clammy and she has vomited; these are signs of cardiac ischemia and indicate that the patient needs immediate medical attention.

6. Identify at least 4 actions you should take next, and state your rationale. **[I/an/S,PI,PSI/ct,ni,tc]**
   - Pull emergency light in the bathroom and call for help. You want additional personnel in case the patient's condition continues to deteriorate.
   - Reassure as well as possible (tone of voice and touch communicate across language barriers), that you'll stay with her and help her. Ask the unit clerk to STAT page anyone who speaks Spanish.
   - Ask the patient about symptoms. Facilitate your questions with nonverbal signs. Gather as much relevant data as possible to determine if the patient is presenting with an MI, pulmonary edema, pulmonary embolus, etc.
   - Move the patient back to bed as quickly as possible, take VS, and complete a brief assessment of the heart and lungs. You want to determine if the patient is having dysrhythmias or has abnormal lung sounds.
   - Initiate oxygen (titrate to maintain O_2 sat >90%), oximeter monitoring, and cardiac monitoring (if available).
   - STAT page the house officer (HO) on call.

Note: If a physician is not immediately available and/or the staffing is such that you can not obtain adequate help, do not hesitate to call a CODE. This is an urgent situation.

7. The physician calls your unit to find out what is happening. What information would you need to convey at this time? **[A/ap/PI,PSI/ct,tc]**
   - Identify yourself, the patient, attending physician, and admitting diagnosis.
   - Briefly report the episode, assessment findings, and your action.

8. The resident is coming to the floor to evaluate the patient immediately. In the meantime she orders Lasix 40 mg IVP STAT. You only have 20 mg in stock. Should you give the 20 mg now, then give the additional 20 mg when it comes up from pharmacy? **[P/c/PI/ct]**
   - Give the 20 mg Lasix to start treatment. However, you should know that response to Lasix is dose related; 20 now + 20 later does not equal the same response as 40 given at one time. You need to make the physician aware that you only gave 20 mg and ask how much more the doctor wants to give when it becomes available.
   - Call the pharmacy and have Lasix brought to the floor STAT.

9. M.M. continues to experience vomiting and diaphoresis that are unrelieved by medication and comfort measures. A STAT 12-lead ECG reveals ischemic changes. The patient is transferred to the coronary care unit. As you give report to the receiving RN, what laboratory value is the most important to report and why? **[PD/AP/S,PI/ct,ni,tc]**
   - Potassium. The K was 3.5 before any Lasix was given and there is no K in the IV fluid; the patient is going to need some K supplement. The order might read K 40 mEq in 100 ml D_5W to infuse over 4 hours. Also indicate serum magnesium level if the report has come back.

10. While recovering in ICU, M.M. slipped in the bathroom and fractured her femur. Because of the surgical risks involved, M. M. was treated conservatively and put in a long leg cast. She is again transferred to your floor. A geriatric nurse practitioner (GNP) has been asked to evaluate M.M.'s home to see if she can be discharged to her own home or will need to stay elsewhere. Identify 8 things that the GNP would assess. **[A/c/S,PI/ct,ni]**
    - Telephone service?
    - Number of steps in the home/apartment?
    - Danger of tripping on throw rugs, loose carpeting, etc.?
    - Presence of hand rails in stairways?
    - Width of doorways?
    - Location of bathrooms (does she have to negotiate steps to get there)?
    - Can toilet seat be raised and railings applied?
    - Adequacy of lighting?
    - What is she going to do for meals, grocery shopping, and laundry?
    - Will someone check on her every day?
    - Does she have sufficient upper body strength to independently and safely ambulate?

11. Since it was determined that M.M. lived in an apartment with poor access, she elected to stay with her daughter and 5 grandchildren in their small home. A home care nurse comes 3 times a week to check on her. M.M. is easily fatigued and the children are quite lively. Suggest some ways the daughter can ensure that her mother isn't overwhelmed and doesn't become exhausted in this situation. **[P/an/PI,PSI/ct,ni,tc]**
    - Even if M.M. can't have her own room, arrange for her to have a quiet corner where she can withdraw prn.
    - Establish a "nap time" every day when she will not be disturbed.
    - Keep the children occupied with a video or something they would like that would keep them quiet for specific times each day (school is out for the summer).
    - Ask the children who are able to follow directions to take turns helping grandma during certain times of the day.
    - Ask if there is a responsible friend or relative with a van or large vehicle who can take M.M. for a brief daily drive or out for a "cup of coffee" to help her get out of the house on a regular basis. This is best followed by a nap.

Case Study 7: Angina

Difficulty: **	*Setting:* Hospital
Index Words: Angina	

R.K. is a 90-year-old woman who lives with her husband of the same age. Two nights before her admission to your cardiac floor, she awoke with heavy, substernal pressure accompanied by epigastric distress. The pain was reduced somewhat when she rolled onto her side but did not completely subside for about 6 hours. The next night she experienced the same chest pressure. The following morning, R.K.'s husband took her to the doctor and she was subsequently hospitalized to rule out myocardial infarction (R/O MI).

You obtain the following information from your nursing history and physical exam: R.K. has no history of smoking or alcohol use; has been in good general health with the exception of osteoarthritis of her hands and knees and some osteoporosis of the spine; and her only medications are ranitidine (Zantac), ibuprofen (Motrin) for bone and joint pain, and "herbs." On admission her VS are 142/84, 88, 16, 37.2°C; weight 52 kg. Trace edema of both ankles is present, but capillary refill and peripheral pulses are 1+. You hear a soft systolic murmur. You place her on telemetry, which shows frequent PACs but no ventricular ectopy. She is not in any discomfort at present.

1. R. K. became fatigued during the admission process and you decide to let her sleep. When she wakes, what additional history and physical information should you obtain related to her admitting diagnosis? **[A/c/PI,PSI/ct,ni,tc]**

   History
   - Medication allergies.
   - Try to identify what "herbs" she takes.
   - General activity level.
   - Sleep patterns.
   - General perceived stress level.
   - Accustomed diet.
   - Help that she or her husband need at home.

   Physical Exam
   - Pain (if present): assess intensity, characteristics, onset, location, duration, factors that make it better or worse, associated symptoms and radiation.
   - Lungs: assess for signs/symptoms of CHF (crackles, dyspnea, cough productive of frothy sputum).
   - Mental status: assess for orientation, alertness, anxiety, confusion, restlessness.

2. List 7 lab/diagnostic tests that you would expect the physician to order, and suggest what each may contribute. **[A/c/Pl/ct]**
   - 12-lead ECG: to determine if R.K. has had a prior myocardial infarction, if she is showing ischemic changes and in what part of her heart, and whether she is having irregular rhythms (the ECG is not a conclusive test for MI).
   - Chest x-ray: to see if the heart is enlarged and whether there are any structural problems or defects that may be contributing to her symptoms.
   - ABGs: to determine whether her symptoms may be related to a respiratory disorder or whether her heart is able to adequately pump blood through her lungs.
   - Cardiac enzymes: CPK and LDH (with isoenzymes if elevated) to determine if she has had a myocardial infarction.
   - CBC.
   - Chemistry panel.
   - Urinalysis.
   - PT/PTT: to examine for basic coagulation disorders.

3. What other source, besides cardiac, might be responsible for her chest and abdominal discomfort (specify)? **[A/c/Pl/ct]**
   - GI: indigestion, gastric ulcer, gastritis, hiatal hernia, esophagitis.
   - Respiratory: pleurisy, pulmonary embolism, pneumonia, pneumothorax.
   - Musculoskeletal: rib fracture, costrochondritis, respiratory muscle strain, vertebral fractures or collapse resulting in nerve impingement.

4. Differentiate between pain of ischemic cardiac origin and that of noncardiac origin. **[A/k/Pl/ct]**

	Ischemic cardiac origin	Non-cardiac origin
• Character:	Constricting, squeezing, burning, dull, pressing, heavy.	Knife-like, stabbing, aggravated by respirations.
• Location:	Precordial, substernal, both arms and hands, shoulders, neck jaws.	Left submammary area, left hemithorax.
• Provoking factors:	Exercise, excitement, stress, cold after meals.	Pain *after* completion of exercise, specific body motion or activities.

5. Define the concept "differential diagnosis" and explain what it means. **[PD/c/Pl/ct]**
   - Differential diagnosis is the medical process of discovering which of two or more possible diseases or conditions is responsible for the symptom the patient is suffering from. The clinical process of making a differential diagnosis involves a systematic comparison and contrast of clinical findings.

6. Explain how the concept of differential diagnosis applies to R.K.'s symptoms? **[PD/ap/Pl/ct]**
   - R.K.'s symptoms could come from several sources, some serious and life-threatening, some less significant. By performing a careful assessment and a series of diagnostic tests, the physician can "rule out" what the diagnosis is *not* by a process of elimination. By narrowing the possibilities, the diagnosis usually is whatever is left.

7. Florence Nightingale frequently emphasized the value of good observation skills in nurses. Explain how a good nursing assessment can contribute to making the differential diagnosis. **[A/c/PI/ct]**
   - Using a systematic method of investigating symptoms such as COLDERRA (C = characteristics, O = onset, L = location, D = duration, E = exacerbation, R = radiation, R = relief, and A = associated signs and symptoms) can help suggest causes of the symptom or conditions that contribute to it. Since nurses spend much more time in direct patient care than physicians, they can make significant contributions to eliminating unnecessary tests by detecting "clues" or discovering *patterns* associated with the distress.

8. Abnormalities on R.K.'s 12-lead ECG were reported as "slight left axis deviation." Serial CPKs are: 27 U/ml, 24 U/ml, 26 U/ml; first LDH is 215 U/ml. A series of tests ruled out a noncardiac cause for her chest pain. On the basis of the information presented so far, do you believe that she has had a myocardial infarction? What is your rationale? **[PD/an/PI/ct]**
   - No: her cardiac symptoms are probably due to angina secondary to CAD rather than an MI based on the following.
     - Cardiac enzymes are within the normal range.
     - ECG did not show ST, T wave, or Q wave changes.
     - Decreased activity and change of position somewhat relieved pain.

9. While you care for R.K. you carefully monitor her. Identify 2 possible complication of CAD and the signs/symptoms associated with each. **[A,I/c/PI/ct,ni]**
   - Cardiac ischemia (see above).
   - Cardiac dysrhythmias, particularly PVCs: dysrhythmias seen on telemetry, syncope, lightheadedness, shortness of breath, palpitations felt by patient.
   - CHF: crackles, dyspnea, confusion, cough productive of frothy sputum, peripheral edema, jugular vein distention.

10. R.K. rings her call bell. When you arrive, she places her hand over her heart and tells you she is "having that terrible heavy feeling again." She is not diaphoretic or nauseated but states she is short of breath. What can you do to make her more comfortable? **[P/an/S,PI,PSI/ct,ni,tc]**
    - Give her supplemental oxygen as ordered (O_2 2-4 L/nc).
    - Give her NTG 0.4 mg SL as ordered (1q5 min prn chest pain x 3 doses) to decrease the venous return to the heart and dilate the coronary arteries to increase the oxygen supply to the heart.
    - Have her rest quietly in bed to decrease oxygen demand.
    - Elevate the head of bed to facilitate lung expansion.
    - Encourage verbalization of concerns to decrease anxiety and oxygen demand.

✍CPK can be reported in terms of U/ml or U/L. Always read laboratory reports carefully to be sure which units are used in your institution.

Case Study 8: Above-the-Knee Amputation

Difficulty: **	*Setting:* Hospital
Index Words: Above-the-knee amputation, coronary artery disease, cardiac transplant, chronic renal failure	

C.C., a 60-year-old single, retired real estate agent, has a long history of cardiovascular disease due to generalized atherosclerosis. He also has hypertension and COPD (with home O_2). Three serious MIs in the past resulted in ischemic cardiomyopathy, necessitating a cardiac transplant 9 years ago. He developed chronic renal failure as a result of the cyclosporine he is taking to prevent rejection. Two years ago he had an axillary-bifemoral graft for peripheral vascular occlusion and ultimately required transmetatarsal amputation of the L foot. Three days ago C.C. had an acute onset of R calf pain with numbness, pain, loss of movement, and coldness of the R lower leg and foot. A vascular scan showed complete occlusion of the R side of the axillary-bifemoral graft, and he was admitted to your SICU in preparation for a R above-knee amputation.

His routine medications include azathioprene (Imuran), furozemide (Lasix), cyclosporine (Sandimmune), prednisone, metholazone (Zaroxolyn), hydrocodone with acetaminophen (Vicodin), Lisinopril (Zestril), warfarin (Coumadin), digoxin (Lanoxin), diazepam (Valium), MgOxide, and KCl. Before the surgery, his VS are 140/72, 115, and 20. Significant abnormal lab values are: K 6.0 mEq/L, BUN 150 mg/dl, creatinine 11.2 mg/dl, PT 42.1 sec, PTT 50 sec, WBCs 16.2 mm^3, cholesterol 295 mg/dl. Chest x-ray shows clear lungs and cardiomegaly. You hear an S_3 gallop and tricuspid regurgitation murmur on cardiac auscultation. His right leg is without pulses by Doppler from the knee down.

1. What critical history information would you need about C.C. to prepare his discharge planning? **[P/c/S,PSI/ct]**
   - Living arrangements: how will he get along at home after his amputation; what facilities/aids does he already have in place in addition to the home O_2?
   - Coping skills: this second amputation will affect his body image; he has already had a heart transplant and partial amputation of his other foot.
   - Support people: he is unmarried; who is available to give him physical and emotional support?
   - Financial needs: his ongoing medical care is extremely expensive.
   - Interdisciplinary team needs: assess his need for PT, OT, dietary, and social work consults.

2. What abnormal lab value is of concern, and what would you expect the physician to order to correct it? **[P/ap/PI/ct]**
   - The physician does not want to take him to surgery with a K of 6.0 mEq/L, so he would order Kayexalate 30 g PO, or order hemodialysis, to decrease the K level.

3. From the above information, what is the reason for the elevated BUN and creatinine? **[PD/c/PI/ct]**
   - Chronic renal failure.

4. From the PT and PTT, what complication might you expect after surgery and why? **[PD/c/S,PI/ct]**
   - You might expect C.C. to develop excessive bleeding after surgery because his current PT (extrinsic clotting mechanism) and PTT (intrinsic clotting system) indicate impaired coagulation.

5. C. C. will return to the SICU after his surgery, as he has after his previous surgeries. He is very apprehensive about the experience. What can you do to allay his fears? **[P/an/PI,PSI/ct,ni,tc]**
   - Investigate the source of his anxiety. What specific features of the SICU experience distress him? Address his specific concerns.
   - Explain how this surgery will be similar to and different from the previous surgeries.
   - Reassure him that he will be kept as comfortable as possible with pain medications.
   - Teach him interventions he can use to control his own pain and anxiety, such as relaxation techniques and imagery.
   - Describe the equipment he will have in the SICU and the reasons he will need them: Swan-Ganz line, arterial line, indwelling urinary catheter, supplemental oxygen by nasal cannula. Assure him that the equipment is there to facilitate his recovery and will be removed as soon as possible.

In the SICU on the third postop day, C.C.'s VS are 122/66, 113, 12. His hemodynamic values are: PCWP 15 mm Hg, central venous pressure (CVP) 11 mm Hg, pulmonary artery pressure (PAP) 28/20 mm Hg, cardiac output 4.5 L/min.

6. From these values, would you describe his condition as hemodynamically stable? **[PD/c/PI/ct]**
   - Yes: his heart rate, CVP and PAP are very slightly elevated, but not enough to worry about.

7. Large amounts of D_5½ NS are given to keep rhabdomyolysis from elevating the BUN. What serious complications might the IV fluid cause, and how would you monitor for that complication? **[P/c/PI/ct,ni]**
   - Fluid overload with resulting CHF.
   - I&O with special focus on urine output; given the renal insufficiency, rhabdomyolysis may prevent excretion of the extra fluid.
   - Listen to heart sounds for increase in murmur and S_3 and S_4 gallops.
   - Weigh patient daily; weight gain is the most accurate measure of fluid retention.
   - Monitor BUN and creatinine daily.
   - Listen to lungs; crackles indicate pulmonary edema.
   - Assess patient for diminished mental status and dyspnea.
   - Watch for tachycardia and tachypnea; they indicate oxygen deficit.

8. Which medications and electrolytes would you expect to be monitor closely and why? **[A/c/PI/ct,ni]**
   - Digoxin: the digoxin level should be monitored appropriately; if the patient is on cyclosporin, decrease the digoxin dose by about 50%.
   - Imuran: monitor the WBC and platelet counts when patients are taking Imuran; notify the physician for WBC $<3.0\ mm^3$ or platelet count $<100\ mm^3$ because the dose may need to be reduced.
   - Cyclosporine: periodically monitor trough levels; maintain the trough level between 250 and 800 ng/ml to minimize both side effects and rejection events. This drug is nephrotoxic so monitor BUN and creatinine levels; it is hepatotoxic, so monitor AST (SGOT), ALT (SGPT), alk phos, amyl, and bilirubin.
   - K, BUN, creatinine (see cyclosporine above).

9. C.C.'s glucose level is 216 mg/dl on the third postop day. It had been 107 mg/dl the day before surgery. How do you account for this elevation? **[PD/c/PI/ct]**
   - Stress hormones, triggered by the physical and emotional trauma of the surgery, cause moderate elevation of the glucose level for a few days. The hormones cause glycogen to be converted to glucose in the liver, and muscle and fat to be catabolized to provide glucose. Epinephrine, norepinephrine, thyroid hormone, glucagon and cortisol are the primary stress hormones involved in this response.
   - Bed rest contributes to glucose intolerance.
   - Prednisone can be a significant contributor to an increased serum glucose level.

10. C.C. tells you he knows he's being silly, but he's experiencing "terrible sharp pain" in his R lower leg. What are you going to do and why? **[P/ap/PI,PSI/ct,ni,tc]**
    - You know that because this is the leg that was amputated, he must be experiencing phantom pain. Phantom pain should be treated just as seriously as any other pain.
    - Reassure him that it is important he tell you about all his pain.
    - Quickly check to see what pain medications are ordered, what specific medication and dose have been effective for him. Don't forget to perform basic assessment including premedication and postmedication levels of pain to determine efficacy of the treatment. It is important not to delay requests for pain medications because many patients wait until they are hurting badly before they "bother the nurse."
    - Check back later to determine the efficacy of C.C.'s analgesia and to reinforce how important it is that he keep you informed on how he is feeling.

    Instructor Note: Remember, C.C. was taking Vicodan before admission and surgery. He may require more pain medication to obtain relief.

Case Study 9: Congestive Heart Failure

Difficulty: ** *Setting:* Hospital

Index Words: Congestive heart failure, sleep disturbance, pneumonitis, hypertension, cultural diversity

J.T. is a 58-year-old Tongan man admitted to your floor with syncope and right-sided heart failure. He was brought to the hospital after "passing out" and "turning blue" for 2 minutes after a severe bout of coughing. Because J.T. speaks very little English, his wife helps you obtain his health history: NIDDM, significant abdominal obesity, hypertension, CHF, chronic hypoxia, frequent pneumonia, hyperlipidemia, and polycythemia. His wife tells you he snores loudly and seems to stop breathing sometimes during the night. He has no history of smoking or alcohol use. His weight is 310 pounds. Over the last week he has had intermittent chest pain with shortness of breath on exertion. The shortness of breath has increased during the last 12 hours. He has been hospitalized in the past for chest pain but has never had an MI. On admission today he has orthopnea, a severe dry cough, palpitations, and shortness of breath. He is not complaining of chest pain or discomfort. His VS are 146/94, 64, 20, 36.7°C. You hear muffled S_1 and S_2 heart sounds and a possible S_3. He has moderate pretibial edema to his knees and a few bibasilar crackles. You place him on oxygen at 3 L/min by nasal cannula and insert a Foley catheter. His blood glucose level is 147 mg/dl and Hct is 50%. Other lab values are normal, including cholesterol and triglyceride levels.

1. What is the relationship of J.T.'s country of origin to his current health problems? **[A/an/PI,PSI/ct]**
   - Tonga is a kingdom consisting of some 170 of the Polynesian Islands. Obesity is a much admired trait among its people, historically considered a sign of prosperity and health. J.T.'s obesity, the source of his health problems, represents something desirable in his culture rather than carrying the stigma associated with body fat in North America.

2. What do you think is the significance of J.T.'s wife's report about his snoring and sleep-related breathing pattern? **[PD/c/PI/ct]**
   - It sounds as if he suffers from sleep apnea, a form of sleep disturbance.

3. Judging from the admission information, do you think he has right-sided CHF, left-sided CHF, or both? Cite your evidence. **[A/c/PI/ct]**
   - Both. The shortness of breath, orthopnea, cough, crackles, and S3 heart sound are signs/symptoms of left-sided failure. The pretibial edema indicates right-sided failure.

4. List 3 other things you could assess to confirm your suspicion of right-sided failure. **[A/ap/PI/ct,ni]**
   - Jugular vein distention: venous pressure is increased as output of the right ventricle decreases and blood backs up into the venous system.
   - Liver enlargement: venous congestion of the liver increases liver size.
   - Ascites: decreased production of albumin by a damaged liver causes ascites and dependent edema.
   - Urine output: increased venous pressure will decrease renal perfusion.
   - Gastric distress/anorexia/nausea: gastric distress is caused by congestion of the bowel.

5. What is a possible explanation for his chronic hypoxia? **[A/c/PI/ct]**
   - Obesity is the most probable explanation. The enlarged abdomen presses against the diaphragm, restricting the lung capacity.
   - Chronic CHF contributes to chronic hypoxia by causing some degree of pulmonary edema and may be related to both obesity and possible sleep apnea.
   - Sleep apnea and hypertension. Sleep apnea, whether central or obstructive, results in cessation of airflow with subsequent hypoxemia and hypercarbia. The decreased PaO_2 and increased $PaCO_2$ lead to widespread pulmonary vascular constriction (pulmonary HTN). Research has shown that this constriction continues for up to 8 hours after waking; conceivably, the patient could suffer from pulmonary HTN for up to 16 hours per day. The chronic hypoxemic state leads to increased RBC production and polycythemia.

6. List 4 priority nursing diagnoses for J. T. **[PD/an/PI,PSI/ct,ni,tc]**
   - Decreased cardiac output related to congestive heart failure.
   - Impaired gas exchange related to congestive heart failure, obesity, and/or chronic sleep apnea.
   - Activity intolerance related to insufficient oxygenation secondary to decreased cardiac output and obesity.
   - Impaired communication related to lack of knowledge of English.
   - Altered nutrition, more than body requirements, as evidenced by weight of 310 pounds.
   - Risk for fluid volume excess related to congestive heart failure.

The night shift nurse confirms the report that J.T. snores loudly ("I could hear him all the way down the hall!") and has 30- to 60-second pauses in his breathing followed by a violent jerk and thrashing as he resumes inspirations. A sleep study is ordered.

7. Define a sleep study and what information can be obtained from it. **[A/c/PI,PSI/ct]**
   - A sleep study usually is conducted in a sleep laboratory to examine pathophysiologic problems related to sleep. An EEG and ECG are connected to record brain wave patterns and cardiac rate and rhythm throughout. Oxygen saturation, respiratory effort, respiratory excursions, and nasal/oral airflow are also recorded. A sleep study can differentiate between central (brain fails to send impulses to initiate respiration) and obstructive (the structures of the throat collapse and obstruct airflow) sleep apnea. A decrease in SaO_2 of greater than 11% from baseline is considered a sleep apnea-related desaturation.

The sleep study showed obstructive sleep apnea with oxygen desaturation as low as 32% for prolonged periods following each apneic episode. During his study, J.T. had over 320 apneic episodes in 1 night.

8. Continuous positive airway pressure (CPAP) is prescribed for J.T. Explain the concept of CPAP and how it will benefit him. **[PD/c/PI/ct]**
   - CPAP is applied through a plastic self-sealing mask that fits over the nose (nasal CPAP) or the nose and mouth (Bipap). The patient breathes a constant flow of air at a pressure that exceeds the patient's inspiratory peak flow demands. This forces the airways to stay open, enabling the patient to breathe and preventing hypoxemia.

On the forth day after admission, J.T. developed chills and fever with a temperature of 38.5°C and an SaO_2 of 88% on 3 L O_2/nc.

9. What are the 2 most likely sources of infection that might be responsible for his fever? **[A/ap/Pl/ct]**
   - Respiratory tract: this is a common source of infection in hospitalized patients; in addition, J.T.'s risk is increased by his decreased lung capacity, severe cough, and history of pneumonia.
   - Urinary tract: this is a common source of infection in hospitalized patients with indwelling urinary catheters.

J. T. was diagnosed with pneumonia and started on erythromycin. During his hospitalization, J.T.'s family has repeatedly brought him food and drinks from home in spite of explanations by the nurses that he is on a 2000-calorie, low-salt, diabetic diet, and on fluid restriction. Because of his obesity and extreme shortness of breath on exertion, he is quite immobilized.

10. Identify the most serious complication of immobility for which he is at risk, and state the reasons for this risk. **[A/c/Pl/ct]**
    - Deep vein thrombosis with possible embolization to the lungs. Leg muscle contraction contributes to venous return of blood from the legs to the heart. With immobility, venous stasis occurs. The right-sided congestive failure also contributes to venous stasis. In addition, his polycythemia increases viscosity of the blood. Stasis and high viscosity predispose to increased blood clotting.

After a week on erythromycin for his pneumonia and diuresis for his CHF, J.T.'s doctor says he is ready to go home. You have developed a list of things that you think he and his family should be taught before he is ready for discharge. After reviewing his history, you have decided that he has many risk factors for coronary artery disease; although he has not had an MI yet, he is at risk for having one. You have placed teaching about cardiac risk factors at the top of your list.

11. List 4 cardiac risk factors that J. T. has and place a check (✓) mark beside the ones that are potentially modifiable through behavioral change. **[A/c/Pl,HP/ct]**
    - ✓ Obesity: male-pattern fat distribution (high WHR).
    - NIDDM: can be controlled, but not cured.
    - ✓ Hypertension.
    - ✓ Lack of exercise.
    - Polycythemia.

Note: Although polycythemia is uncommon and is not on the list of usual coronary risk factors, it increases the tendency for clot formation and increases the risk for MI.

12. Identify 2 major pathologic conditions J.T. has for which he needs teaching. **[PD/c/S,Pl/ct,ni,tc]**
    - CHF: his failure to maintain his fluid restriction indicates a lack of understanding about the disease (certainly a possibility because of his language barrier) or willful noncompliance.
    - Diabetes: again, his failure to stay on his diabetic diet indicates a need for teaching or encouragement or both.

13. What do you think is the likelihood J.T. will be motivated to exercise and diet to lose weight and why? **[A/an/S,PI,PSI/ct]**
    - It is highly unlikely J.T. will be interested in exercise and dieting. From the above information, it appears that his whole social support system is committed to "sabotaging" a restrictive diet. The idea of risk factor reduction reflects North American values and ideals, especially with respect to weight loss. Health care professionals need to recognize that not everyone values risk factor reduction or idealizes a slender body. Patients have a right to select their own lifestyles and live accordingly without suffering judgment or prejudice by health care professionals.

Case Study 10: Heart Transplant

Difficulty: ** *Setting:* Hospital

Index Words: Heart transplant

Three years ago, M.Y., a 50-year-old building contractor from Montana, consulted his physician for shortness of breath, fatigue, swelling of his legs, and syncopal episodes. An echocardiogram done at the time revealed an ejection fraction of 25% to 30% with mild mitral regurgitation. M.Y. refused a cardiac catheterization and other invasive tests and procedures, instead choosing to be treated for his CHF with medications (furosemide [Lasix], enalapril [Vasotec] and aspirin). He did well until 3 to 4 months ago when he developed increasing pedal edema, generalized fluid retention, dramatic decrease in activity level, severe dyspnea, and cough. Another echocardiogram showed his ejection fraction had decreased to 12% and that he also had 4-chamber dilation. He was diagnosed with idiopathic dilated cardiomyopathy, hospitalized, and started on dobutamine (Dobutrex) and lidocaine drips. His PCWP was 26 mm Hg and cardiac index 1.8. He was transferred by plane to a large regional medical center because of the seriousness of his condition to await a heart transplant.

M.Y. lives alone. His only living family members are a brother and a sister who both reside in distant states. M.Y. spent 2 weeks in the MICU while his cardiac output and blood pressure were supported by dopamine (Intropin) and dobutamine. The transplant surgery was successful, and he is now recovering on the telemetry unit.

1. You talk with M.Y. about his presurgery experience. Name at least 6 changes in everyday functioning you would you expect a person with advanced CHF to experience. **[A/c/PI,PSI/ct]**
   - Unable to maintain employment.
   - Overwhelming fatigue, leading to decreased capacity for everyday activity.
   - Decreased ability to socialize with others.
   - Decreased ability to take care of residence.
   - Decreased ability to engage in supportive tasks of living (grocery shopping, paying bills, doing laundry, making meals, etc.).
   - Decreased ability to take care of oneself.
   - Decreased ability to engage in social roles.
   - Difficulty sleeping, leading to disrupted everyday activities.

2. Name at least 5 emotional issues you might expect in an individual with advanced CHF and explain your rationale. **[PD/c/PSI/ct]**
   - Difficulty concentrating: CHF results in decreased blood supply to the brain and profound fatigue from decreased blood flow and nutrient supply.
   - Fear of death or disability: this is a very realistic fear and would be considered quite normal in a situation like this.
   - Depression: the potential for depression depends on prior experiences in life and how hopeless the situation is perceived.
   - Grieving or loss: again, this is a normal response to loss of vitality and life.
   - Anxiety: inability to pay medical bills, uncertainty about the future, focusing on one's feelings that fluctuate widely due to disease and medications all contribute to a generalized feeling of anxiety. Also, anxiety from wondering what will happen to one's loved ones.
   - Feelings of hopelessness and helplessness.
   - Anger from feeling helplessness and impotent.

3. Formulate a question to help M.Y. talk about his present feelings. **[A,P/ap/ct,ni,tc]**
   - Almost any way of communicating permission to him, in addition to letting him know that emotional turmoil is common in posttransplant patients, may help him talk about his own feelings. A good starting sentence may be, "I'm concerned about how you are feeling. After their transplants, a lot of people tell me they feel confused about what has happened. Have you had any experiences or feelings like that?"

The transplant team prepares M.Y. for discharge. The social worker is checking into the financial aspects of care in M.Y.'s home community. As the transplant nurse, you have been asked to talk with him about issues relating to his discharge readiness. You decide to start with a psychosocial evaluation to determine problem areas, identify strengths, and determine need for further evaluation and treatment.

4. What are some potential problem areas related to M.Y.'s transplant you will want to investigate? **[A,P/an/S,PI,PSI/ct,ni]**
   - How does he feel about his illness before the transplant? He has refused cardiac catheterization and other aggressive treatment. Was he denying the seriousness of his disease, or did he have realistic reasons for his decision? What did the fatigue and loss of physical endurance mean as far as his work and personal life were concerned? What was his emotional response to the sudden deterioration of his condition 3 months ago? Patient's feelings about their illnesses often affect their response to treatment and their ability to achieve their optimum level of health.
   - How does he feel about the transplant? Is he hopeful of returning to a good quality of life or is he depressed about his future? Are his expectation about the impact of the surgery on his life realistic? After a transplant, he will be required to follow a difficult and demanding medical regimen. This will require multiple visits to the hospital, biopsies, and taking medication despite multiple negative side effects. It may also mean having to cope with medical complications such as rejection episodes and infections.
   - What are his potential support systems? You know that his only family, the brother and sister, live some distance from him. Does he have close friends in his town in Montana? Is he accustomed to coping with problems alone, or is the assistance of others very important for him? Are there any formal support groups available, such as those associated with a cardiac rehabilitation program or the American Heart Association?
   - How does he feel spiritually about having the heart of another individual in his body keeping him alive? Some people view the heart as more than a physical pump. It has meaning for them as a site of their "self" or "soul." Sometimes, the recipient of a heart also feels some guilt about living at the expense of another's loss of life. How M.Y. feels about these issues will affect his emotional adjustment. Most transplant programs encourage the cardiac recipient to write a letter to the family of the donor. Anonymity is promised for both donor family and the recipient.
   - How does he feel about the interruption in his life imposed by the necessity of living close to the medical center or traveling there for a period of time after the surgery? Checkups after discharge depend on individual needs, but clinic visits are normally 2 to 3 times per week for several weeks, then weekly for 2 months.
   - Is he grieving the loss of his health and normal lifestyle?

5. What can you do to help him if he has problems in any of the above psychosocial areas? **[P/an/PSI/ct,ni,tc]**
   - Arrange a consultation with the cardiac transplant team social worker. Cardiac transplant programs have social workers who are trained to work specifically with the problems of cardiac transplant patients.
   - Arrange for him to meet other transplant recipients; they really know what he is experiencing.
   - Allow him to express his feelings and concerns freely and acknowledge the appropriateness of the feelings (anger, doubt, sadness, guilt).
   - Help provide adequate rest and comfort, including pain control, to facilitate his ability to cope.
   - Allow him as much control of his activities as possible. Lack of control is a particular problem for heart transplant patients because their medical regimen is quite inflexible and fixed. For instance, immunosuppressive medications must be taken regularly and on time.
   - Give him accurate information as needed based on his ability to understand and cope.

6. In order to plan his discharge teaching, you evaluate his understanding of the physical implications of his transplant surgery and the treatments required. List 6 important areas of knowledge you will investigate. **[A,P/an/S,PI,PSI/ct,ni]**
   - Anatomy and physiology of cardiac transplantation.
   - Clinic visits (schedule and procedures).
   - Record keeping (daily weights, vital signs, and medications).
   - Medications (immunosuppressants, antibiotics, antihypertensives, cholesterol-lowering drugs, H_2 blockers).
   - Graft rejection.
   - Prevention of infection.
   - Activity.
   - Diet.

You discover that he understands the anatomy and physiology, record keeping and clinic visits, and medications well after extensive teaching by his physician. However, he has many questions about rejection, infection, activity, and diet. You address these latter issues.

7. During the first 3 to 6 months after a transplant, most patients experience an episode during which their body tries to reject the new heart. You teach M.Y. that he must contact his physician if he experiences any signs and symptoms of rejection. List 4 signs and symptoms. **[A,P/c/PI/ct,ni,tc]**
   - Flulike symptoms: chills, aches, tiredness, headache, dizziness, nausea and vomiting.
   - Change in pulse rate or heart rhythm.
   - Fluid retention or sudden weight gain.
   - Sudden decrease in blood pressure (systolic pressure under 100).
   - Shortness of breath.

8. List 5 guidelines he should know to guard against infections. **[P/c/S,Pl/ct]**
   - Stay away from large congested crowds.
   - Stay away from individuals who are actively sick.
   - Use good handwashing frequently.
   - Report any cough, fever, nausea or vomiting.
   - If he cuts himself, he should clean the wound promptly and keep it dry.
   - Avoid close contact with soil, plants, animals, and small children at least for the first few months.
   - Practice good oral hygiene and see his dentist regularly since the mouth is a major source of infection. Take antibiotics before and after dental procedures.

9. What should M.Y. be taught about diet? **[P/k/Pl/ct]**
   - A common problem after transplant is excessive weight gain, which can lead to high blood pressure, coronary artery disease, and diabetes.
   - He should receive counseling from a registered dietitian about diet modifications.

10. M.Y. will begin a regular exercise program shortly after surgery. What should he be taught about activity? **[P/k/S,Pl,HP/ct]**
    - It is important to warm up slowly before beginning exercise and to cool down afterward. The donor heart has no sympathetic nervous system innervation to speed the heart rate.
    - Exercises should be a low-impact type, such as swimming, walking, and bicycling.
    - No heavy lifting should be done for at least 6 weeks.
    - Contact sports should be avoided.
    - Permission from the transplant team should be received before commencing to drive.

Case Study 11: Endocarditis

Difficulty: ** *Setting:* Hospital, home care

Index Words: Endocarditis, coronary artery disease, home care

J.F. is a 50-year-old married homemaker with a genetic autoimmune deficiency who has suffered from recurrent bacterial endocarditis. The most recent episodes were a *Staphylococcus aureus* infection of the mitral valve 16 months ago and a *Streptococcus mutans* infection of the aortic valve 1 month ago. During this latter hospitalization, an echocardiogram showed aortic stenosis, moderate aortic insufficiency, chronic valvular vegetations, and moderate atrial enlargement. Two years ago she received an 18-month course of TPN therapy for malnutrition caused by idiopathic, relentless nausea and vomiting. She has also had CAD for several years, and 2 years ago suffered an acute anterior wall MI. In addition, she has a history of chronic joint pain.

Now, after being home for only a week, J.F. has been readmitted to your floor with endocarditis, nausea and vomiting, and renal failure. Since yesterday she has been vomiting and retching constantly, and has had chills, fever, fatigue, joint pain, and headache. As you admit her, you note that she wears glasses and has dentures. She was immediately started on TPN at 125 ml/h and on penicillin 2 million units IV q4h, to be continued for 4 weeks. Other medications are Lasix 80 mg PO qd, amiodipine (Norvasc) 5 mg PO qd, metoprolol 25 mg bid, and droperidol (Inapsine) 0.25-0.5 ml IVP prn for N/V. Admission VS 172/48 (supine) and 100/40 (sitting), 116, 20, 37.9°C. As you assess her, you find a grade II/VI holosystolic murmur and a grade III/VI diastolic murmur; 2+ pitting tibial edema but no peripheral cyanosis; clear lungs; orientation x 3 but drowsiness; soft abdomen with slight tenderness in the L upper quadrant; hematuria; and multiple petechiae on skin of arms, legs, and chest.

1. What is the significance of the orthostatic hypotension, the wide pulse pressure, and the tachycardia? **[PD/c/PI/ct]**
   - These phenomena indicate hypovolemia secondary to the intractable nausea and vomiting.

2. What is the significance of the abdominal tenderness, hematuria, joint pain, and petechiae? **[PD/c/PI/ct]**
   - Embolization of vegetations from damaged heart valves, with resulting infarction of various organs, is a common complication of endocarditis. Infarction of the spleen can present as abdominal tenderness. Infarction of the kidneys causes hematuria and reduced urine output. Petechiae result from microembolization to small skin vessels, and arthritis from embolization to joints.

3. As you monitor your patient throughout the day, what other signs and symptoms of embolization will you watch for? **[A/ap/Pl/ct,ni]**
   - Cerebral embolization manifested by changes in levels of consciousness, visual changes, headache, TIAs, and stroke.
   - Embolization to the extremities manifested by decreased or absent arterial pulses, cool fingers and toes with delayed capillary refill, and cyanosis.
   - Coronary artery embolization manifested by signs of angina, MI, CHF, or cardiac dysrhythmias.
   - Embolization to the bowel manifested by abdominal pain, cramping, nausea, and vomiting.

4. Three important diagnostic criteria for infectious endocarditis are anemia, fever, and cardiac murmurs. Explain the cause for each sign. **[A,PD/an/Pl/ct]**
   - Anemia: chronic glomerulonephritis is caused by embolization of vegetations to the kidneys. The renal failure results in the decreased production of erythropoietin, a hormone secreted by the kidneys that stimulates growth and development of RBCs.
   - Fever: inflammatory mediators, released in response to the infectious organisms, produce fever.
   - Cardiac murmurs: turbulent blood flow through the damaged valves produces murmurs. In J.F.'s case, the holosystolic (throughout systole) murmur is caused by blood being forced through the stenotic aortic valve during systole, and the diastolic murmur by backflow of blood from the aorta into the L ventricle through the incompetent aortic valve during diastole (aortic regurgitation).

5. On the day after admission, you review J.F.s laboratory test results: Na 138 mEq/L, K 3.9 mEq/L, Cl 103 mEq/L, BUN 85 mg/dl, creatinine 3.9 mg/dl, glucose 185 mg/dl, WBCs 6.7 mm^3, Hct 27%, Hgb 9.0 g/dl. Identify the values that are not within normal ranges, and explain the reason for each abnormality. **[A,PD/an/Pl/ct,ni]**
   - BUN and creatinine: elevated because of the renal failure.
   - Glucose: elevated in response to the release of stress hormones, particularly catecholamines.
   - Hct and Hgb: decreased secondary to renal failure (see above) and bleeding into skin and other organs.

6. What is the greatest risk for J.F. during the process of rehydration and what would you monitor to detect its development? **[P/c/Pl/ct,ni]**
   - Increased intravascular volume combined with aortic stenosis and regurgitation can cause severe CHF. Monitor for crackles, dyspnea, cough with frothy sputum, increased pedal edema, jugular vein distention, confusion, anxiety, increased drowsiness and lethargy, increased intensity of murmurs, and new S_3/S_4 heart sounds.

As you admitted J.F., you were aware that as soon as she is stable, she will be going home in a few days on TPN and IV antibiotics. Therefore, you plan to initiate discharge preparations and teaching as soon as possible.

7. List 5 questions you might ask in assessing her home health care needs. **[A/an/S,PI,PSI/ct,ni,tc]**
   - Is her husband able to help care for her physical needs? Is he home during the day, or does he work? Is he comfortable with nursing tasks such as TPN administration, pain management, activities of daily living assistance?
   - Is her husband a good source of emotional support for her?
   - Does she have any other friends or relatives living nearby who would be available for help with physical care or emotional support?
   - What additional assistance will she need from a home health care agency? Regular visits from and RN for antibiotic and TPN administration and IV maintenance, pain control? Home health aide? Housekeeper? Occupational or physical therapist?
   - What is the physical setup of her home? Are there stairs she might be too weak to climb? Are there any changes that would make things easier for her, such as converting a downstairs room into a bedroom?
   - What is the family's financial situation? Should a social worker be brought in for consultation?
   - What are J.F.'s emotional and coping needs? Should you involve a psychotherapist in her care?

Fortunately, J.F. has a supportive husband and 2 daughters who live nearby who can function as caregivers when J.F. is discharged. They, as well as the patient, will also need teaching about endocarditis. Although J.F. has been ill for several years, you discover that she and her family have received little education about the disease. You prepare a teaching plan for the family.

8. List 2 predisposing causes of bacteremia that you will explain. **[P/c/S,PI/ct,ni,tc]**
   - Poor oral hygiene and dental work: J.F. wears dentures, and it is very important that they are kept clean and properly fitting. Explain the reason that prophylactic antibiotics will be necessary before any dental work is performed.
   - Invasive procedures: J.F. will have central IV line access for her TPN and antibiotics. Careful handwashing and aseptic technique must be used in caring for the line to prevent bacterial infection, particularly of *Staphylococcus* and *Streptococcus* organisms.
   - Skin and mucous membrane infections and abrasions: boils, blisters, scrapes, burns, and other injuries should be prevented if possible and treated if necessary to prevent infection.

9. List 3 other things you would teach. **[P,I/c/S,PI/ct,ni,tc]**
   - Explain the disease process and the purpose of treatment procedures. Include the anatomy and physiology of the disease.
   - Teach her to read a thermometer accurately and to consult a physician for a temperature greater than 101 °F.
   - Teach the importance of informing dentists and other health care personnel about her history of endocarditis before having any procedures performed and to notify her dentist at the first signs of oral infection or gum disease.
   - Instruct her to carry emergency identification at all times.

10. Your hospital discharge planner facilitates J.F.'s transition to home care. During the initial home visit, the home health nurse evaluates J.F.'s IV site for implementation of the IV therapy program, and interviews the family members to determine their willingness to be caregivers and their level of understanding, and enlists the patient's and family's assistance to identify 10 teaching goals. What topics would be included on this list? **[P/c/S,Pl/ct,ni]**
    - Teach J.F. and family proper handwashing technique.
    - Teach about signs and symptoms of medications.
    - Teach signs and symptoms of infection at the IV site and infiltration of the IV.
    - Teach signs and symptoms of impeded or rapid flow of medication solutions.
    - Teach accurate calculation of milliliter per minute and regulation of IV drip rate.
    - Teach care of heparin lock for intermittent antibiotic medications.
    - Teach flush of heparin lock with NS solution to ensure patency.
    - Teach family to document date and time of all infusions started and completed.
    - Teach J.F. and family regarding positioning of site with IV.
    - Teach J.F. and family signs and symptoms of infection, phlebitis.
    - Teach J.F. and family when to contact an on-call RN and/or physician.
    - J.F. is on TPN and will either have a central catheter or PICC (peripherally-inserted central catheter). The TPN will be administered using an infusion pump; teach J.F. and her family about TPN and how to use the infusion pump.

      (From Marrelli, 1994.)

11. The home health nurse also writes short- and long-term goals for J.F. and her family. Identify 2 short- and 3 long-term goals. **[P/ap/S,Pl/ct,ni]**

    <u>Short-term</u>
    - J.F. receives ordered solution and medications without complications.
    - J.F. has a patent IV.
    - J.F.'s family is able to support her care at home.

    <u>Long-term</u>
    - VS are normal.
    - Infection is resolved.
    - Adequate hydration is achieved.
    - Fluid and electrolyte status is within normal limits for J.F.

      (From Marrelli, 1994.)

Mr. F. and his 2 daughters learned to administer her TPN during the 18-month treatment. Be aware that IV cases are usually covered by most insurers on a case-by-case basis and with clear documentation.

12. What documentation would be required in order to obtain reimbursement? **[P/c/S,Pl/ni,tc]**
    - Positive outcomes regarding teaching.
    - Type of IV catheter used and purpose.
    - Dates of insertion and/or site change.
    - Frequency of site change or site care given.
    - Specific orders for frequency of site care.
    - Schedule and rate of infusion.
    - Schedule for flushing.
    - Progress noted since admission.
    - Site of infection and symptoms.
    - Exacerbation of symptoms or side effects of antibiotics.
    - Dehydration symptoms.
    - Unstable VS.
    - Projected date of discharge.
    - Change in medication or solution.
    - Change in rate and frequency of therapy.
    - All charges.

    (From Marrelli, 1994.)

Case Study 12: Cardiac Arrest

Difficulty: **	*Setting:* Hospital
Index Words: Cardiac arrest, sudden death, cardiomyopathy	

L.M. is a 60-year-old woman who is admitted to your telemetry unit in a major medical center after being successfully resuscitated by medics from a cardiac arrest due to ventricular fibrillation. L.M., a divorced housewife, had her sudden death experience in the small rural community where she lives and was transported to your facility for evaluation and treatment after she was stabilized. At the time of her arrest her K level was 2.8 mEq/L and Mg level was low. As you continue to review her medical history, you learn that she had rheumatic fever as a child and over the years has developed severe rheumatic heart disease with mitral and aortic valve involvement and dilated cardiomyopathy. Four years ago she had a commissurotomy for mitral valve prolapse. She also has probable aortic valve stenosis. During the past year she has experienced increasing problems with chest pain, shortness of breath, and dyspnea on exertion. Two months ago she developed a severe cough and increasing fatigue. She has been on furosemide (Lasix) 40 mg PO qd, digoxin (Lanoxin) 0.25 mg PO qd, captopril 50 mg PO q8h, potassium (K Dur) 20 mEq qd, and warfarin (Coumadin) 5 mg PO qd. In addition, during the week before her cardiac arrest, she was taking erythromycin 500 mg q6h for a lower respiratory tract infection. Although she stopped smoking 4 years ago, she had a 40 pack/year smoking history.

1. What organism causes rheumatic fever? **[PD/k/Pl/ct]**
   - Group A beta-hemolytic *Streptococcus*.

2. What medication is commonly used prophylactically to prevent development of rheumatic heart disease when an individual has rheumatic fever? **[I/c/Pl/ct]**
   - Oral penicillin (or erythromycin). A 10-day regimen of oral antibiotic medication is aimed at eradicating the streptococcal infection. The patient must take the antibiotic for a full 10 days. To prevent recurrence of acute rheumatic fever, continuous prophylactic antibiotic therapy is necessary. L.M. probably has not received this therapy.

3. Why would someone like L.M. be given Coumadin? **[P/c/S,Pl/ct]**
   - Blood flow through damaged heart valves is not laminar; there are areas of turbulence and areas of stasis of blood in the cardiac chambers. This can result in thrombus formation and embolization of clots to the brain. Coumadin inhibits clot formation and is usually taken for life by individuals with valve problems or who have had valve replacement.

4. Reviewing the above health history, what factors do you think contribute to her current symptoms of chest pain, shortness of breath, dyspnea on exertion, cough, and fatigue? Explain your rationale for each. **[PD/c/PI/ct]**
   - Valvular disease: mitral valve prolapse causes regurgitation of blood through the mitral valve during systole (increasing the amount of blood returning to the L ventricle during the next diastole). Aortic stenosis causes decreased ejection of blood during systole. Both increase the volume of blood remaining in the heart at the end of diastole (preload). This extra volume adds to the workload of the already weak heart.
   - Dilated cardiomyopathy: because of years of excessive chamber enlargement, the L ventricle becomes dilated resulting in impairment of contractile function. Cardiac decompensation occurs, accompanied by pulmonary congestion and the other signs and symptoms of CHF.
   - Lower respiratory tract infection: pulmonary infection has contributed to the difficulty her heart has meeting the demand of the tissues for oxygen. This results in exacerbation of the CHF. The cough and fatigue are also due to the infection itself, as well as to the worsening CHF.

5. What factors in the above health history may have precipitated L.M.'s cardiac arrest? **[PD/c/PI/ct]**
   - Hypokalemia and hypomagnesemia: both are well-known to trigger increased automaticity and reentry, mechanisms that initiate ventricular dysrhythmias; decreased levels of K and Mg can also cause prolongation of the QT interval, precipitating ventricular dysrhythmias.
   - Cardiomyopathy: ventricular dysrhythmias are common in all kinds of cardiomyopathies.

L.M.'s admission VS are 102/60, 84, 16, and 36°C. Her telemetry monitor shows atrial fibrillation and frequent PVCs. When you listen to her heart, you hear an S_3 gallop, a grade III/VI systolic murmur, and a soft, blowing diastolic murmur. Her PMI is displaced laterally. She has no pedal edema. You hear crackles in her lungs. Other assessment findings are normal. She is transferred to the coronary care unit and is placed on continuous heparin and lidocaine IV infusions, and started on O_2 at 40% by face mask. Her lab values are drawn. Later in the day during a cardiac catheterization, her cardiac output was found to be 2.3 L/min and her mean pulmonary artery pressure 29 mm Hg.

6. Based on the above assessment, do you believe that L.M. is experiencing some heart failure? Why or why not? **[PD/an/PI/ct,ni]**
   - Yes. The S_3 gallop and crackles in the lungs are signs of CHF.

7. L.M.'s lab tests return. Her PT is 23.4 seconds, PTT 30 seconds. What other lab tests would you especially want to monitor? **[P/c/S,PI/ct,ni]**
   - K, Mg, and digoxin levels: because she is still having ventricular dysrhythmias, it is very important to have the K and Mg levels within the normal (even the high end of normal) range.
   - Lidocaine level: the toxic effects of lidocaine can be severe; aggravation of cardiac dysrhythmias (blocks), difficulty breathing or swallowing, convulsions, respiratory depression, and cardiac or respiratory arrest. The therapeutic range for lidocaine is 1.5 to 5.0 mg/L.
   - ABGs: because of L.M.'s CHF and lung infection, all of her blood gases need to be followed, especially the PO_2, O_2 sat, and PCO_2.

8. Why is it important to monitor L.M.'s PTT? Is her PTT within the therapeutic range? Is the PT within the normal range? **[P/c/S,PI/ct,ni]**
   - Heparin inhibits the intrinsic clotting cascade, and its effects on clotting are monitored by the PTT. PTT levels are always followed when an individual is receiving heparin therapy.
   - L.M.'s PTT of 30 seconds is not in the therapeutic range. Normal range for activated PTT is 25 to 35 seconds. Therapeutic range is 1.5 to 2.5 times the normal (control) level.
   - The PT is elevated because she has been on Coumadin. The PT is used to monitor the inhibiting effects of Coumadin on the extrinsic clotting cascade. Normal PT range is 11 to 13 seconds, and therapeutic range is 1.5-2.0 times greater than control.

9. List 4 relevant nursing diagnoses for L.M. **[PD/an/PI/ct]**
   - Decreased cardiac output r/t valvular disorders and weakened cardiac muscle. Her cardiac output is 2.3 L/min (normal is about 4-6 L/min, depending upon the patient's size and individual metabolic requirements).
   - Activity intolerance r/t decreased oxygen-carrying capacity.
   - Fatigue r/t decreased K and Mg levels, decreased oxygen-carrying capacity, and decreased activity over time.
   - Risk for pain (cardiac) r/t hypoxic cardiac tissue.
   - Risk for fluid volume excess r/t inability of the heart to adequately pump.
   - Risk for altered tissue perfusion (cardiac) r/t decreased oxygen-carrying capacity.

10. In order to prevent serious complications, you will assess and monitor for potential problems. List 3 significant potential physiologic problems for which L.M. is at risk. Explain. **[A/c/PI/ct,ni]**
    - Cardiogenic shock: she has CHF, and it is important that her heart failure not be allowed to progress to the point where organ perfusion and cellular oxygenation are impaired.
    - Ventricular tachycardia and fibrillation: she has recently had a cardiac arrest due to VF and is now on lidocaine for frequent PVCs.
    - Hypoxemia: decreased cardiac output, pulmonary edema, and lower respiratory tract infection all predispose her to potential hypoxemia.
    - Right-sided CHF: if her pulmonary vascular pressures continue to rise, the R ventricle may fail, causing an increase in systemic venous pressure. If this occurs, systemic edema and organ congestion will result.

11. The technologic monitoring and care L.M. receives demands so much time that there has been little opportunity to talk with her about her feelings related to her sudden death experience. As you plan to approach her, you remind yourself to be sensitive to communication limitations imposed by her pathologic condition. What are 2 of these, and how will they affect your interaction? **[P,I/an/PI/ct,ni,tc]**
    - Shortness of breath: talking will place additional stress on her heart and lungs and will be evidenced by short, choppy sentences.
    - Fatigue: affects attention span and ability to concentrate or focus.
    - Amnesia or repression: L.M. may not remember anything relating to the event at all.

Case Study 13: Myocardial Infarction

Difficulty: **	*Setting:* Hospital cardiac intensive care
Index Words: Myocardial infarction, substance abuse	

T.G. is a 40-year-old woman who was admitted to your CCU with a positive anterior wall - MI secondary to cocaine use. Upon arrival in the unit, she still has the nitroglycerine (NTG) drip infusing that had been started in the ambulance and maintained in the ED. You are instructed to titrate the drip for relief of her chest pain. Her maintenance IV is D_5½ NS at 100 ml/h. Oxygen by nasal cannula is to be titrated to keep her O_2 sat >90%. As you assess her, you find that the NTG has relieved her chest and L arm pain, but that a dull chest pressure persists and that her chest is tender to pressure. Her cardiovascular and pulmonary assessments are otherwise normal. She has a headache and is drowsy, but alert and oriented. Admission VS are 136/97, 79, 20, 37.2°C. Weight 222 pounds; height 5′2".

The report from the ED nurse is as follows: "T.G. is a single woman supporting her 3 children by working as a clerk in a small grocery store. The family is on Medicaid and lives with T.G.'s boyfriend. She has smoked 1½ packs of cigarettes a day for 15 years and has chronic hepatitis B. She also has an 18-year history of cocaine and IV heroin addiction. When using heroin, she injects the drug 2 to 3 times per day. Last night she administered the cocaine by intravenous injection for the first time in an attempt to 'stop the heroin habit.' She felt all right when she went to bed just before midnight, but woke about 0500 with severe chest pain radiating to her L arm and hand, neck, and both sides of her jaw. She also had nausea, vomiting, shortness of breath, diaphoresis, and dizziness. Her boyfriend called 911 and she was taken to the hospital by ambulance."

1. What nursing diagnoses would you choose for T.G.? List your 3 top priority diagnoses and evidence for the need for each. **[PD/an/PI,PSI/ct]**
   - Pain r/t myocardial ischemia. She reported acute pain (up to 9/10).
   - Risk for decreased cardiac output r/t dysrhythmias and myocardial ischemia. A patient with a positive MI is at risk for dysrhythmias and cardiogenic shock, both of which can cause hypoxia and decreased cardiac output.
   - Risk for sleep pattern disturbance r/t pain, the noisy CCU environment, and her chronic cocaine abuse.
   - Altered nutrition *less* than body requirements. Her weight is 222 pounds, height 5′2". Obesity alone is never an indicator of *nutrition* greater than body requirements.
   - Altered health maintenance r/t history of tobacco, cocaine, and heroin use.
   - Health seeking behaviors r/t statement trying to "stop the heroin habit." Since she stated that she injected cocaine to "stop the heroin habit," this may be capitalized on in her rehabilitation phase.

   Instructor Note: Interventions for the first 4 diagnoses must be initiated immediately, particularly if the nutritional imbalance features hypomagnesemia. Interventions for the last 2 would better be postponed until she is stable and out of the CCU.

Note: Obesity indicates only *energy* intake greater than body requirements. Patients presenting as obese effect have nutritional imbalances and deficits, particularly low-income patients or substance abusers who frequently have significant nutritional problems. Finally, body weight alone tells nearly nothing about nutritional status.

You look up the effects of cocaine and find that the 2 primary acute effects on the cardiovascular system are (1) blocking of the reuptake of catecholamines, resulting in increased stimulation of both alpha-adrenergic receptors (vasoconstriction) and beta-adrenergic receptors (increased heart rate and increased cardiac automaticity); and (2) blocking of the fast-sodium channel in the myocardium, resulting in depression of depolarization and a slowing of conduction velocity (local anesthetic effect). In addition, myocardial contractility is suppressed. Chronic cocaine leads to acceleration of atherosclerosis and increased tendency for platelet aggregation.

2. Based on this information, what possible ECG changes due to cocaine toxicity would you monitor for? **[P/ap/Pl/ct,ni]**
   - Sinus tachdysrrhythmias.
   - Prolongation of the PR, QRS, and QT intervals (similar to the effects of type I antidysrhythmic agents).
   - Ventricular dysrhythmias.

3. What physiologic complications of cocaine toxicity would you monitor for? Identify 3. **[P/ap/Pl/ct,ni]**
   - Systemic hypertension.
   - Decreased coronary artery flow resulting in further cardiac ischemia and pain.
   - Increased oxygen demand due to increased heart rate and blood pressure.
   - Deep vein thrombosis with possible pulmonary embolization.
   - Congestive heart failure due to decreased myocardial contractility, increased heart rate and increased afterload.
   - Cardiogenic shock (hypotension and shock may follow the initial hypertension and tachycardia as oxygen demand exceeds supply).
   - Cardiac arrest secondary to ventricular dysrhythmias.

4. Review the data on the effects of cocaine above. Propose mechanisms by which cocaine might lead to myocardial infarction. **[PD/k/Pl/ct]**
   - Acceleration of atherosclerosis.
   - Acute coronary vasospasm causing ischemia.
   - Coronary vasospasm causing stasis of blood with subsequent thrombus formation.
   - Increased heart rate and blood pressure increasing oxygen demand.
   - Increased platelet aggregation resulting in coronary artery thrombus.

5. Two days after she was admitted, T.G. began to appear anxious, depressed, restless, and irritable. She is doubled over and complains of abdominal cramping. You also notice new muscle twitching and tremors. She refuses to eat. To what do you attribute these symptoms? **[A,PD/c/Pl/ct]**
   - She probably is in cocaine and heroin withdrawal. This should have been anticipated by nurses and physicians.

6. The physician ordered methadone 10 mg PO tid for T.G. What is the rationale for prescribing methadone in this instance? **[P/c/Pl/ct]**
   - Methadone is a synthetic narcotic with properties similar to those of morphine, but it produces less sedation and euphoria than morphine. It is addictive, but withdrawal symptoms are less intense than for street drugs. Methadone is frequently used for temporary maintenance and treatment of hospitalized patients to prevent severe drug withdrawal from abused substances.

7. Before T.G. is transferred to the telemetry floor, you consult with the social worker to identify her discharge needs. Together you list 3. **[PD/an/S,PI,PSI/ct,ni,tc]**
   - Drug abuse rehabilitation: she needs teaching and intensive help for this problem. Her cardiac problems and possibly her chronic hepatitis B are due to drug use. It is possible that the hepatitis B is the result of intravenous use of street drugs.
   - Financial needs: she is a single parent of 3 children with a low-paying job whose only insurance is Medicaid.
   - Cardiac teaching needs: she needs teaching about her cardiac risk factors (obesity, smoking, cocaine use) and necessary lifestyle changes. She will also need to understand the normal recovery process after an MI.

8. Shortly after T.G. is moved back to your telemetry unit, you find her disconnected telemetry unit and leads on her bed and she is nowhere to be found. When she returns about an hour later, she is very mellow and easy-going, almost lethargic. She immediately falls asleep and is difficult to arouse. To what do you attribute her absence and her present behavior? **[PD/an/PSI/ct]**
   - T.G. probably left the unit to meet her drug contact. Her behavior and physiologic response indicate that she is under the influence of illicit drugs.

Note: Nearly every large hospital in the country is covered by one or more drug dealers. Hospital personnel and patients who are abusing drugs need their "fix" or "hit" and are willing to pay well for it. Drug dealers are willing to oblige with personalized service.

9. What is going to be your response to the above situation? **[A,PD,P/an/PI/ct,ni,tc]**
   - Notify the physician immediately.
   - Notify the nursing supervisor and hospital security services.
   - Chart what you have observed, and document any actions you take.
   - Monitor her vital signs and neurologic status q15min during the next several hours. You do not know how "pure" the drugs were, what she took, or what her response will be. If her condition starts deteriorating, call for help immediately.
   - Call for a team consultation that includes hospital security services. If T.G. stays on your unit, it is likely she will have to find a way to pay for her continued drug deliveries. Theft and prostitution are 2 ways drug money can be obtained, and they occur within the walls of hospitals, too.

Case Study 14: Coronary Artery Disease

Difficulty: **	*Setting:* Outpatient clinic
Index Words: Coronary artery disease, congestive heart failure	

You are working in the internal medicine clinic of a large teaching hospital. Today your first patient is 70-year-old J.M., a man who has been coming to the clinic for several years for management of CAD, hypertension, and anemia. A cardiac catheterization done a year ago showed 50% occlusion of the circumflex coronary artery. He has had episodes of dizziness for the past 6 months and orthostatic hypotension, shoulder discomfort, and decreased exercise tolerance for the past 2 months. On his last clinic visit 3 weeks ago, a chest x-ray and 12-lead ECG were done, showing cardiomegaly and a L bundle branch block. Results of blood studies drawn at this time were chemistries: Na 136 mEq/L, K 5.2 mEq/L, BUN 15 mg/dl, creatinine 1.8 mg/dl, glucose 82 mg/dl, and Cl 95 mEq/L. CBC: WBC 4.4 mm^3, Hgb 10.5 g/dl, Hct 31.4%, and platelets 229 mm^3. This morning his daughter has brought him to the clinic because he has had increased fatigue, significant swelling of his ankles, and shortness of breath for the last 2 days. His VS are 142/83, 105, 18, and 36.6°C.

1. Knowing his history and seeing his condition this morning, what further questions are you going to ask J.M. and his daughter? **[A/ap/S,Pl/ct,ni,tc]**
   - Activity: What activities make you tired? Do you sometimes feel like you can't get your breath (SOB)?
   - Diet: Do you use salt in your cooking or at the table? Are there any foods like chips, peanuts, pizza, turkey dressing, ham (fill in local or ethnic salt-rich favorites) that you like? Have you eaten any of these recently (try to relate salt intake to symptoms that started 2 days ago).
   - Sleep. How many pillows do you sleep on? Do you wake up during the night with shortness of breath?
   - Fluid retention. Have you gained weight or has your urine output decreased over the past few day? Have you had trouble getting your shoes on?
   - Lungs. Do you have a cough? Do you cough anything up (is it productive)? (If so, have him describe the sputum.)
   - Cardiac rhythm. Are you having any strange feelings in your chest? Do you feel like there's a bird flipping around in your chest (palpitations)? Have you been feeling lightheaded or dizzy in the past 2 days?
   - Chest pain. Are you having any discomfort or numbness in your chest, back, shoulders, arms, hands, or jaws? (If so, have him describe the sensations.)
   - Smoking history. Have you ever smoked? Do you smoke now? If so, how many packs a day do you smoke? (J.M. stopped smoking 10 years ago.)
   - Occupational history. This question is critical with respect to smoking history. Watch for occupational (or wartime) experience in mining, toxin, or pulmonary irritant exposure (e.g., asbestos, Agent Orange). Combined with smoking, these make a lethal combination for the heart as well as lungs.

   Instructor Note: This is a good time for students to practice asking questions in "every-day people-talk" whether in English or another language as a basis for obtaining diagnostically useful answers as well as promoting therapeutic communication. This also is a great time to detect where people are confused and address knowledge deficits; hence, assessment by a good nurse always potentially features nursing interventions and therapeutic communication.

J.M. tells you he becomes exhausted and short-of-breath climbing the stairs to his bedroom and has to lie down and rest ("put my feet up") at least an hour twice a day. He has been sleeping on 2 pillows for the last 2 weeks. He has not salted his food since the doctor told him not to because of his high blood pressure. But he admits having had peanuts and ham 3 days ago. He denies having palpitations but has had a constant, irritating, nonproductive cough lately.

2. You think it likely that J.M. has congestive heart failure. From his history, what do you identify as probable causes for his CHF? **[A/c/Pl/ct,ni]**
   - Hypertension: chronic hypertension can require the heart to pump hard against the resistance of the vessels. This results in cardiac muscle hypertrophy (the cardiomegaly seen on his chest x-ray).
   - Coronary artery disease: ischemic myocardium is not able to produce adequate stroke volumes.
   - Anemia: increases the demand for oxygen of the tissues and, therefore, the demand on the heart, while at the same time contributing to myocardial ischemia.

3. You are now ready to do your physical assessment. List at least 9 things you would assess to confirm your suspicion about the CHF. Also indicate with an "L" or an "R" whether the sign is due to left-sided or right-sided heart failure or both. **[A,PD/c/Pl/ct,tc]**

   <u>L,R</u> Heart sounds: increased fluid volume in the heart can produce cardiac murmurs and S_3 and S_4 gallops.
   <u>L</u> Vital signs: heart rate may be elevated and blood pressure decreased from baseline. Increased respiratory rate may result from pulmonary edema.
   <u>L,R</u> Heart rhythm: dysrhythmias can result from cardiac ischemia (and to a lesser degree from his marginally elevated K level).
   <u>L,R</u> Weight: rapid increase in weight is a sign of fluid retention.
   <u>L</u> Lung sounds: bilateral crackles, a sign of pulmonary edema, are commonly heard as blood backs up into the lungs.
   <u>L</u> Peripheral circulation: cyanosis, coolness, decreased pulses, and capillary refill of fingers and toes indicate decreased peripheral perfusion secondary to decreased cardiac output.
   <u>R</u> Jugular vein distention: increased venous pressure causes blood to distend the jugular vein.
   <u>R</u> Liver size: increased venous pressure can result in liver engorgement.
   <u>R</u> Pitting peripheral and sacral edema: fluid retention and increased venous pressure result in edema in dependent areas of the body.
   <u>R</u> Abdominal tenderness; due to congestion of abdominal organs.
   <u>R</u> Ascites: decreased liver function, secondary to liver congestion, can decrease the hepatic production of blood proteins.
   <u>L,R</u> Mental status: poor cerebral perfusion and cerebral edema can result in confusion, restlessness, lethargy, sense of impending doom.
   <u>L,R</u> Skin moisture and temperature: damp, cool skin can be signs of sympathetic nervous system response to hypoxemia.

   <u>Instructor Note</u>: Again, this is a good time for students to teach patients about signs and symptoms to watch for related to their disease.

4. The doctor confirms your feelings that J.M. is experiencing some CHF. What classes of medications might the doctor prescribe? **[P/k/PI/ct]**
   - Diuretic to decrease fluid volume (preload).
   - Inotrope to increase cardiac contractility and cardiac output.
   - Vasodilator to increase organ perfusion and coronary artery perfusion.
   - Iron to treat the anemia.

Note: The Hgb and Hct might be falsly decreased because of hemodilution of the CHF.

5. This is J.M.'s first episode of significant CHF. Before he leaves the clinic you want to teach him about lifestyle modifications he can make and monitoring techniques he can use to prevent or minimize future problems. List 5 suggestions you might make and the rationale for each. **[P,I/ap/S,PI,HP/ct,ni,tc]**
   - Gradually increase and pace your activities to decrease the work requirements and oxygen demand of the heart.
   - Minimize stress to reduce sympathetic nervous system response with increased work load of the heart.
   - Avoid hot/cold environments; both increase cardiac demand.
   - Learn to take your pulse and call your doctor if your pulse is less than 50, greater than 100 or is very irregular. Irregular, very rapid, or very slow heart rates can exacerbate CHF.
   - Weigh yourself daily to monitor for fluid retention. Report a 2- to 5-pound weight gain over 1 to 4 days to your doctor. Sudden weight gain indicates fluid retention.
   - Carefully follow your salt-restricted diet to minimize fluid retention.
   - Take your medications faithfully and call me immediately if you don't want to take them anymore.

6. You tell J.M. the peanuts and ham he had 3 days ago probably set off his present episode of CHF. He looks surprised. J.M. says, "But I didn't add any salt to them!" What health care professional could he be referred to help him understand how to prevent future crises? State your rationale. **[P,I,E/an/S,PI,PSI/ct,ni,tc]**
   - They obviously do not understand that many foods contain high amounts of salt. They need help in understanding what foods are "safe" for J.M. A registered dietician could help them with suggestions for a diet low in salt and techniques for making low-salt meals tasty.

7. J.M. receives a prescription for furosemide with a potassium supplement. He wrinkles his nose at the suggestion of potassium and tells you he "hates those horse pills." He tells you a friend of his said he could eat bananas, instead. He says he would rather eat a banana everyday than take one of those pills. How will you respond? **[P/c/S,PI/ct,ni,tc]**
   - With empathy and humor. Tell him that sounds good, but in order to get as much banana-potassium as pill-potassium, he would have to eat a banana 6 feet long!
   - Tell him there are other ways the doctor can order his potassium, such as in a drink.

Case Study 15: Abdominal Aortic Aneurysm

Difficulty: ** *Setting:* Hospital, home care

Index Words: Abdominal aortic aneurysm, coronary artery disease, hypertension, sleep disturbance, depression

J.M. is a 70-year-old retired construction worker who has experienced epigastric pain, nausea, and upset stomach for the past 6 months. He has a history of CHF, atrial fibrillation, dyspnea, hypertension, and depression, and he is on supplemental oxygen at night for sleep apnea. J.M. has just been admitted to the hospital for surgical repair of a 6.2 cm abdominal aortic aneurysm (AAA), which is now causing him constant pain. Upon arrival on your floor his VS are 109/81, 61, 16 and 98.3°F. When you perform your assessment, you find that his apical heart rhythm is irregularly irregular and his peripheral pulses are strong. His lungs are clear, and he is alert and oriented. Except for the atrial fibrillation, there are no abnormal physical findings; however, he has not had a bowel movement for 3 days. His electrolytes and other blood chemistries and clotting studies are within normal range, but his Hct is 30.1% and Hgb 9.0 g/dl.

J.M. has been depressed since the death of his wife 9 years ago. He has no children. His height is 6'2" and weight 210 pounds. His chronic medical problems have been managed over the years by medications: captopril 25 mg PO tid, digoxin 0.25 mg PO qd, fluoxetine (Prozac) 40 mg PO qd, furosemide (Lasix) 40 mg PO qd, trazodone 50 mg PO qhs, KCl 20 mEq PO bid, and lovastatin 20 mg PO bid.

1. J.M. has several common risk factors for AAA, which are evident from his health history. Identify and explain 3 factors. **[A/c/Pl/ct]**
   - Atherosclerosis: this is inferred because he is taking lovastatin, a drug used to reduce serum lipid levels. Atherosclerosis injures vessel walls, causing weakness.
   - Hypertension: the elevated blood pressure puts a continuous strain on weakened arterial walls.
   - Advanced age.: hypertension and atherosclerosis are more common in the elderly.
   - Male gender: the incidence of AAA is 7 times higher in men than in women. Part of this may be due to the abdominal fat characteristic of male-pattern obesity which places increased pressure on all abdominal organs.

2. Pain is the most common symptom of AAA. J.M.'s epigastric pain, accompanied by nausea, is typical. List 2 other common signs/symptoms of AAA that J.M. did not have and explain their significance. **[A/c/Pl/ct]**
   - Intermittent claudication: can occur if blood flow to the extremities in decreased by leaking of the aneurysm.
   - Lower extremity edema: if the aneurysm puts pressure on the large abdominal veins, venous pressure increases.

While J.M. awaits his surgery, it is important that you monitor him carefully for decrease in tissue perfusion.

3. Identify 5 things you would you would be sure to assess, and state your rationale for each. **[A/c/S,Pl/ct,ni]**
   - Urine output: a decrease in kidney perfusion will result in decreased urine production.
   - Abdominal pain: an increase in abdominal pain can mean enlargement of the aneurysm.
   - Bowel sounds: increased or absent bowel sounds can indicate decreased perfusion to the GI tract.
   - Peripheral circulation: decrease in pedal pulses, coolness, cyanosis, or mottling of the skin of the feet, or increase in capillary refill time indicate impaired peripheral circulation.
   - Chest pain: if perfusion to the myocardium is decreased, the heart can become ischemic.
   - Vital signs: hypotension, tachycardia, and tachypnea are signs of hypovolemia or hemorrhagic shock.
   - Level of conscious: if cerebral perfusion is diminished, the patient may become confused and anxious.

4. What is the most serious, life-threatening complication of AAA and why? **[PD/c/Pl/ct]**
   - Rupture of the aneurysm. A ruptured aneurysm (as opposed to one with a slow leak) is usually rapidly fatal.

The resection of J.M.'s aneurysm was successful, but for the first 3 postop days he was delirious and required one-to-one nursing care and soft restraints before he became coherent and oriented again. He was still somewhat confused when he was transferred back to your floor.

5. List 5 nursing diagnoses that you think are high priority for J.M.'s postoperative care. **[PD/an/S,Pl,PSI/ct,ni]**
   - Pain r/t surgery.
   - Altered thought processes: confusion/disorientation r/t surgical intervention.
   - Risk for infection r/t to surgery.
   - Risk for altered systemic tissue perfusion r/t to leak, rupture or occlusion of the aortic graft.
   - Risk for ineffective breathing pattern r/t to pain and history of sleep apnea and abdominal surgery.
   - Risk of constipation r/t prior history of constipation and abdominal surgery.
   - Impaired physical mobility related to surgery.

   Instructor Note: The question that immediately comes to mind in reference to J.M.'s delirium and confusion is whether his sleep apnea, which has been treated by nocturnal O_2, has gotten worse after his surgery (e.g., anesthesia effects, pain). The assumption is that he is receiving postop oxygen anyway. Confusion is a common daytime phenomenon in older adults with untreated or inadequately treated sleep apnea.

6. Postoperative care of the patient undergoing aneurysectomy includes preservation of the graft, preservation of tissue perfusion, and prevention of infection. List 3 nursing interventions that would address these issues and explain each. **[P/c/S,PI/ct,ni]**
   - Elevation of the head of bed should not exceed 30 to 40 degrees because sharp hip flexion could cause the graft to kink.
   - Knees should not be gatched because knee flexion compresses popliteal vessels, restricting venous return.
   - Careful and regular assessment for decreased tissue perfusion (see above) should be done to detect leak, rupture, or occlusion of the graft.
   - Dressing changes should be done with careful aseptic technique.
   - Monitoring for signs/symptoms of infection should be done each shift.

When J.M. is being prepared for discharge, you talk to him about health promotion and lifestyle change issues that are pertinent for him.

7. Identify 4 health-related issues you might appropriately address with him and what you would teach in each area. **[P,/c/S,PI,PSI,HP/ct,ni,tc]**
   - Hypertension: importance of low-sodium diet, proper use of antihypertensive medications, weight loss, and exercise. With his history of AAA, he will need to keep his blood pressure under control.
   - Weight loss: rationale and methods. Weight loss will lower his risk for atherosclerosis.
   - Exercise: rationale and methods. Exercise is valuable in the treatment of atherosclerosis and depression, but it is essential that patient receive prescriptive exercise guidelines. Exercise carries great benefit but it also carries great risk if it is done inappropriately.
   - Diet: importance of low-sodium, low-cholesterol, high-fiber diet.
   - Constipation: importance of high fluid/fiber intake and exercise.
   - Psychosocial support needs: discuss resources available in his community for meeting psychosocial support needs.

8. J.M. will be receiving follow-up visits from the home health care nurse to change his dressing and evaluate his incision. What can you do with J.M. before discharge that will help him understand what she will be doing? **[P,I/ap/S,PI,PSI/ct,ni,tc]**
   - Explain to J.M. that he will be having a home health care nurse visit him after he goes home. She will take care of his wound and dressing.
   - Ask him if he would like to look at his incision. This will give you an opportunity to teach him about signs and symptoms of infection or dehiscence. Get a mirror so he can get a good look while you point out (with a sterile, gloved hand) the incision line, "normal" healing tissue color, that it is not puffy, and that there is nothing oozing from the incision.

Case Study 16: Premature Ventricular Contractions

Difficulty: *** *Setting:* Hospital

Index Words: Premature ventricular contractions, cardiac arrest, implantable cardioverter defibrillator

J.C., a 40-year-old married college professor, has just been admitted to your telemetry floor with a diagnosis of "benign ventricular ectopy." He suddenly began experiencing frequent episodes of palpitations 2 years ago. These were accompanied by lightheadedness, weakness, dizziness, and decreased ability to concentrate. Holter monitoring revealed very frequent PVCs exacerbated by caffeine and exertion. On admission, he appears trim, muscular, and physically fit. As you are assessing him, he tells you that he played football in college and has lived a very active lifestyle ever since. He confides that his symptoms seriously interfere with his activities and his marital relationship, and cause him a lot of anxiety and depression, to the point where he almost "took his life" a year ago. He has been taking clonazepam (Klonopin) for his anxiety for about 18 months. His physician tried 4 different beta-blockers and the antidysrhythmic drug, mexiletine (Mexitil), to control his PVCs, but none was successful and all had unpleasant side effects. In desperation, J.C. has agreed to try another antidysrhythmic, flecainide (Tambocor), and was admitted for cardiac monitoring. His physical assessment, laboratory values, and cardiac catheterization were normal in all areas.

1. Identify 4 relevant nursing diagnoses for J.C. **[PD/c/S,PI,PSI/ct]**
   - Anxiety/fear r/t threat of sudden death, deteriorating marital relationship, inability to perform usual activities (e.g., concentration at work).
   - Risk for decreased cardiac output r/t his frequent PVCs. Frequent PVCs decrease the time for diastolic filling for each premature beat, therefore, decreasing the volume of blood ejected and the cardiac output.
   - Activity intolerance r/t lightheadedness and weakness accompanying the PVCs. As the cardiac output is impaired, perfusion and oxygenation of the brain are impaired.
   - Altered family process r/t problems with his wife.
   - Grieving r/t actual loss of physical capabilities which have always been exceedingly important to him

2. Of the above problems, which is potentially life-threatening? **[PD/c/S,PI/ct]**
   - Risk for decrease in cardiac output, including possibility of sudden death. Frequent PVCs, particularly if multifocal or paired, can lead to ventricular tachycardia and/or ventricular fibrillation (in which the there is effectively no cardiac output). Without rapid detection and successful resuscitation (CODE), this is fatal.

3. When the heart threatens to stop working without notice, there is an understandably incredible feeling of loss of control and panic. The first objective should be to restore some sense of control to J.C. What are 5 things you could do to help relieve some of his anxiety? **[P/ap/PSI/ct,ni]**
   - Teach him about the effects of flecainide. Flecainide is a Class I antidysrhythmic agent, which represses PVCs by slowing the velocity of impulse conduction through the heart and increasing ventricular refractoriness. It usually does not alter cardiac function. Review the dosage and side effects with him. A serious side effect of flecainide is a prodysrhythmia effect, particularly in patients with ischemic cardiac disease or poor left ventricular function. Reassure him that he has neither of these problems and should have no serious side effects.
   - Assure him that his heart rhythm is being continuously monitored by telemetry and that should any serious rhythms occur during his flecainide trial, the staff would immediately intervene to stop the dysrhythmia.
   - Investigate with him how much technical detail he wishes to know about his problem. Many individuals use self-education as a means of gaining a sense of control.
   - Encourage him to walk around the floor and, when professional supervision is available, to use the exercise equipment in the cardiac rehabilitation room down the hall for moderate exercise. Maintaining physical fitness if very important to him and is known to have a calming and mood-lifting effect.
   - Provide opportunities for him to express his frustrations and concern and listen with empathy if he confides in you. Keep in mind that *you* may not always be in a good mood if your heart were threatening to stop at any moment!
   - If your hospital has social workers, psychiatric clinical nurse specialists, or clergy trained in psychotherapy, you might ask one of these individuals to talk with him.

4. Review each of the following admit orders. If the order is appropriate, place an "A" in the space provided. If it is inappropriate, specify why and correct it. **[A/ap/S,PI/ct]**

- ___ Continuous telemetry monitoring.
- ___ Routine VS.
- ___ Activity ad lib.
- ___ Cardiac enzymes on admission and q8h x 3 then q AM.
- ___ NTG 1 0.4 mg SL prn chest pain.
- ___ Call physician for PVCs >6/min.
- ___ Low-cholesterol diet.
- ___ IV lock.
- ___ Chem 27, CBC in AM.
- ___ 12-lead ECG q AM.
- ___ Lasix 40 mg PO qd.
- ___ Monitor flecainide level as appropriate.

Answers:

- A Continuous telemetry monitoring.
- A Routine VS.
- A Activity ad lib.
- I Cardiac enzymes on admission and q8h x 3 then q AM. Cardiac enzymes are to determine myocardial damage usually associated with trauma or an MI. J.C. has no indication of this at this time.
- I NTG 0.4 mg SL prn chest pain. J.C. has not indicated that there is any chest pain associated with his problem.
- A Call physician for PVCs >6/min.
- A/I Low-cholesterol diet. Depends on rationale.

  Instructor Note: Many people have the belief that "animal fat and cholesterol are bad" but are unaware that just substituting polyunsaturated fats in the diet is also unhealthy. The research supports an overall reduction in fat intake rather than just reducing cholesterol. There are no lipid levels on J.C. to establish that hyperlipidemia is a problem for him. However, given the probability of long-term decreased activity, the focus on low-fat, healthy eating may be a good preventive measure.
- A IV lock.
- A Chem 27, CBC in AM.
- A 12-lead ECG q AM.
- I Lasix 40 mg PO qd. There is no indication that J.C. requires a diuretic
- A Monitor flecainide level as appropriate.

5. List 3 appropriate nursing interventions related to J.C.'s dysrhythmia. **[P/ap/S,PI,CT,NI,TC]**

- Have access to appropriate medication (e.g., lidocaine, procainamide).
- Observe for changes in heart rhythm associated with activity, sleep, pain, medications.
- Document rhythms routinely and with change in activities.
- Suggest distraction therapy for him. If he focuses on his heart, it results in an increased stress response. Ask him to choose things he thinks will help keep his mind busy. Because intense concentration may be difficult due to the hospital environment and situational fatigue, suggest that he might read something he's wanted to read for a long time but thought he was too busy for.

J.C. has just returned to his room from an exercise session in the cardiac rehab room when he collapses on the floor. You witness his fall.

6. What are the appropriate emergency actions that you should take? **[I/k/PI/ct,ni]**
   - Assess the patient: unresponsiveness, airway, breathing, and circulation (pulse).
   - If unresponsive, call for help and begin Basic Life Support: if patient is not breathing, open the airway and initiate rescue breathing by mouth to mask method; if pulseless, initiate cardiac compressions per protocol.

According to the cardiac monitor, J.C.'s collapse was due to a sudden episode of ventricular fibrillation. Thanks to a quick response by the hospital's CODE Team, he was successfully defibrillated and resuscitated, then transferred to the CCU (coronary care unit).

7. What important information would you include in your report to the CCU nurse who will be caring for J.C.? **[P/an/PI,PSI/ct,tc]**
   - Brief history of his dysrhythmia, including associated signs/symptoms.
   - Patient's anxiety response to the dysrhythmia problem, including coping strategies and the troubled relationship with his wife.
   - VS, lab, and test results (cardiac catheterization).
   - Hospital course, including activities that appear to increase the incidence of PVCs and those preceding his cardiac arrest, his response to the flecainide to date.

You approach J.C. saying "I think we should notify your wife about your condition." J.C. tells you she is out-of-town on a business trip but calls in regularly for messages. He asks you to call her. Note, that if he were unconscious or cognitively impaired, you *must* notify her since she is the next of kin.

8. J.C.'s wife receives the CCU nurse's message on her answering machine to call the unit. When she returns the call, what information should the nurse tell her? **[P/c/PSI/ct,ni,tc]**
   - Since she is next of kin and J.C. has given his permission, you may tell her everything. This includes admitting condition, diagnosis, any test results, course of hospitalization, prognosis, and location (he's been transferred to CCU for observation).

9. She hisses into the telephone "What the heck do you expect *me* to do about it. There's no way I'm going to drop a good business deal to run home and hold his hand. He's sure got *you* fooled....there's nothing wrong with him that a good psychiatrist couldn't fix." As the nurse, how should you respond? **[P/an/PSI/ct,ni,tc]**
   - Keep cool. You are the professional. You tell her you don't know anything about their relationship and you are not there to judge anyone or to interfere in their issues. You wanted to notify her that her husband experienced multiple abnormal heartbeats; one of these episodes led to a medical emergency. He was transferred to the CCU where they could monitor him more closely. Her husband asked you to call; you are simply telling her what has transpired since he was admitted. If she has specific questions, you would encourage her to contact the physician.

Note: In some places, the physician would make this call.

10. After J.C.'s condition has stabilized, he is referred to the cardiac rehabilitation and prevention program for an exercise prescription. A clinical exercise physiologist helps him develop individualized guidelines for safe exercise. Identify and explain the major components of an exercise prescription. **[P/ap,an/S,PI,HP/ct]**
    - Exercise should be individualized and prescribed by professionals with specialized training. Therapeutic exercise should, above all, be nonviolent. The components of the exercise prescription should include:
        - Status of the person. What specific pathologic conditions or risk factors exist? Age, gender, diagnosis, medication regimen, and level of functioning are also considered.
        - Type of exercise. Aerobic, cardiorespiratory exercise should involve rhythmic, repetitive movement of large muscle groups. Walking, swimming, and cycling usually are best for most people. Rope jumping is terrible for most people.
        - Intensity of exercise. How hard the person should work is best indicated by heart rate. A moderate exercise heart rate "training" range is calculated. Patients are taught how to monitor their pulse to see if their exercise intensity is in the training range.
          Instructor Note: Individuals on beta-blockers will show a blunted heart rate response and cannot use the normal heart rate calculations.
        - Frequency of exercise. Therapeutic exercise programs suggest patients start with exercise sessions three times a week, preferably on alternating days. People may eventually work up to 6 to 7 days/week if they wish.
        - Duration of exercise. How long should the person exercise? The rule is start slowly and build up gradually. A person in poor condition may start out at 5-10 minutes/day and increase this time per session by 1 to 2 minutes each week.

11. J.C. is used to a much more "macho" approach to exercise: "No pain, no gain." What would be the advantage to him in following an individualized plan drawn up by the exercise physiologist? **[E/an/S,PI,PSI,HP/ct]**
    - The individualized exercise program will provide safe, effective levels of activity that are commensurate with his cardiac status and medications at minimal risk.
    - It will help alleviate his fear about his heart and not being able to exercise.
    - It might help alleviate his anxiety about looking "wimpy."

The flecainide did not work for J.C. He suffered 3 more significant episodes of ventricular fibrillation over the next 2 months and had to be defibrillated. It was decided that he would receive an implantable cardioverter defibrillator (ICD).

12. Briefly describe what an ICD is and how it works. **[A/c/PI/ct]**
    - The ICD is an electronic implantable device used to detect and terminate potentially lethal ventricular dysrhythmias through the delivery of electrical shocks to the heart. A tiny power system and electronic circuitry generate appropriately timed shocks and pacing stimuli. An electrode and wire system connected to the heart complete the circuit. The device senses a disruption in rhythm and delivers a shock to the heart to depolarize all the cells so the heart has the opportunity to recover a conducted rhythm.

13. If a patient with an ICD collapsed in the shower on your unit, what safety precautions would you take before assisting him/her? **[P/ap/S/ct,ni]**
    - Put rubber gloves on, turn off the shower, make sure you are *not* standing in water, and pull the patient out.

Case Study 17: Coronary Artery Disease

Difficulty: ***	*Setting:* Hospital
Index Words: Coronary artery disease, congestive heart failure, coronary artery bypass graft	

Your patient, 60-year-old K.W., has a significant cardiac history. He has long-standing coronary artery disease (CAD) with occasional episodes of congestive heart failure (CHF). One year ago he had an anterior wall MI. In addition, he has chronic anemia, hypertension, chronic renal insufficiency, and a recently diagnosed 4-cm suprarenal abdominal aortic aneurysm. Because of his severe CAD, he had to retire from his job as a railroad engineer about 6 months ago. This morning he is being admitted to your telemetry unit for a same-day cardiac catheterization. As you take his health history, you note that his wife died a year ago (about the same time that he had his MI) and that he does not have any children. He is a current cigarette smoker with a 50-pack/year smoking history. As you talk with him, you realize that he has only minimal understanding of the catheterization procedure. His VS are 158/94, 88, 20 and 36.2°C.

1. Before he leaves for the cath lab, you briefly teach him the important things he needs to know before having the procedure. List 5 priority topics you will address. **[P/c/PI,PSI/ct,ni,tc]**
   - Why he is to have the procedure.
   - How he will be prepared for the procedure.
   - What to expect during the catheterization itself.
   - What routine monitoring to expect after the procedure.
   - What staff members will be present to support him.
   - Possible complications and how they will be prevented or managed.

Several hours later, K.W. returns from his catheterization. The cath report shows 90% occlusion of the proximal left anterior descending coronary artery (LAD), 90% occlusion of the distal LAD, 70% to 80% occlusion of the distal right coronary artery, an old apical infarct, and an ejection fraction of 37%. About an hour after the procedure was finished, you perform a brief physical assessment and find that he now has a carotid bruit, a grade III/VI systolic ejection murmur at the cardiac apex, crackles bilaterally in the lung bases, and trace pitting edema of his feet and ankles. Except for a soft systolic murmur, these findings were not present before the catheterization.

2. What is your evaluation of the catheterization results? **[PD/an/PI/ct,ni]**
   - He has severe occlusion of 3 major coronary arteries, meaning that much of his ventricular muscle is without adequate blood supply. The old apical infarct is now tough, noncontractile scar tissue. Both the coronary occlusions and scar tissue contribute to the low ejection fraction (EF). Normally about 58% to 70% of the blood present in the L ventricle at the end of diastole (preload) is ejected with each cardiac contraction. An EF of 37% indicates that his L ventricle has lost almost half of its ability to pump blood.

3. What problem do the changes in assessment findings suggest to you and identify what led you to your conclusion? **[PD/c/PI,PSI/ct,ni,tc]**
   - K.W. is developing congestive heart failure. He has crackles in bilateral bases, pitting edema in his lower extremities, and a systolic ejection murmur.

   Instructor Note: Patients usually express statements like, "Something is wrong..I just don't feel right." The nurse needs to be alert to this and reassure them that she is listening to them and monitoring their status.

4. List 4 actions you would take as a result of your evaluation of the assessment and state your rationales. **[P/an/PI,PSI/ct,ni,tc]**
   - Take his VS and continue taking them every 15 minutes. K.W. is experiencing some sudden changes in his cardiovascular status that require close monitoring.
   - Ask the patient about symptoms relevant to CHF such as shortness of breath, anxiety. Data about subjective symptoms add the patient's sensations to your objective assessment.
   - Note the patient's mental status. Is he restless, confused, lethargic? Mental status is a good indicator of cerebral perfusion. Watch for changes!
   - Determine his need for supplemental O_2. Initiate O_2 therapy if needed. The crackles indicate the development of pulmonary edema and potential need for O_2.
   - Call the physician immediately, and report the above findings.

After assessing the patient, K.W.'s doctor admitted him with a diagnosis of CAD and CHF for coronary artery bypass graft (CABG) surgery. Significant lab results drawn at this time were Hct 25.3%, Hgb 8.8 g/dl, BUN 33 mg/dl and creatinine 3.1 mg/dl. K.W. was diuresed with Lasix and given 2 units of packed red blood cells (PRBCs).

5. Review K.W.'s health history. Can you identify a probable explanation for his chronic renal insufficiency and anemia? **[PD/c/PI/ct]**
   - If the perfusion to the kidneys is poor over a prolonged period of time, renal insufficiency develops. In addition, poorly perfused kidneys are not able to produce adequate amounts of erythropoietin, an important stimulus for red blood cell production. This contributes to a chronic anemic condition.

Five days later, after his condition was stabilized, K.W. was taken to surgery for bypass of 3 coronary arteries (CABG x 3). When he arrived in the SICU he had a Swan-Ganz catheter in place for hemodynamic monitoring and was intubated and on a ventilator at FIO_2 .70 and PEEP 5 cm H_2O. His first hemodynamic readings were: pulmonary artery pressure (PAP) 41/23 mm Hg, CVP 13 mm Hg, PCWP 13 mm Hg, cardiac index (CI) 1.88 L/min/m^2. ABGs drawn at this time were: pH 7.36, PCO_2 46 mm Hg, PO_2 61 mm Hg, and SaO_2 85%, with a Hgb 10.3 mg/dl.

6. What is your evaluation of his hemodynamic status based on the above parameters? **[A/an/PI/ct]**
   - PAP is slightly high (normal 15-30/1-12 mm Hg).
   - CVP is high (normal 2-6 mm Hg).
   - PCWP is slightly high (normal 1-10 mm Hg) but many physicians like to keep the PCWP closer to 15 mm Hg to ensure adequate cardiac output). The PCWP is an indication of the preload.
   - CI is low (normal 2.8-4.0 L/min/m^2).

Clinically, these values show that the pressures within his heart and lungs are a little high and that his cardiac output is a little low, indicating that his heart is still having difficulty pumping out all the blood that is returned to it and/or that he is a little fluid overloaded. His condition will require careful monitoring.

7. K.W. is receiving continuous IV infusions of nitroprusside (Nipride) and dobutamine (Dobutrex). He also has just received 2 units of fresh frozen plasma (FFP) and 500 ml of albumin IV. Given this information, do you think the hemodynamic values reported above reflect poor L ventricular function or fluid overload and why? **[A,PD/an/PI/ct,ni]**
   - Poor L ventricular function. If K.W. was fluid overloaded and had adequate ventricular function, all the numbers would be elevated. The fact that the CI was decreased while the rest of the values were elevated indicates poor left ventricular function.

8. Why is K.W. receiving the nitroprusside and dobutamine? **[PD/c/PI/ct]**
   - To increase cardiac output. Nitroprusside produces peripheral vasodilation. Because more blood remains in the peripheral cardiovascular system, cardiac preload and afterload are decreased. Dobutamine stimulates myocardial adrenergic receptors, thereby increasing CO without significantly increasing heart rate. Dobutamine, when used with nitroprusside, has a synergistic effect to increase CO.

9. What is your responsibility when administering nitroprusside and dobutamine to your patient? **[A/c/S,PI/ct,ni]**
   - Monitor for side effects of both drugs. The major side effects of Nipride are HA, vertigo, nausea, and abdominal pain. Also, because Nipride is rapidly metabolized to cyanide and thiocyanate, patients receiving prolonged infusions >3 μg/kg/min should be monitored for thiocyanate toxicity. Levels should not exceed 1 mmol/L. The major side effects of dobutamine are tachycardia, HTN, and PVCs.

10. Why did he receive the FFP and albumin? **[PD/c/PI/ct]**
    - FFP is a volume extender. Plasma normally makes up 45% to 60% of blood volume. Albumin is a plasma protein, which provides colloidal oncotic pressure (COP) within the CV space. Kidney disease is associated with decreased levels of plasma protein. The COP serves to mobilize fluids from the extravascular to the intravascular space, thereby reducing tissue edema and maintenance of CV volume. Together, FFP and albumin expand intravascular volume, boost BP, and augment CO.

11. Explain whether or not it is possible for K.W. to experience a transfusion reaction when receiving albumin or FFP infusion. **[A/k/S,PI/ct]**
    - Yes, it is possible for him to suffer a transfusion reaction from FFP. ABO compatibility is necessary, but Rh compatibility is not. Albumin administration is safe for K.W.

12. What is your interpretation of his ABGs on 70% O_2? **[PD/c/PI/ct]**
    - His acid/base balance is normal, but he is not oxygenating adequately. His PO_2 and O_2 sat are both below normal and should be much higher on 70% O_2 and PEEP. In addition, the oxygen-carrying capacity of his blood is low, as evidenced by the low Hgb level.

After 3 days in the SICU, K.W.s condition was stable and he was returned to your telemetry floor. Now, 5 days later, he is ready to go home, and you are preparing him for discharge.

13. List at least 5 general areas related to his CABG surgery in which he should receive instruction before he goes home. **[P/ap/S,PI,PSI,HP/ct,ni,tc]**
    - Signs and symptoms of problems: what to watch for, what to do if he has them, and when to call the doctor.
    - Medications: how to use them, why he needs them, and what possible side effects to be aware of.
    - Diet: guidelines for lifestyle changes.
    - Activity: guidelines for lifestyle changes.
    - Resources: what is available in his community, particularly cardiac rehabilitation centers and smoking cessation programs. Community resources will be particularly important for K.W. because he is without wife and children for support.
    - Mental status: what to expect in mood swings and changes in short term memory.

Case Study 18: Coronary Artery Disease

Difficulty: ***	*Setting:* Hospital, outpatient cardiac rehabilitation
Index Words: Coronary artery disease, hypertension, angina	

It is midmorning on the cardiac unit where you work and you are getting a new patient, G.P. G.P., a 60-year-old retired businessman, is married and has 3 grown children. As you take his health history, he tells you that he began feeling changes in his heart rhythm about 10 days ago. He has hypertension and a 10-year history of angina pectoris. During the past week he has had more frequent episodes of midchest discomfort. The chest pain has awakened him from sleep but does respond to NTG, which he has taken sublingually about 8 to 10 times over the past week. During the week he has also experienced increased fatigue. He states, "I have lost my sensation of well-being." A cardiac catheterization done several years ago revealed 50% occlusion of the right coronary artery (RCA) and 50% occlusion of the left anterior descending (LAD) coronary artery. He tells you that both his mother and father had CAD. He is taking amlodipine and metoprolol.

1. What other information are you going to ask about his episodes of chest pain? **[A/c/PI,PSI/ct,ni,tc]**
   - Are they accompanied by other signs/symptoms, such as nausea, vomiting, diaphoresis, shortness of breath, anxiety?
   - Do they occur during exercise, after eating a large meal, in cold weather, or during periods of stress? It is less common for angina to occur during sleep than during exertion when the heart's demand for oxygen is increased. Resting angina is often caused by spasm of the coronary arteries.
   - What is the quality of the pain? Ask him to describe the sensation in his own words.
   - How long do the episodes last?
   - Does the pain radiate to other areas of the body?

2. What are common sites for radiation of ischemic cardiac pain? **[A/k/PI/ct]**
   - Epigastric area, arms and hands (especially left), back (intrascapular area), shoulders, jaws.

3. You know that G.P. has atherosclerosis of the coronary arteries but he has not told you about his risk factors. You need to know his risk factors for CAD in order to plan teaching for lifestyle modifications. What questions will you ask him? **[A/c/,PI,PSI/ct,ni]**
   - Weight: obesity is a serious risk factor; obtain his WHR.
   - Smoking history.
   - Diet: ask about his usual fat and caloric intake and if he knows his cholesterol and triglyceride levels.
   - Stress: find out what stressors he has in his life and his usual methods for controlling stress.
   - Exercise: does he have a regular exercise program. If so, what kind of exercises does he do? Does he have angina or become short of breath when he exercises or does yard work?

4. Although he has been taking SL NTG for a long time, you want to be sure he is using it correctly. What information would you make sure he understands about the side effects, use, and storage of sublingual NTG? **[A,,P,I/an/S,PI/ct,ni,tc]**
    - Tablets should be kept tightly sealed in brown bottle to protect them from moisture and light. A bottle of tablets should not be kept longer than 6 months.
    - He should carry the tablets with him at all times for emergency use.
    - The antihypertensive medications he is taking may compound the hypotensive effects of NTG.
    - He should sit or lie down upon first indication of anginal pain and place tablet under tongue or in buccal pouch. Lying down will reduce hypotensive effects.
    - He should allow the tablet to dissolve naturally and not swallow until the drug is entirely dissolved.
    - Pain not relieved by 3 sublingual tablets over a 15-minute period may indicate acute MI or severe coronary insufficiency. He should call an ambulance to take him to an emergency department.

When you first admitted G.P., you placed him on telemetry and observed he was in atrial fibrillation converting frequently to atrial flutter with a 4:1 block. His VS and all of his lab tests were within normal range, including LDH and CPK levels; K was 4.7 mEq/L. He was converted with medications (quinidine and diltiazem) from atrial fib/flutter to tachy/brady syndrome with long sinus pauses that caused lightheadedness and hypotension.

5. What risks does the new rhythm pose for G.P.? **[E,AE/c/S,PI/ct]**
    - Syncope and falls due to the hypotension.
    - Increased anginal episodes and more serious dysrhythmias because of decreased perfusion to the heart.
    - Confusion, altered level of consciousness due to decreased perfusion to the brain.
    - CHF due to inadequate heart rate during bradycardia and inadequate ventricular filling during tachycardia.

Because G.P.'s dysrhythmia was causing unacceptable symptoms, he was taken to surgery and a permanent DDI pacemaker was placed and set at a rate of 70/minute.

6. What does the code "DDI" mean? **[A/k/PI/ct]**
    - The first "D" indicates the heart chamber paced; meaning dual pacing because both the atrium and ventricle are paced.
    - The second "D" indicates the chamber sensed; meaning dual sensing because both the atrium and ventricle are sensed.
    - The "I" indicates how the pacemaker will respond to the patient's own activity, meaning pacemaker activity is inhibited by the patient's activity.

7. The pacemaker insertion surgery places G.P. at risk for several serious complications. List 3 potential problems that you will monitor for as you care for him. **[P,E,A/an/S,PI/ct,ni]**
   - Infection: to prevent infection, prevent stricture, pressure, or irritation of the pacemaker site. Use sterile technique with dressing changes.
   - Pacemaker dysfunction: the pacemaker can fail to pace (initiate an electrical impulse), fail to sense (be responsive to the patient's own cardiac activity), or fail to capture (stimulate a ventricular contraction). All of these problems can result in dysrhythmias, ineffective cardiac function, and symptoms for the patient.
   - Perforation of the endocardium: the result could be cardiac tamponade. The patient might experience sharp chest pain on inspiration and excessive hiccups, increased heart rate, decreased blood pressure, and shortness of breath.
   - Hematoma at the incision site: you would see evidence of increased ecchymosis, swelling, and tenderness at the incision site.
   - Pneumothorax: the patient would experience sudden, sharp, chest pain and shortness of breath.

8. G.P. will need some education regarding his new pacemaker. What information will you give him before he leaves the hospital? **[P/c/S,PI,PSI/ct,ni,tc]**
   - Call the doctor if you have signs/symptoms of infection, such as excessive redness, swelling, unusual pain, or drainage at the incision site, fever.
   - Restrict arm lifting movements/exercises for 2 to 3 weeks following surgery.
   - Call the doctor if you have any of the following signs/symptoms of pacemaker malfunction: dizziness, palpitations, chest pain, unusual weight gain.
   - Observe safety precautions by avoiding contact sports, avoiding pressure to the incision, wearing a Medic Alert tag, carrying a pacemaker ID card, and avoiding high-voltage electrical and magnetic equipment.

Note: Information about the Medic Alert emergency identification system can be obtained by calling 1-800-432-5378.

9. G.P.'s wife approaches you and anxiously inquires, "My neighbor saw this science fiction movie about this guy who got a pacemaker and then he couldn't die. Is that for real?" How are you going to respond to her? **[P/c/PSI/ct,ni,tc]**
   - Do not laugh! Patient's and their families sometimes hear bizarre stores about "high-tech" health care issues. It is fortunate she felt she could ask you this question; be sure that if she asked you about it, she probably worried about it a great deal.
   - Reassure her that it might have made a great plot for a movie but it's not a "for real" situation.
   - Explain to her the pacemaker only gives off "mini-electrical signals" to make the heart beat regularly.
   - This might be a good time to ask if she and G.P. have discussed and done anything about health care power-of-attorney and advanced directives for each other.

After discharge, G.P. is referred to a cardiac prevention and rehabilitation center to start an exercise program. He will be exercise tested, and an individualized exercise prescription will be developed for him based on the exercise test.

10. What information will be obtained from the graded exercise (stress) test (GXT) and what is included in an exercise prescription? **[A,PD,P,I,E/an/S,PI,PSI,HP/ct,]**
    - G.P.'s cardiorespiratory responses (heart rate, blood pressure, respiratory gases (O_2 and CO_2, and perceived exertion) to specific workloads will be evaluated to ensure that he can safely exercise in the intensity range that will be prescribed for him.
    - His resting (lowest) and peak (highest) exertional heart rate will be incorporated into the exercise prescription.
    - The exercise prescription will start him at a workload that is not dangerous or emotionally threatening to him (e.g., slow and easy).
    - Just as medications are prescribed (type, dose, time, route), exercise for cardiac patients should be prescribed in these terms:
        - Type of exercise (what kind?).
        - Intensity of exercise (how hard?), usually measured in terms of pulse or perceived exertion.
        - Frequency of exercise (how often?), usually beginning 3 days per week.
        - Duration of exercise (how long?), usually measured in minutes or distance.

Case Study 19: Hypovolemia

Difficulty: ***	*Setting:* Hospital ED, hospital ICU
Index Words: Hypovolemia, hypertension, cardiomyopathy	

C.W., a 70-year-old man, was brought to the ED at 0430 this morning by his wife. She told the ED triage nurse that he had dysentery for the past 3 days and last night he had a lot of "dark red" diarrhea. When he became very dizzy, disoriented, and weak this morning, she decided to bring him to the hospital. C.W.'s VS were systolic BP 70 mm Hg, diastolic BP inaudible (70/-); 110, 20. A 16-gauge IV catheter was inserted and a LR infusion was started. The triage nurse obtained the following history from the patient and his wife. C.W. has had idiopathic dilated cardiomyopathy (IDCM) for several years. The onset was insidious but the cardiomyopathy is now severe, as evidenced by a L ventricular ejection fraction of 13% found during a recent cardiac catheterization. He experiences frequent problems with CHF because of the IDCM. Two years ago he had a cardiac arrest that was attributed to hypokalemia. He also has a long history of hypertension and arthritis. Fifteen years ago he had a peptic ulcer.

An endoscopy showed a 25 x 15 mm duodenal ulcer with adherent clot. The ulcer was cauterized and C.W. was admitted to the MICU for treatment of his volume deficit. You are his admitting nurse. As you are making him comfortable, Mrs. W. gives you a paper sack filled with the bottles of medications he has been taking: enalopril (Vasotec) 5 mg PO bid, warfarin (Coumadin) 2 mg PO qd, digoxin 0.125 mg PO qd, KCl 20 mEq PO bid, and tolmetin (an NSAID) 400 mg PO tid. As you connect him to the cardiac monitor, you note that he is in atrial fibrillation. Doing a quick assessment, you find a pale man who is sleepy but arousable and oriented. He is still dizzy, hypotensive, and tachycardic. You hear S_3 and S_4 heart sounds and a grade II/VI systolic murmur. Peripheral pulses are all 2+ and trace pedal edema is present. Lungs are clear. Bowel sounds are present, midepigastric tenderness is noted, and the liver margin is 4 cm below the costal margin. A Swan-Ganz catheter and an arterial line are inserted.

1. What medications probably precipitated C.W.'s GI bleeding? **[A,D/c/Pl/ct]**
   - Tolmetin: C.W. has been taking tolmetin for his arthritis. Overwhelming evidence has linked NSAIDs to gastroduodenal ulcers and bleeding. NSAIDS irritate the gastric mucosa and decrease the mucosa's ability to protect the stomach lining from HCl.
   - Coumadin: Coumadin inhibits the extrinsic pathway of the coagulation cascade.

2. What is the most serious potential complication of C.W.'s bleeding? **[PD/c/Pl/ct]**
   - Hypovolemic shock that could lead to renal failure or even death.

3. From his history and assessment, identify 5 signs/symptoms (direct and/or indirect) of GI bleeding and loss of blood volume. **[A/c/Pl/ct,ni]**
   - 3-day history of diarrhea.
   - Dark red blood visible in the stool.
   - Dizziness and disorientation because of inadequate perfusion of the cerebral cortex.
   - Weakness because of inadequate oxygen delivery to the tissues.
   - Very low blood pressure; a direct result of volume loss.
   - Tachycardia; compensation for low blood pressure.
   - Increased respiratory rate; compensation for inadequate oxygen delivery to the tissues.

C.W. received a total of 8 units of PRBCs, 5 units of fresh frozen plasma (FFP), and many liters of crystalloids to keep his systolic BP above 90 mm Hg. On the second day in the MICU, his total fluid intake was 8.498 L and output 3.660 L for a positive fluid balance of 4.838 L. His hemodynamic parameters after fluid resuscitation were PCWP 30 mm Hg, cardiac output 4.5 L/min.

4. Why will you want to monitor his fluid status very carefully? **[A,P,I,E/c/Pl/ct,ni]**
   - C.W. needs fluids and blood products to replace the lost blood volume, but because of his history of CHF it would be very easy to overload him with fluids and push him into pulmonary edema.

5. List 6 things you will monitor to assess C.W.'s fluid balance. **[A,P,E/an/S,Pl/ct,ni]**
   - Urine output; with inadequate volume to perfuse the kidneys, the urine output will drop below 30 ml/h.
   - Fluid intake; compare output and intake.
   - Daily weight: fluid weight is lost or gained very rapidly and is an excellent indicator of changes in fluid volume.
   - VS; as the intravascular volume rises in response to IV fluids, the BP can be expected to increase and the heart rate decrease.
   - Cardiac output (CO) and PCWP: both are good measures of L ventricular function and preload. The PCWP is already high; an increase could be a first indication of fluid overload.
   - Mental status: a good indication of cerebral perfusion.
   - Lungs: crackles and dyspnea are indicators of pulmonary edema.
   - Heart sounds: an increase in the baseline murmur and gallops could indicate fluid overload.

6. Explain the purpose of the fresh frozen plasma for C.W. **[P/c/Pl/ct]**
   - Replacement of intravascular fluid. FFP also contains plasma proteins and clotting factors. The albumin will pull interstitial fluid into the intravascular compartment. The clotting factors will help control the bleeding.

As soon as you get a chance, you look at his admission lab results. The K is 6.2 mEq/L, BUN 90 mg/dl, creatinine 2.1 mg/dl, Hgb 8.4 g/dl, Hct 25%, WBC 16 mm^3, and PT 18.3 sec. Other results are within the normal range.

7. Are you worried by the elevated K? Why, or why not? Explain your answer. **[E/an/PI/ct]**
   - You are not very concerned right now because the fluid resuscitation will probably bring it down. You will watch for ventricular dysrhythmias, however. You will also want to request an order for C.W.'s magnesium level.

8. Why do you think BUN and creatinine are elevated? **[A,PD/c/PI/ct]**
   - Inadequate renal perfusion due to hypovolemia.

9. What do the low Hb and Hct levels indicate about the rapidity of his blood loss? **[A,PD/an/PI/ct]**
   - Because The Hb and Hct are low, the bleeding has probably taken place over several days. Interstitial fluid has had time to move into the vascular compartment, diluting the RBCs. In an acute bleed, the Hb and Hct would be normal (undiluted).

10. What is the explanation for the prolonged PT? **[PD/c/PI/ct]**
    - It is being influenced by Coumadin therapy.

11. How do you account for the elevated WBC count? **[A,PD/an/PI/ct]**
    - Physical stress and inflammation caused by the severe bleeding and tissue hypoxia can increase the neutrophil count.

Mrs. W. has been with her husband since he arrived at the ED and is very worried about his condition and his care.

12. List 4 things you might do to make her more comfortable while her husband is in the MICU. **[P/ap/PSI/ct,ni,tc]**
    - Tell her that a nurse is watching her husband very closely, and that his heart rhythm is being monitored at all times.
    - Explain the equipment (monitoring devices, tubes, wires, alarms) used for his care. Familiarity with them may make them seem less intimidating to her.
    - Explain all procedures and treatments before they are performed.
    - Report her husband's condition to her regularly. This demonstrates caring if the report is unsolicited.
    - Encourage her to take care of herself while her husband is in the hospital by eating well and getting enough rest.
    - Let her know that if she goes home for brief periods, she can call the MICU at any time to inquire about her husband.
    - Encourage her to seek support from friends, family, or clergy.

Case Study 20: Cardiac Arrest

Difficulty: ***	*Setting:* Hospital ICU, telemetry unit
Index Words: Cardiac arrest, implantable cardioverter defibrillator	

K.K., a 40-year-old administrative secretary, lost consciousness and slumped to the floor while eating dinner with her husband. He initiated CPR. Paramedics arrived within 4 to 5 minutes and found her in ventricular fibrillation. After successful defibrillation, she was transported to the hospital. In the MICU her nurse obtained K.K.'s health history from her husband. She has a long history of RHD (rheumatic heart disease) with MVP (mitral valve prolapse) and severe L ventricular dysfunction. She has had atrial fibrillation/atrial flutter for 6 years. She also has had ventricular dysrhythmias for several years being treated with various antidysrhythmic drugs; furosemide, however, she was not taking her medications at the time of the arrest because of their unpleasant side effects. Her doctor feels she has been noncompliant with her medications and that she is denying her need for mitral valve replacement. For the past 2 months she has had CHF with greatly decreased activity tolerance. Medications she was taking at the time of the arrest were: furosemide (Lasix) 80 mg PO qd, KCl 20 mEq PO bid, digoxin 0.125 mg PO qd, lisinopril (Zestril) 5 mg PO qd, verapamil (Verelan) 120 mg PO qd, and warfarin (Coumadin) 2.5 mg PO qd. On the day of her arrest she had diarrhea.

1. From K.K.'s history, what factors probably contributed to her cardiac arrest? **[A/c/PI/ct]**
   - Mitral valve prolapse (MVP): commonly associated with both atrial and ventricular dysrhythmias.
   - CHF: L ventricular dysfunction and CHF can cause cardiac ischemia, triggering ventricular dysrhythmias.
   - Not taking needed antidysrhythmic medications.
   - Diarrhea: can decrease the serum K level; this probably precipitated the arrest.

On admission to the MICU, K.K. was hypotensive and unresponsive to voice commands. She was intubated and placed on mechanical ventilation. A central line was inserted, and dopamine and lidocaine drips started. For the first day in the MICU she remained unresponsive to commands, pupillary reaction was sluggish, eyes deviated slowly to the right, upper extremities had increased tone, and lower extremities were flaccid. Painful stimuli elicited withdrawal and decorticate posturing. Her 12-lead ECG showed atrial fibrillation at a rate of 136/min, ST segment depression in leads II, III, AVF and V_1-V_6 and T wave inversion in leads V_3-V_5.

2. What is the probable cause for her neurologic deficits? **[PD/an/PI,ct]**
   - Cerebral hypoxia secondary to the cardiac arrest.

3. Explain how rapid atrial fibrillation can cause a decrease in cardiac output and contribute to CHF. **[PD/c/PI/ct]**
   - The rapid, irregular rate decreases the time available for ventricular filling. This can dramatically decrease the blood volume in the ventricles at the end of diastole (the blood available for the next ejection). In atrial fibrillation the "atrial kick" is also lost. Atrial kick is the ejection of the last 25% of blood in the L atrium into the L ventricle at the end of diastole. In addition, the rapid rate increases the workload of the heart and exhausts the cardiac reserve of energy.

4. What is the significance of the ST segment depression and T wave inversion in her 12-lead ECG? **[PD/c/PI/ct]**
   - Myocardial ischemia with possible injury and necrosis. The physician will want to rule out MI.

5. List 8 lab results that the MICU nurse should check as soon as possible. **[A/an/PI/ct,ni]**
   - CPK and LDH levels with accompanying isoenzymes if elevated: released by injured heart muscle. Elevated levels are present if an MI has occurred, and the degree of elevation is an indication of the extent of myocardial damage.
   - Lidocaine level: toxicity is serious. Serum levels should not be above 5.0 mg/L.
   - Digoxin level: toxicity is a common cause of both atrial and ventricular dysrhythmias. Toxic levels are >2 ng/ml.
   - K level: normal serum K range is very narrow, 3.5 to 5.1 mEq/L. Both hyperkalemia and hypokalemia can trigger ventricular dysrhythmias.
   - Mg level: hypomagnesemia can also cause ventricular dysrhythmias.
   - BUN and creatinine: elevated during hypoperfusion of the kidneys. The BUN and creatinine are an indication of the degree of hypoxic damage to the kidneys suffered during the arrest and hypotensive period following the arrest.
   - Lactate level: levels are elevated during cardiac arrest and hypoperfusion states as cells convert from aerobic to anaerobic metabolism. This test is the best indication of perfusion and oxygenation at the cellular level.
   - PT: she has been on Coumadin to prevent clot formation secondary to her valvular disease. Coumadin prolongs the PT. Her PT was 31 seconds, which is elevated as you would expect.
   - Cholesterol level: although she has no history of coronary artery disease (CAD), with her already severe L ventricular dysfunction, development of CAD is to be avoided. Keep in mind that in postMI, both cholesterol and triglyceride levels can be elevated.
   - Antidysrhythmic drug: to find out what her drug level currently is.

   Instructor Note: Although all chemistries and CBCs would be checked, some of the most important tests are listed above.

After 4 days in the MICU, K.K.'s condition was stabilized and she was transferred to your telemetry floor. When you first assess her, you find jugular vein distention at 10 cm and hear a grade II/VI systolic murmur and an S_3 sound. A thrill is felt over the precordium, and the S_1 and S_2 can be seen on the chest. She no longer has sensory or motor deficits, and her long-term memory is good. However, she is confused, oriented only to name, and has poor short-term memory. Her lidocaine level in the MICU the day before the transfer (the day the lidocaine was discontinued) was 16.8 mg/L; digoxin level was normal. A cardiac catheterization and ECHO cardiogram showed that K.K. has irreversible heart valve, L ventricle, and L atrium damage and is no longer a candidate for mitral valve replacement. She states she is very fearful about her memory loss and the inoperable heart damage.

6. List 3 factors that might be contributing to K.K.'s confusion and disorientation. **[A,PD/an/PI,PSI/ct]**
   - Residual effects of her hypoxic episode.
   - Lidocaine toxicity.
   - Stay in the MICU. Disorientation and confusion are common in ICU patients because of many factors, among them sleep and sensory deprivation, and the frightening and complex environment.
   - Fatigue.

7. List 4 nursing interventions you might implement to relieve K.K.'s fear. **[PD/c/PI,PSI/ct,ni]**
   - Monitor her level of mental activity/memory and assess contributing factors.
   - Give her accurate, daily feedback on the progress of her memory recovery.
   - Provide opportunity for her to verbalize feelings, concerns, anxiety.
   - Explain to her that emotional and cognitive disturbances are not uncommon during stressful periods.
   - Include K.K.'s husband in planning interventions and in discussions of her progress. Encourage his support.
   - Assist her with coping strategies (e.g. relaxation, imagery, meditation).

After 2 weeks in the hospital, K.K. is scheduled for placement of an internal cardioverter defibrillator (ICD) to prevent future cardiac arrest from ventricular fibrillation. You will do her preoperative teaching about ICDs.

8. What is an ICD and how does it work? **[A,PD/c/PI/ct]**
   - An ICD is an electronic device that is implanted in the body. It is designed to monitor the heart's rhythm. If the ICD senses that the rhythm is ventricular tachycardia or ventricular fibrillation, it will deliver an "internal" shock to the heart to correct the abnormal rhythm.

9. List 4 discharge instructions related to the ICD that you will give K.K. **[P/c/S,PI,PSI/ct,ni,tc]**
   - Warn her that patients are often distressed by lack of warning of shocks, multiple shocks, and progressively increased sensations with multiple shocks. She may need support for this problem.
   - Instruct her to:
     - Keep her incision dry for 2 days.
     - Call her doctor if she notices redness, swelling, or other indication of infection at her incision site.
     - Call her doctor if she has symptoms of irregular heart rhythm (lightheadedness, palpitations, shortness of breath, fatigue).
     - Inform her doctor if she receives a shock and to keep a log of date/time shocks are received and the preceding events and associated symptoms.
   - Wear Medic Alert identification and carry her ICD ID card at all times.
   - Warn her family that if she becomes unconscious in the shower or tub, they should put on rubber gloves, keep their feet out of standing water, turn off any running water, and then lift her out. This prevents their being shocked.

Case Study 21: Cardiac Aneurysm

Difficulty: ***	*Setting:* Hospital, home care
Index Words: Cardiac aneurysm, chronic renal failure, dialysis, home care	

During a routine checkup, D.A.'s doctor heard 2 new heart murmurs: a grade II/VI diastolic flow murmur heard at the R sternal border and a prominent grade IV/VI systolic ejection murmur heard over the entire precordium but best at the L sternal border. The murmurs are asymptomatic. D.A. is a slender, active 50-year-old engineer, married with 2 teenage children. He has polycystic kidney disease with renal failure and has been on dialysis for 5 years. His mother also had polycystic kidney disease. Besides frequent UTIs, he has no other significant medical problems, no history of cardiac disease, and no cardiac risk factors. A transthoracic/transesophageal ECHO showed a "high pressure jet from the R atrium or R ventricle." Cardiac catheterization showed an "aortic to R ventricle connection through a R coronary sinus of Valsalva leak." The catheterization also showed normal coronary arteries, normal L ventricular function, and no aortic regurgitation.

D.A. was admitted to the hospital for surgical repair of a ruptured sinus of Valsalva aneurysm. During the surgery a 4-mm hole from the R coronary sinus to the R atrium was discovered and repaired with a patch. There were no complication. You are caring for D.A. in the SICU after the surgery. On the first postop day his VS are 90/54, 87, 12, 37.8°C. Central venous pressure averages 10 mm Hg. He has a temporary pacemaker set at 87/min, which is functioning correctly. Lungs are clear. He has been extubated and is on O_2 at 2 L/min by nasal cannula with an SaO_2 of 99%. He has a chest tube and indwelling urinary catheter. You review his lab results, noting BUN 120 mg/dl, creatinine 8.5 mg/dl, and K 6.2 mEq/L. His preop Hct was 32%; today it is 22.1% and Hgb is 9.0 g/dL. Other lab values are within normal ranges.

1. Which of the physiologic data reported above should cause you concern and prompt careful monitoring on your part? **[A/an/Pl/ct,ni]**
   - Low blood pressure: he may be at risk for CHF with poor organ perfusion or even shock.
   - Elevated BUN and creatinine: expected because of his renal failure, but indicative of a need for dialysis soon.
   - Elevated K: puts him at risk for heart blocks and ventricular dysrhythmias.
   - Low Hct and Hgb: he lost a lot of blood during the surgery, and he was given a cell-saver transfusion to minimize blood loss.

2. When you perform your physical assessment, you should pay special attention to signs/symptoms related to D.A.'s problems. List at least 5 priority assessment areas, and explain why they are important. **[A/c/PI/ct,ni]**
   - Heart sounds: you want to know if the patch is holding. After the surgery, D.A. had a grade I/VI systolic ejection murmur; this is your baseline. If the murmur gets louder, notify the surgeon immediately.
   - Cardiac rhythm: D.A.'s heart is being paced. You will want to check his rhythm strip to make sure the pacer is functioning correctly. Also, after cardiac surgery, increased cardiac irritability can lead to dysrhythmias.
   - Peripheral perfusion: check distal pulses; assess for edema; check color, temperature, and capillary refill of fingers and toes. BP is low. If cardiac output in inadequate, vessels in the extremities may be vasoconstricted to shunt blood flow to vital organs.
   - Level of consciousness: confusion, lethargy, and disorientation are signs of decreased cerebral perfusion, in this case probably secondary to decreased cardiac output.
   - Urine output: D.A. does not have normal urine output because of his renal failure, so this cannot be used as an indicator of organ perfusion as it can in a patient with normal kidneys.
   - Lungs: crackles and shortness of breath are early indications of CHF, which might occur with patch failure.

3. Mrs. A. is present at the bedside, supportive and anxious. Considering her apprehension, what can you do to make her more comfortable? **[A,PD,P/an/PSI/ct,ni,tc]**
   - Assess her coping reserves. Is she eating and sleeping well? Does she have any personal support systems? Find resources to help her if necessary.
   - Encourage her questions and keep her informed about the goals for her husband's care and his condition and progress.
   - Explain the SICU environment, equipment, and procedures. The lines, tubes and monitors can be confusing and create a barrier between the patient and family members.
   - Encourage her to talk with her husband or just be with him. Allow them private time alone together.
   - If she would like to participate in his care, find small tasks and comfort measures that she can do for him.
   - Provide the SICU phone number for her, and assure her she can call at any time to talk to her husband's nurse.

On the third postop day, D.A. had an infectious disease consult. The consulting physician wrote in the chart, "The *Enterobacter* infection of the sinus of Valsalva is the likely cause of the aneurysm. The heart was probably seeded from a renal source. If the patch continues to harbor organisms, the patient may have future problems." D.A. was started on IV antibiotics (gentamicin, ticarcillin, and cefuroxime [Zinacef]).

4. List at least 3 problems D.A. might have as a result of the heavy-duty antibiotic therapy. What will you monitor for each? Consider his renal failure and common side effects of the medications. **[A,PD,P/ap/ct,ni]**
   - Ototoxicity: gentamicin is known to cause hearing loss and vestibular problems. Monitor his hearing and check for dizziness and vertigo. Ototoxicity can cause permanent deafness. Monitor gentamicin peak and trough serum levels.
   - Renal failure: gentamicin, particularly, but also ticarcillin and cefuroxime can cause renal failure. This will be difficult to assess because of D.A.'s preexisting renal failure. Monitor BUN and creatinine levels, and creatinine clearance. D.A. received dialysis throughout his hospitalization.
   - Opportunistic infections: many antibiotics can cause bacterial overgrowth resulting in diarrhea, anogenital itching, and stomatitis. One of the most serious infections is pseudomembranous colitis due to an overgrowth of *C. difficile*. Cephalospurins and broad-spectrum antivbiotics are especially known to cause pseudomembranous colitis.
   - Allergic reaction: all of the antibiotics prescribed for D.A. could cause an allergic reaction. People who are more likely to suffer allergic reactions are those with asthma, hayfever, or penicillin hypersensitivity. Be alert for fever, chills, rash, pruritus, and an anaphylactic reaction.

5. Mrs. A. confides in you, "You know, my 15-year-old son refuses to talk about his dad's illness. He won't even come to see him in the hospital. The guidance counselor called from school yesterday and said he's been acting out in school. I'm exhausted trying to work family life from both ends." How are you going to respond? **[A,P/an/PSI/ct,ni,tc]**
   - Acknowledge the frustration and conflict she must be suffering in trying to deal with her husband's and her children's needs. It's a pretty good bet there is nothing left for her.
   - Suggest that the son is afraid his father is going to die and is engaging in denial. Tell her denial is very common in children of parents who are very ill or dying. This may help her understand his behavior in the context of fear rather than rebellion or rejection.
   - Ask her if she would like to talk to one of the cardiac unit social workers about the problem. They may be able to offer some concrete suggestions about how to work with her son.
   - Remind her that the son's behavior may also reflect fear for himself. If he knows that his father's polycystic kidney disease is inherited, he may be afraid what is happening to his father may happen to him.

6. In preparation for discharge, a peripherally inserted central catheter (PICC) is placed. What is a PICC, and what are the advantages and disadvantages of this type of catheter? **[PD/c/PI/ct]**
    - It is a silicone-rubber catheter approximately 20 inches long that is percutaneously placed. It is usually inserted above the antecubital fossa, preferably in the basilic vein.
        - Advantages: easily inserted at bedside with minimal complications
        - Disadvantages: catheter may occlude smaller peripheral vessels and can be a source of phlebitis and thrombus formation.

D.A. is being discharged to home, where a home care nurse will continue to monitor the IV site and teach the wife how to administer the IV antibiotics.

7. Identify 2 nursing diagnosis that would apply to IV antibiotic administration in the home? **[PD/an/S,PI,PSI/ct]**
    - Fear r/t medication side effects and progression of disease.
    - Knowledge deficit r/t home IV administration.
    - Risk for injury.
    - Risk for infection.
    - Impairment of skin integrity.

Case Study 22: Percutaneous Transluminal Coronary Angioplasty

Difficulty: *** *Setting:* Hospital CCU

Index Words: Percutaneous transluminal coronary angioplasty, myocardial infarction, dysfunctional family

You are in the middle of your shift in the CCU of a large urban medical center. Your new admission, C.B., a 47-year-old woman, has just been brought by Life Flight to your institution from a small rural community over 100 miles away. She is unstable after an acute MI. C.B.'s VS are 100/60, 86, 14. After you make C.B. comfortable, you receive this report from the AirMed nurse: "C.B. is a full-time homemaker with 4 children. She has had episodes of 'chest tightness' for several years but this is her first documented MI. She has elevated cholesterol and triglyceride levels and has smoked 1½ packs of cigarettes per day for 30 years. Besides this and recent night sweats and hot flashes, she doesn't have any other medical problems. Yesterday at 2000 she began having substernal chest pain that radiated to her neck bilaterally and down both arms. She rated the pain as '9' on a scale of 1 to 10. She lay down with a heating pad but the pain didn't go away. Her husband then took her to the local ED where a 12-lead ECG showed hyperacute ST elevation. They were about to give her some t-PA when she went into V fib (ventricular fibrillation) and arrested. She was successfully defibrillated with 2 shocks. Then she was given the t-PA and put on lidocaine, heparin, and nitroglycerin drips. They also gave her some metoprol. This morning when her systolic pressure (BP) dropped into the 80s, she was put on a dopamine drip and flown here for a possible PTCA (percutaneous transluminal coronary angioplasty). Right now the lidocaine is going at 2 mg/min, the heparin at 1200 μ/h, and the dopamine at 5 μ/kg/min. The nitroglycerin is off."

The Life Flight nurse hands you a copy of yesterday's 12-lead ECG that shows normal sinus rhythm with ST elevation in leads II, III, AVF, and V_5-V_6. She also gives you a copy of yesterday's lab work: Na 145 mEq/L, K 3.6 mEq/L, HCO_3 19 mEq/L, BUN 9 mg/dl, creatinine 0.8 mg/dl, WBC 14.5 mm^3, Hct 44.3%, and Hgb 14.5 g/dl.

1. Given her diagnosis of acute MI, what other lab results are you going to look at? **[A,PD/an/S,PI/ct,ni]**
   - CPKs, LDH, and their isoenzymes.
   - Cholesterol and triglyceride levels.
   - ABGs.
   - PT and PTT.
   - Lidocaine level.
   - Mg.

2. You found the following lab results in the patient's chart. For each, interpret the result, and evaluate the meaning for C.B. **[PD/an/S,PI/ct,ni]**
   a. CPKs drawn upon admission to the ED and at 4 hour intervals were: 95 U/L, 1931 U/L, and 4175 U/L. CPK-MB isoenzymes were: 5%, 79%, and 216%.
      - The normal CPK varies somewhat from lab to lab but is usually considered to be <200 U/L; the CPK-MB isoenzymes should be <5%. CPK is released from several tissues after damage. The MB isoenzyme is specific for damaged cardiac muscle. Since the CPK level is proportional to the amount of myocardial injury, CPKs give a good indication of the severity of the MI. C.B. has had a massive MI.
   b. Cholesterol: 180 mg/dl.
      - Normal cholesterol is <200 mg/dl. In spite of a history of high cholesterol, this is a normal result.
   c. SaO_2 on O_2 at 6 L/min by nasal cannula: >90%.
      - Normal SaO_2 is 91% to 95% (depending on altitude). Her oxygen saturation on 6 L/min is barely adequate.
   d. PT was 11.9 secs and PTT was 26.9 secs (before heparin infusion).
      - Both are within the normal range.
   e. Mg level was 2.2 mg/dl.
      - Normal level is 1.5-3.0 mg/dl. Hypomagnesemia can cause cardiac dysrhythmias.

3. Why wasn't the LDH reported on the blood drawn in the ED? **[A/c/PI/ct]**
   - LDH is not released into the blood until 12 to 48 hours after the myocardial cells become ischemic, and blood level does not peak until 2 to 3 days.

4. The 12-lead ECG can tell you the location of the infarction. Look at the leads that show ST elevation (see above). What areas of C.B.'s heart have been damaged? **[A/k/PI/ct]**
   - Leads II, III, and AVF "look at" the heart from below. ST elevation in these leads indicates inferior wall damage. Leads V_5 and V_6 view the heart from the left side. ST elevation in these leads indicates lateral wall damage.

5. What is t-PA? Why is it given and when is it given to a patient having an MI? How is it administered? **[PD,P/c/PI/ct]**
   - t-PA (tissue-type plasminogen activator), called accelerated t-PA, is a thrombolytic agent used to lyse the clot in the coronary artery that is causing occlusion and infarction. Treatment must be started within the first 4 to 6 hours after onset of chest pain in order that the clot may be lysed before death of tissue occurs. The pharmacy will mix t-PA 100 mg/100 ml sterile H_2O. For patients weighing less than 65 kg, administer 15 mg rapid bolus, then administer 40 mg over the next 30 minutes, and an additional 25 mg over the following 60 minutes (total t-PA = 80 mg). This protocol may vary according to location.

6. An hour after her admission, you are preparing C.B. for her PTCA. Evaluate her readiness for teaching and her learning needs. What would you tell her? **[P,I/an/PI,PSI/ct,ni,tc]**
   - Be brief in your explanation because she is still in some pain and in unstable condition. This is not the time to go into lengthy anatomy and physiology discussions. Her biggest problem right now probably is fear.
   - Briefly explain the procedure. Tell her that the purpose is to restore blood flow to her stenosed coronary artery by dilating the artery with a balloon-tipped catheter. She will be taken to the cardiac cath lab where the angioplasty will be performed under local anesthesia.
   - Briefly explain what she might experience. Tell her she may feel a warm, flushed sensation, a sudden burning feeling (like a flash fire), or feel a need to urinate as the dye is injected. She will experience chest pain during dilation of the vessel. During or after the procedure she may feel irregular heart beats or temporary numbness and tingling of the extremity used for the procedure. Some patients tell you it felt as if they were having an MI all over again.
   - Reassure her that doctors and/or nurses will be with her at all times to assist her with pain control and give support and information as she requires it.
   - If you feel comfortable doing so, explore whether she would like someone to pray with her. This can be extremely powerful in relief of fear.

The following day you care for C.B. again. During her PTCA procedure yesterday a circumflex coronary lesion was found and the artery was successfully dilated. She is still on the lidocaine and heparin drips. The dopamine has been discontinued. VS are stable. PCWP is 20 mm Hg and cardiac output is 7.3 L/min. You check her lab results for lidocaine and PTT levels.

7. The lidocaine level is 2.5 μg/ml, and the PTT is 61 seconds. Analyze the results and state any actions you would take. **[A,P/an/PI/ct,ni]**
   - Therapeutic lidocaine levels are between 1.5 and 6 μg/ml; >7 μg/ml is toxic. Her lidocaine level is therapeutic. Continue to follow daily levels and watch for signs of neurotoxicity (drowsiness, dizziness, confusion, visual disturbances, and behavioral changes). Evaluate the antidysrhythmic effectiveness of lidocaine; also evaluate C.B. for signs and symptoms of lidocaine toxicity.
   - PTT is followed to assess effectiveness of heparin, inhibiting the intrinsic clotting pathway in the clotting cascade. Therapeutic PTT is 1.5 to 2.5 times the normal range of 25 to 35 seconds. Her PTT is in the therapeutic range. Continue to follow the daily PTT levels.

As you work with C.B., you notice that she is extremely anxious. You had observed some anxiety yesterday which you had attributed to the strange CCU environment, pain, and anticipation of the PTCA procedure. You know that the PTCA was successful and that she is physically stable. You wonder what is wrong. She tells you that her MI occurred right in the middle of a move with her family from her rural community to an even smaller and unfamiliar town some 500 miles away in a neighboring state. She is dreading the move. Her husband "becomes angry easily and starts lashing out" toward her and the children. She is afraid to move to a community where she will have no friends and family to support her.

8. How can you help your patient? Evaluate the situation and describe possible interventions. **[P,I/an/S,PI,PSI/ct,ni,tc]**
   - The reasons for C.B.'s anxiety are much more complicated than you had thought. You need to decide if you have the experience and background to help her or if you should involve another member of the interdisciplinary team. Possible actions:
     - Support the patient with your presence and active listening. Assure her that physically she is doing well.
     - If spousal abuse is involved, a social worker or psychiatric nurse specialist who specialize in abuse would be important resources.
     - If child abuse is involved, investigate the possibility of having this case reported to the authorities. C.B. should be given the number of a "safe house" or a community resource.

9. C.B.'s husband comes to visit. He is a handsome, well-dressed man who appears to be loving and attentive toward C.B. He brought a bouquet of roses for her and a box of chocolates for the nurses, "Because I appreciate how good you girls have been to my wife." One of your younger colleagues comments to you, "Why, what a nice guy! What is her problem? Every woman would love to be married to a man like that!" How are you going to respond? **[P/an/PSI/ct,ni,tc]**
   - You have very little information on which to base your judgment.
   - She has expressed fear for herself and the children.
   - Abusive spouses are often very charming and personable outside the home. This often contributes to the reluctance of abused wives and children to tell anyone because, "No one would ever believe me."
   - Do not allow your professional judgment to be clouded by gifts or impressive personalities.

CHAPTER 2: PULMONARY DISORDERS

Case Study 1: Asthma

Difficulty: *	*Setting:* Outpatient clinic
Index Words: Asthma, exercise-induced asthma	

A.K. is a 38-year-old woman who runs 3 miles every morning. She comes to the Family Nurse Practitioner Clinic with complaints of a burning feeling in her throat and upper airway that begins shortly after she starts running. She states that she gets increasingly more winded and sometimes has to stop running to catch her breath.

1. As the intake nurse working in the clinic, what routine information would you want to obtain from A.K.? **[A/k/PI,PSI/ct,ni,tc]**
   - VS.
   - Personal and family history.
   - Medications.
   - Allergies.
   - Description of her symptoms: location, quality, quantity, timing, setting, factors that aggravate or relieve, associated manifestations.

2. What two body systems do you suspect might be involved in A.K.'s problem? **[PD/k/PI/ct]**
   - Cardiovascular and respiratory.

3. What would you do to differentiate between problems in the two body systems? **[A/c/PI/ct,ni]**
   - Auscultate heart for adventitious sounds. Pay particular attention to the mitral valve for a murmur or click.
   - Auscultate and percuss the lungs.

You assess A.K. and note the following: S_1S_2 with no murmurs, clicks, or rubs; on inspiration her heart rate speeds up and you think you hear a split S_2; and on expiration her heart rate slows down and you don't hear the split.

4. Discuss the significance of these findings. **[PD/c/PI/ct]**
   - The respiratory cycle-related variation in heart rate is called a respiratory-dependent sinus dysrhythmia and can best be heard at the 2nd or 3rd L intercostal space. It is commonly detected in younger adults and athletically fit individuals. The split S_2 heard only on inspiration is called physiologic splitting and also is considered normal.

Her lungs are clear throughout and percuss resonance. You measure height and weight to calculate her *estimated* peak expiratory flow rate (PEFR). You then measure A.K.'s *actual* PEFR using a peak flow meter (PFM).

5. Explain the purpose of the PEFR measurement. **[P/k/S,Pl/ct,ni]**
   - PFM measures the maximum flow rate that can be generated during a forced expiration with fully inflated lungs. The PEFR is measured in liters/minute and requires a maximal effort on the part of the individual being tested.

   Instructor Note: PEFR measurement is a valuable clinical tool to assess degree of airflow obstruction and severity, for monitoring response to therapy, for diagnosing exercise-induced asthma (EIA), and for detecting asymptomatic deterioration due to normal aging. It is recommended that patients take PEFR measurements using the PEF meter in the morning and evening, both before and after inhaled medication, for 2 to 3 consecutive weeks. The individual's personal best is established as the highest PEFR measurement achieved in the PM after inhaled medication. Use the PFM to relate objective physiologic status (PEFR) to subjective symptom perception. The PFM is a valuable but often overlooked safety and educational tool.

6. You record A.K.'s PEFR measurement and note that it is within 5% of estimated normal PEFR. Discuss the significance of her pulmonary evaluation and these findings. **[I/c/Pl/ct,ni]**
   - A.K.'s lung assessment and peak expiratory flow rate are normal.

The FNP confirms your examination findings and, after reviewing A.K.'s PEFR measurements, discusses the possibility of exercise-induced asthma (EIA) with A.K. She directs A.K. to record her PEFR then go for her usual morning run. If she experiences the burning feeling in her throat and upper airway and/or becomes short of breath, she should stop running and immediately measure and record her PEFR. Repeat measurements should be taken at 5 minute intervals for 20 to 30 minutes. Ask A.K. to bring her PEFR record with her next time.

7. What is the FNP hoping to learn from the presymptom to postsymptom PEFR measurement? **[A/c/Pl/ct]**
   - A preexercise to postexercise drop in PEFR of $\geq$15% suggests EIA. Exercise-induced asthma usually peaks in 5 to 10 minutes after stopping the exercise and usually resolves within 30 minutes of stopping.

A.K. returns in 1 week for a follow-up visit. She hands you a list of PEFR measurements. You calculate that A.K.'s postrun measurements range from 75% to 85% of her prerun values and her PEFR returned to normal within 25 minutes of stopping activity.

8. What does this patterns of change indicate? **[PD/an/Pl/ct]**
   - This pattern is consistent with EIA.

The FNP gives A.K. an albuterol (Ventolin) metered-dose inhaler (MDI) with a spacer and instructs her to take 2 puffs 15 minutes before she exercises. The FNP is called to see another patient and asks you to complete the discharge teaching with A.K.

9. What information should you discuss with her? **[I/ap/PI/ct,ni,tc]**
   - Explain that albuterol is a bronchodilator that relaxes smooth muscles around the large airways. Inform A.K. that an MDI has fewer side effects than oral medication but she may experience some anxiety or slight tremors.
   - Instruct A.K. in the proper use of the MDI with the spacer: (1) remove the protective cap, attach the spacer, and shake the inhaler well; (2) breathe out normally, put the opening of the spacer in your mouth and close your lips around it; (3) spray 1 puff into the spacer then slowly breathe in as deeply as you can over a period of 3 to 4 seconds, The spacer will whistle if you breathe in too quickly; and (4) remove the spacer from your mouth and hold your breath for 10 seconds, wait 1 minute between puffs.
   - Have A.K. demonstrate the use of the inhaler with spacer and correct her technique.
   - Instruct A.K. to rinse her inhaler and spacer in warm water once daily and allow to air dry.
   - Demonstrate how to approximate how much medication is left in her MDI. *Instructor Note:* MDI canisters contain between 120 to 240 puffs depending on the medication. To find out how much medication is left, place the canister in a bowl of water. If the canister is full, it remains at the bottom; ¾ full floats off the bottom; ½ full floats to the top but remains vertical; ¼ full starts to list to one side; and almost empty floats on its side.
   - Stress the importance of keeping the MDI with her when she exercises.
   - Stress the importance of reporting any symptoms she experiences during nonexercise periods.

10. A.K. says she doesn't like to be dependent on medication. How would you respond to her statement? **[I/ap/S,PI,HP/ct,ni,tc]**
    - Inform A.K. that the goal of management is to allow her to engage in any activity she chooses without experiencing asthma symptoms. Tell her that EIA frequently indicates an underlying asthma problem. Stress the importance of monitoring her PEFR between exercise periods to determine if she is experiencing constriction during nonexercise periods.

11. A.K. asks if it is possible for her to develop full-blown asthma. How would you respond? **[PD/ap/PI,PSi/ct,tc]**
    - Yes it is possible but nobody can predict the likelihood of that happening.

A.K. was motivated to take her MDI so she could maintain her exercise regimen. At a follow-up visit, she tells you she saw, "Lots of folks using an MDI at last Saturday's race."

Case Study 2: Atelectasis

Difficulty: *	*Setting:* Hospital
Index Words: Atelectasis	

M.N., age 40, is admitted with acute cholecystitis, elevated WBC, and a fever of 102°F. She has undergone a cholecystectomy and has been transferred to your floor from ICU the second day postop. She has an NGT to continuous low wall suction, one peripheral IV, and a large abdominal dressing. Her orders are as follows: progress diet as tolerated; D_5¼ NS with 40 mEq KCl at 125 ml an hour; turn, cough, and deep breathe q2h; incentive spirometer (IS) q2h while awake; dangle in AM, ambulate in PM; morphine sulfate 10 mg IM q4h for pain; ampicillin (Omnipen) 2 g IVPB q6h; chest x-ray (CXR) in AM.

1. Are these orders appropriate for M.N.? State your rationale. **[A/c/Pl/ct]**
   - M.N. should not receive a diet order until she resumes bowel sounds.
   - M.N. would be NPO. It usually takes 48 to 72 hours for the bowels to resume peristalsis following abdominal surgery.
   - Morphine sulfate should be given in very small doses (1-2 mg) IV more frequently (q2h prn).

2. Identify the two most common respiratory-related complications for patients with abdominal or thoracic surgery. **[PD/k/Pl/ct]**
   - Pneumonia/pneumonitis.
   - Atelectasis.

3. What information and assessments would help you differentiate between the two complications in Question 2? **[A/c/Pl/ct,ni]**

	Atelectasis	Pneumonia
• Time of onset	Usually occurs within hours. to a few days after surgery.	Usually requires several days to develop.
• VS	Both may have increased BP,P,R, and T.	
• Signs	Diminished lung sounds.	Bronchovesicular sounds, "gurgling."
• Symptoms	Patients may complain of dyspnea with both problems.	

4. What procedure is necessary to differentiate between atelectasis and pneumonia? **[PD/k/Pl/ct]**
   - A chest x-ray is necessary to diagnose atelectasis or pneumonia.

5. You are assigned to take care of M.N. Her VS are 148/82, 118, 24, 101°F. Her SaO_2 is 88%. Based on these numbers, what do you think is going on with M.N. and why? **[A/c/Pl/ct]**
   - Her BP, HR, and RR are high and may be because of incisional pain, fever (inflammatory process), or hypoxemia.
   - T is elevated, may be due to inflammatory response from infection (cholecystitis on admission) or may be a normal postop reaction.
   - Her SaO_2 is decreased because of incisional pain, atelectasis, and hypoxemia.

6. You know M.N. is at risk for postop atelectasis. What is atelectasis? **[A/c/PI/ct]**
   - Atelectasis is a collapsed or airless state of the lung, which may be acute or chronic and may involve all or part of the lung.
   - Pain-related inhibition of respiration is a significant cause of postop atelectasis.

After morning report you do an assessment and auscultate decreased breath sounds and crackles in the R base posteriorally. Her RML and RLL percuss slightly dull. She splints her R side when attempting to take a deep breath. You suspect that she is developing atelectasis.

7. What most likely accounts for M.N.'s inspiratory-related behavior? **[PD/c/PI/ct]**
   - M.N. may be splinting because of incisional pain.

8. What effect will M.N.'s splinting have on potential atelectasis? **[PD,E/c/PI/ct]**
   - Splitting will exaggerate or promote atelectasis.

9. Identify and clarify 5 actions you would take next. **[P/ap/PI/ct,ni]**
   - Administer pain medication and tell her that you are going to let her rest for 20 minutes until the morphine has time to take effect. Then you will be back to help her cough and deep breathe.
   - Demonstrate cough and deep breathing techniques. Coach her while she coughs, dangles at the side of the bed, and walks around the room.
   - Explain and demonstrate the correct use of the incentive spirometer (IS).
   - Encourage early ambulation.
   - Check the AM CXR results and keep M.N. informed about her progress.
   - Explain your assessment and CXR findings and elicit the patient's cooperation with the plan of care.

10. What 4 interventions might be used for pulmonary hygiene? **[I/k/S,PI/ct,ni]**
    - Have the patient turn frequently.
    - Have the patient cough and deep breathe.
    - Percuss over the patient's lung fields.
    - Have the patient use an incentive spirometer.
    - Give fluids to thin secretions.
    - Assist the patient to ambulate.

11. Identify 3 outcomes that you expect for M.N. as a result of pulmonary hygiene and increased activity? **[PD/ap/PI/ct]**
    - Decreased resting RR.
    - Auscultate increased breath sounds over the RLL.
    - Clearing crackles.
    - SaO_2 >90%.
    - Ileus prevention.

12. M.N.'s sister questions you, saying, "I don't understand. She came in here with a bad gallbladder. What has happened to her lungs?" How would you respond?
[E/an/PSI/ni,tc]
    - The sister and perhaps M.N. are concerned that something may have gone wrong with M.N. during her hospitalization. They need to be reassured. State everything in positive terms.
    - Inform them that M.N. was very sick when she was admitted and that her incision site is painful. Explain that you are giving M.N. pain medication so that she will be able to cough and breathe deeply, move around in bed, and walk so that she will not develop atelectasis or pneumonia.
    - Assure them that M.N. is recovering well from surgery.
    - Show M.N.'s sister how to help M.N. with ambulation.

13. Radiology calls up with a report from the radiologist on the AM CXR. M.N. has atelectasis. Will that change anything from what you have already planned for M.N.? Explain what you would do differently if M.N. had pneumonia.
[PD,P,I/an/ct,ni]
    - No. You should continue your above plans and monitor effectiveness.
    - If M.N. had pneumonia, you would still carry out the same plan and monitor the outcomes; the only thing that might change would be to add new antibiotics to her treatment plan.

Case Study 3: Tuberculosis

Difficulty: *	*Setting:* Public health clinic
Index Words: Tuberculosis	

You are a public health nurse working at a county immunization and TB clinic. B.A. is a 61-year-old woman who wishes to obtain a food handler's license and is required to show proof of a negative Mantoux (PPD) test before being hired. She came to your clinic 2 days ago to obtain a PPD test for tuberculosis. She has returned to have you evaluate her reaction.

1. The CDC recommends screening people at high risk for TB and provide preventive therapy for those at high risk for developing active disease. List 5 populations at high risk. **[A/k/S/ct]**
   - Medically underserved populations.
   - Foreign-born, from countries with high prevalence.
   - Domestic or occupational contacts of infectious TB cases.
   - Alcoholics and IV drug abusers.
   - Residents and staff of acute and long-term facilities, prisons, detention facilities, and homeless shelters; some employers may require proof that a person does not have TB before they are hired.
   - Individuals with chronic disease who are immunosuppressed.

2. What is the preferred method for TB screening? **[A/k/S/ct]**
   - The preferred method is a TB skin test (Mantoux) performed by injecting 5 tuberculin units of purified protein derivative (1/10th ml) intradermally in the midvolar region of the left arm. A discrete pale elevation of the skin (wheal) should be produced.

3. When should the individual return to have the test interpreted? **[A/k/Pl/ct]**
   - The test should be read 48 to 72 hours after injection.

4. How do you determine if the test is positive or negative? **[A/k/Pl/ct]**
   - You measure the area of *induration* (not erythema), which is defined as a hardened area under the skin. The area is measured transverse to the long axis of the forearm.

<u>Note</u>:The American Thoracic Society and Center for Disease Control have adopted the following guidelines for positive Mantoux reaction:

- A PPD induration $\geq$5 mm is considered positive for persons with or at-risk for HIV infection; those who have had close, recent contact with someone who has infectious tuberculosis; or persons who have CXR that show old, healed TB.
- A PPD induration $\geq$10 mm is considered positive for foreign-born persons from high prevalence countries; IV drug users; medically underserved, low income populations; residents of long-term care facilities; people with chronic illnesses; and all children and adolescents.
- A PPD induration $\geq$15 mm is considered positive for all other persons.

5. What additional information would you want to obtain from B.A. before interpreting her skin test result as positive or negative? **[PD/c/Pl/ct]**
   - Obtain a social history (ETOH ingestion; prescription or illegal drug use; smoking history); domestic and occupational conditions.
   - Medical history: exposure to TB, signs or symptoms of active TB infection, medications, PMH, has she had regular access to health care?

Although B.A. was reluctant to give information, she stated that she was exposed to TB as a child, acknowledges consuming 3 to 4 oz ETOH/day, and has smoked 1½ packs per day for 40 years. She lives with her daughter and becomes angry at the suggestion that she might have TB.

6. Three days later, you measure B.A.'s skin test and note that the area of erythema measures 30 mm in diameter and the area of hardness measures 20 mm in diameter. Determine if B.A.'s skin test is positive or negative. **[A/k/Pl/ct]**
   - Although B.A. is not included in any of the CDC's high-risk groups, her test is positive because the area of induration is greater than 15 mm.

7. What does a positive PPD result mean? **[A/k/S,Pl/ct]**
   - B.A. has been exposed to infectious TB.

8. How would you determine if someone like B.A. has active tuberculosis? **[P/k/Pl/ct]**
   - It is necessary to have a CXR.

The physician in your TB clinic determines that B.A.'s CXR is clear (shows no signs of any TB). The CDC recommends preventive therapy for adults with evidence of infection but no active disease.

9. According to the American Thoracic Society/Centers for Disease Control (1990) guidelines, what constitutes usual preventive therapy? **[A/k/Pl/ct]**
   - The patient is instructed to take isoniazid (INH) PO for 6 to 12 months.

10. What are the age-related side effects of preventive therapy? **[A/k/Pl/ct]**
    - For people 35 years of age or older, a major side effect of INH is hepatitis. This risk increases with age and concommitent alcohol use. Another side effect is peripheral neuropathy.

11. Based on the information B.A. gave about her history, identify what public health follow-up would be warranted? **[P/ap/S,Pl/ct,ni]**
    - Skin-test all household members to determine if any of them are the source of B.A.'s infection.

Because of her age, ETOH consumption, negative CXR, and resistance to discussing TB, the physician decides not to discuss the option of preventive therapy with B.A.

12. What information should B.A. receive before leaving the clinic? **[I/ap/S,Pl/ct,ni,tc]**
    - She should understand the signs and symptoms of active TB (in case her TB becomes active) (e.g., fever, night sweats, fatigue, anorexia, and weight loss).
    - She should be told that she will always have a positive TB skin test because she has been exposed. The only way to determine if she has active disease is by CXR.

B.A. was hired under the condition that she must immediately report any signs and/or symptoms of active disease to the county health department or her physician and have a yearly CXR.

Case Study 4: The Mechanically-Ventilated Patient

Difficulty: *	*Setting:* Home care
Index Words: Guillain-Barré syndrome	

P.R., a 31-year-old woman, contracted an upper respiratory tract infection, developed a high fever, and began to experience progressive ascending paralysis. She was admitted to the local hospital, diagnosed with Guillain-Barré syndrome, and 10 days later was discharged to home with home health care nurses, from your agency, around the clock. She is intubated and mechanically ventilated. Her VS are 112/68, 134, 12, 101 °F. The placement of her nasal-duodenal tube was confirmed by abdominal x-ray. Her total parenteral nutrition (TPN) was discontinued yesterday and she was started on enteral nutrition (EN). The consulting dietician calculated P.R.'s caloric need at 2800 calories/24 hours because of her fever.

1. Identify and discuss 3 factors that would influence the physician's decision to place P.R. on EN. **[PD/c/PI/ct]**
   - P.R. is intubated, so oral feeding is not an option.
   - TPN requires a central line and has an associated risk of infection.
   - If the gut is not used, it will lose its competency and allow bacteria and toxins to translocate into the vascular system. This translocation activates the inflammatory response.

2. Absolute medical contraindications to enteral feeding (EN) are few, and it is preferable to demonstrate failure of EN than to assume that the GI tract is nonfunctional and initiate TPN. Give 3 examples of medical diagnoses for which EN would be contraindicated. **[PD/c/PI/ct]**
   - Complete bowel obstruction.
   - Recent gastric or duodenal surgery.
   - Malabsorption syndromes.
   - Secretory diarrhea due to chemotherapy or abdominal radiation.

3. Pulmonary aspiration is a risk with enteral feedings, although the risk is substantially reduced with duodenal placement. Identify 4 measures that can be taken to minimize the risk of aspiration. **[P/k/S,PI/ct,ni]**
   - Accurately determining the feeding tube position.
   - Temporarily insert an NG tube to check for gastric residuals every 4 hours for several days.
   - Start the feeding slowly (10 to 20 ml/h) and advance by 20 ml q12-24h if tolerated.
   - Elevate the head of the bed between 30 and 45 degrees.
   - Insert green food coloring into the EN so aspiration into the lungs can be detected early. Some agencies use blue food coloring, which can result in a positive guaiac reading.
     Instructor Note: Be aware that food coloring is neither clean nor sterile and can contribute to contamination of tube feeding.

4. Identify 5 strategies for preventing bacterial contamination of the feeding formula and tubing. **[PD/k/PI/ct,ni]**
   - Good handwashing when working with formula.
   - Hang only as much formula as can be infused in 8 to 12 hours.
   - Clean the tops of the cans with alcohol before opening.
   - Rinse bag and tubing before adding new formula.
   - Avoid adding medications to hanging formula.
   - Change tubing setup every 24 hours.

5. Identify 2 indicators that an EN infusion rate is too rapid. **[A/k/PI/ct,ni]**
   - Obtain residuals >100 to 150 ml per hour.
   - N&V.
   - An increase in abdominal distension and/or discomfort.

6. The nurse needs to monitor P.R.'s GI response to EN and steroid therapy. Identify 2 observations that need to be recorded, and explain the significance of each. **[A/c/PI/ct,ni]**
   - Number and consistency of stools every 24 hours. The stool of patients on tube feeding are normally soft, pasty, and number less than 3 per day.
   - Determine if her stools are guaiac-positive. Steroids are ulcerogenic, and any patient on steroids needs each stool guaiaced. If stools are guaiac-positive, notify the physician to obtain a prescription for H_2 receptor-blockers or sucralfate (Carafate).
   - Presence of diarrhea or constipation.

7. It is a common belief that diarrhea (defined as >3 liquid stools/day) is a natural consequence of EN administration. Discuss whether this is a true statement. **[PD/c/S,PI/ct]**
   - Diarrhea is not normal with enteral feedings and should be investigated and the cause identified. Systematically remove one offending agent at a time, and observe P.R.'s response to the change in treatment. Diarrhea may lead to problems in the areas of skin care, fluid and electrolyte balance, and nutritional deficits.

8. Identify 3 factors that could cause diarrhea. **[A/k/PI/ct]**
   - Rate and type of formula.
   - Medications (e.g., type, proper administration).
   - Contamination of feeding bags and formula. The bacteria *Clostridium* is frequently a causative agent. Obtain a stool specimen for *Clostridium difficile (C. difficile)* toxin assay.
   - Sterilization of the bowel r/t antibiotic therapy.

   Instructor Note: Expected nutritional outcomes include an albumin of $\geq$3.5 and a prealbumin (PAB) of $\geq$18 (normal is 18 to 45). Albumin and prealbumin are both proteins produced by the liver. Because prealbumin has a short half-life (2 days), it serves as an extremely sensitive marker of nutritional status. PAB levels rapidly decrease in the presence of protein caloric malnutrition and return to normal in as few as 3 days after repletion. (From *Dietetic Currents, 51*[1], 1994, Ross Laboratories, Columbus, Ohio.)

As P.R.'s nurse, you are concerned about meeting her needs for fluids, oral hygiene, skin integrity, and activity.

9. Discuss 5 indicators that would help you assess fluid status. **[A/k/PI/ct]**
   - VS.
   - Lung sounds.
   - Consistency of sputum.
   - Skin turgor.
   - 24 h I&O trends.
   - Urine specific gravity.
   - Presence or absence of edema.

10. The goal related to P.R.'s mouth care is to preserve the oral mucosa and dentition. Identify 3 strategies for providing oral hygiene with an oral endotracheal tube (ETT) in place. **[A/k/PI/ct,ni]**
    - Use artificial saliva (normal pH for mouth) tid and prn to decrease the risk of an oral infection.
    - Perform mouth care q2-4h while awake and q6h at night. Use a soft pediatric-size toothbrush to prevent tissue damage. Use half-strength H_2O_2 and follow by normal saline rinse if unable to brush the teeth.
    - Use nystatin swish and swallow prophylactically with antibiotic therapy to decrease the risk of developing a *Candida* infection in the mouth; put it in with sponge or syringe and suction nystatin if the patient cannot swallow.
    - Reposition the ETT every 24 hours.

11. What is the rationale for not taking an oral temperature in the vicinity of an ETT? **[A/k/PI/ct]**
    - The air passing through the ETT is warmed and humidified. The heat is conducted to the anatomical structures around the ETT and results in a falsely elevated temperature reading.

12. You assess P.R.'s skin every 4 hours. Identify 3 treatment goals in relation to skin/positioning. **[PD/c/PI/ct]**
    - Relieve pressure on the skin.
    - Improve pulmonary ventilation.
    - Enhance comfort.
    - Prevent contractures such as foot drop.

13. What 4 strategies will facilitate the expected outcome of maintaining skin integrity? **[P/ap/PI/ct,ni]**
    - Therapeutic positioning for return of functioning (e.g., a pad under the shoulder to affect normal body position).
    - Regular turning.
    - Use elbow and heel pads to prevent skin breakdown.
    - Use moon boots or high-top shoes to prevent foot drop.
    - Evaluate appropriateness of overlay mattress (an air mattress that lays on top of the regular mattress).

14. You approach P.R. to begin ROM exercises. You ask her if she is experiencing muscle pain at this time and she nods "yes." You tell P.R. that you will wait until she is pain-free to perform the exercises. Why? **[PD/c/S,PI/ct,ni,tc]**
    - Exercising painful muscles may promote demyelination.

It took 4 months for P.R. to make a full recovery.

Case Study 5: Asthma

Difficulty: **	*Setting:* Outpatient clinic
Index Words: Asthma	

M.N., a 22-year-old man, is highly allergic to dust and pollen; anxiety appears to play a role in exacerbating his asthma attacks. His wife drove M.N. to the clinic when his wheezing was unresponsive to beclomethasone (Vanceril) and ipratropium bromide (Atrovent) inhalers. Upon arrival, his VS are 152/84, 124, 42, 100.4°F. M.N. is started on 4 L O_2/nc, an IV of D_5W at KVO, and ABGs were pH 7.31, $PaCO_2$ 48 mm Hg, HCO_3 26 mEq/L, PaO_2 55 mm Hg, SaO_2 86%.

1. Explain the pathophysiology of asthma. **[A/k/Pl/ct]**
   - Asthma is a disease characterized by hyperactivity of airways to various stimuli that results in widespread airway narrowing.

2. Identify pathophysiologic responses during an asthma attack. **[A/k/Pl/ct]**
   - Activated immunologic response: stimulates production of IgE.
   - Increased airway resistance: mucus production fills the airway and inhibits the movement of air.
   - Decreased lung compliance: increased swelling of tissue makes it more difficult to expand lungs with inspiration.
   - Impaired mucociliary function: increased mucus production covers cilia and inhibits their sweeping motion.
   - Altered gas exchange: decreased V_T means air doesn't reach alveoli and cannot take part in gas exchange, resulting in decreased PaO_2 and may result in increased $PaCO_2$.

3. Are M.N.'s VS acceptable? State your rationale. **[A/c/Pl/ct]**
   - No. His systolic BP is too high (152/84), he is tachycardic (124) and tachypneic (42), and his temperature is elevated (100.4°F). M.N. is anxious and experiencing shortness of breath. His respiratory muscles are working very hard to breathe, thereby increasing his metabolic rate, temperature, and stress.

4. Identify the drug classifications and actions of Vanceril and Atrovent. **[A/k/Pl/ct]**
   - Vanceril is a corticosteroid that reduces mucus production, inflammation, and swelling in airways. It decreases sensitivity of airways to irritants and allergens. There are few systemic effects because there is minimal systemic absorption. This drug should be used regularly and should *not* be used for fast relief of shortness of breath.
   - Atrovent (ipratropium bromide) is an anticholinergic that relaxes smooth muscles (bronchodilation) but takes effect more *slowly* than fast-acting, beta-2 agonists, such as albuterol, terbutaline, metaproterenol, or pirbuterol. Atrovent may cause headache, nervousness, or dry mouth.

5. Are Vanceril and/or Atrovent appropriate for use during an asthma attack? **[A/k/Pl/ct]**
   - No, neither of these inhalers is fast-acting.
   - Vanceril should not be used during an acute attack.

6. The physician orders albuterol 3 mg nebulization treatment STAT. What is the rationale for this order? **[P/c/PI/ct]**
   - Albuterol (e.g., Ventolin, Proventil, metaproterenol, pirabuterol) is a fast-acting, beta-2 agonist that acts to relax and open airways and increase ciliary movement to help clear secretions. It may cause shakiness, nervousness, tachycardia, and/or increased blood pressure, so M.N. should be closely monitored.

7. What is the rationale for immediately starting M.N. on oxygen? **[A,P/c/PI/ct]**
   - Bronchoconstriction has caused an increase in airway resistance and decrease in V_T. The goal of therapy is to compensate by increasing the concentration of inspired oxygen.

8. List 5 short-term interventions that may help relieve M.N.'s symptoms. **[P/ap/PI/ct]**
   - Initiate albuterol treatment as ordered to relieve bronchoconstriction and increase ciliary efficiency.
   - Give albuterol with warmed, humidified, aerosolized particles to help thin secretions
   - Elevate the head of the bed or have M.N. sit in a chair to promote maximum lung expansion.
   - Give supplemental O_2 to relieve hypoxemia.
   - Hydration will help thin pulmonary secretions and facilitate expectoration. This can be achieved by increasing the IV rate and encouraging PO fluids.
   - Coach M.N. to cough effectively to facilitate airway clearance.
   - Coach M.N. in pursed lip breathing to increase pressure throughout the airways and facilitate expiration.

After several hours of IV and PO rehydration and a second albuterol treatment, M.N.'s wheezing and chest tightness resolve, and he is able to expectorate his secretions. The doctor discusses M.N.'s asthma management with him, and he tells him that his inhalers meet his needs on a day-to-day basis but fail him when he has an asthma attack. The doctor discharges M.N. with a prescription for Proventil MDI and a "spacer" and recommends that he call the pulmonary clinic for follow-up with a pulmonary specialist.

9. What issues would you address in discharge teaching with M.N.? **[P,I/an/PI,PSI/ct,ni,tc]**
   - Have his wife join him before giving M.N. any instructions.
   - Review and reinforce the information given by the physician for the benefit of M.N. and his wife. The physician told M.N. that his inhalers are OK for day-to-day control but they act slowly and are not adequate to open his airways during an asthma attack. The physician gave M.N. a prescription for a fast-acting inhaler to help him open his airways and advised him to see a pulmonary specialist in the clinic.
   - Encourage M.N. and his wife to make and keep the pulmonary clinic appointment.
   - Ask M.N. to demonstrate the use of his MDI.

You ask M.N. to demonstrate the use of his MDI. He vigorously shakes the canister, holds the aerosolizer at an angle (pointing toward his cheek) in front of his mouth, and squeezes the canister as he takes a quick, deep breath.

10. What common mistakes has M.N. made when using the inhaler? **[A/an/PI/ct]**
    - Lack of coordination between activating the inhaler and initiating the deep breath.
    - Angling the inhaler to spray the tongue or side of the mouth.
    - Failing to hold his breath for 10 seconds postinhalation.
    - Failure to clean the inhaler after each use results in crystallization of medication around orifice and failure to deliver entire dose.
    - Failure to rinse mouth after using steroid inhalers can result in *Candida* infection in the oropharynx (M.N. is on Vanceril, a steroid inhaler).

11. How would you council M.N. about the use of his MDI? **[E/an/S,PI/ct,ni,tc]**
    - Tell M.N. that he did pretty well but you have a few pointers to help him get more medication into his lungs. Demonstrate how to point the inhaler straight toward his mouth. Tell him to depress his tongue (get it out of the way) so that he doesn't spray it. And remind him to hold his deep breath for 10 seconds before breathing out.
    - Instruct him in the use of the spacer (such as an aerochamber). Research shows that spacers let patients get more medicine and they don't have to worry about timing their breath with the discharge of the canister.
    - Instruct him to clean the spacer in warm soapy water and place it on a paper towel to air dry. This should be done daily.
    - Give him written instructions about follow-up with the pulmonary specialist, and instruct him, in writing, to ask the pulmonary doctor about a "peak flow meter" (PFM).

12. What is the function of a peak flow meter (PFM) and how are they used? **[A/c/PI/ct]**
    - A PFM as an objective measure of expiratory air flow and is measured in L/min. The patient is instructed to inhale maximally, seal their lips around the mouthpiece, and expire as quickly and as forcefully as possible. A nomogram (based on the patient's age and height) is used to determine predicted values; that is, how forcefully the person should be able to exhale. After establishing a baseline, patients are instructed to test their peak flow rate (PFR) whenever they experience chest tightness or become SOB. The PFR becomes an objective number to gauge the severity of their constriction. Patients are taught that if the PFR is below a certain number, they are to seek immediate medical attention.

13. M.N.'s wife asks about the possibility of M.N. having another attack. How would you respond? **[PD/k/PI/ct,ni,tc]**
    - Yes. It is very likely that M.N. will have another asthma attack in the future. Inform them that there is no way to predict when an attack will occur, and stress the importance of proper management. Explain that pulmonary doctors specialize in pulmonary problems, such as asthma, and are knowledgeable about the latest treatments and drug therapy.

14. Identify 4 nursing diagnoses that apply to M.N. **[PD/an/S,PI/ct]**
    - Impaired gas exchange r/t decreased V_T.
    - Ineffective breathing pattern r/t bronchoconstriction.
    - Ineffective airway clearance r/t increased mucus production.
    - Altered tissue perfusion r/t hypoxemia.
    - Knowledge deficit r/t proper use of inhaler.

Case Study 6: Restrictive Lung Disease/Pleural Effusion

Difficulty: **	*Setting:* Hospital
Index Words: Pleural effusion, restrictive lung disease	

J.D., a 38-year-old man, is admitted to your medical floor with a diagnosis of pleural effusion. He complains of shortness of breath, pain in his chest, and weakness. His VS are 142/82, 118, 38 labored and shallow, 102°F. His chest x-ray (CXR) shows a large pleural effusion and pulmonary infiltrates in the right lower lobe (RLL) consistent with pneumonia.

Instructor Note: Discuss the difference between cardiac and pleural pain. Explain that it is necessary to ask questions to determine the difference.

1. Given his diagnosis, are J.D.'s admission vital signs expected? State your rationale. **[A/c/S,PI/ct]**
   - Yes. J.D.'s SBP is slightly elevated and is tachycardiac and tachypneic with shallow, labored breathing. His temperature is elevated due to an inflammatory response (pulmonary infection) and increased work of breathing. Because of the increased metabolic rate, his body has to work harder to deliver oxygen and nutrients to the cells.

2. What is pleural effusion? **[A/k/PI/ct]**
   - Pleural effusion is an accumulation of fluid (serous fluid or purulent material) in the pleural space (between lung and chest wall).

3. List 3 common causes of pleural effusion? **[A/k/PI/ct]**
   - Congestive heart failure.
   - Cancer.
   - Pulmonary edema.
   - Pneumonia.

4. Review the pathophysiology and consequences of pleural effusion and pulmonary infiltrates. **[A/k/PI/ct]**
   - The inflammation of the pleura alters capillary membrane permeability and impairs lymphatic drainage resulting in excess pleural fluid. As the amount of exudate increases, it compresses lung tissue and reduces lung volumes. Ventilation to the affected area is decreased, but perfusion remains fairly normal, resulting in a ventilation-perfusion mismatch and hypoxemia. His effusion freely moves to dependent areas of the lung; the fluid moves to the lower lobes when he is in an upright position and to the posterior lung fields when he is supine.
   - Pulmonary infiltrate is the accumulation of fluid in the pulmonary tissues (parenchyma). The tissues become heavy and less elastic, thereby making it more difficult to move air in and out of the lungs and slowing diffusion of gases across the alveolar/capillary membrane. Also, as fluid accumulates in the pleural space, there is less room for lung expansion, and V_T decreases.

5. What is the difference between exudate and transudate? **[A/k/Pl/ct]**
   - Exudate is a fluid with a high content of protein and cellular debris that has escaped from blood vessels and has been deposited in tissues or on tissue surfaces, usually as a result of inflammation.
   - Transudate is a fluid substance that has passed through a membrane or has been extruded from a tissue. In contrast to an exudate, a transudate is characterized by high fluidity and a low content of protein, cells, or solid matter derived from cells.

6. How does the underlying pathophysiology give rise to the presenting signs and symptoms? **[PD/ap/Pl/ct]**
   - Shallow, labored breathing is due to pulmonary infiltrates and fluid accumulation in the pleural space.
   - Weakness is due to hypoxemia r/t fluid accumulation in the parenchyma (pulmonary infiltrates).
   - Pain in his chest is due to pleural irritation (pleuritic pain); the pleura are full of pain sensors.

The physician performs a thoracentesis and drains 1500 ml fluid. A specimen for C&S is sent to the laboratory, and the patient is started on cefuroxime 1 g IVPB q8h.

7. What is a thoracentesis? **[A/k/Pl/ct]**
   - It is the removal of fluid from the pleural space using a needle or thin catheter. The fluid is sent for pathologic examination, C&S, cell count, glucose, and total protein. The thoracentesis can be repeated several times if fluid continues to accumulate in the pleural space.

8. What maneuvers would promote the clearance of pulmonary secretions? **[P/c/Pl/ct]**
   - Cough and deep breathing promotes expectoration of secretions, lung expansion, and prevents atelectasis.
   - Incentive spirometry (IS) promotes lung expansion and provides a visual feedback for J.D. For example, is he taking in enough air to expand his lungs. IS also provides an objective indicator to determine if and when expected outcomes are achieved (appropriate volume for J.D.).

9. You enter the room to reposition J.D. If J.D. is supine, what side would you turn him to and why? **[P/k/Pl/ct,ni]**
   - Position J.D. with his "good lung" (L) down to improve ventilation-perfusion matching. Perfusion is gravity dependent; when in an upright position, the apex of the lung receive no blood flow and the blood flow increases as you approach the bases. Dependent areas of the lung have better ventilation and perfusion than nondependent lung zones (i.e., improved gas exchange in dependent lung areas).

10. The pleural fluid C&S results indicate large amount *Klebsiella* growth that is sensitive to cefuroxime. What action should you take next? **[P/ap/S,Pl/ct,ni,tc]**
    - Although you realize that the physician probably will not change antibiotics (*Klebsiella* is sensitive to cefuroxime) you would notify J.D.'s physician of the C&S results.

11. Because fluid continues to collect in the pleural space, the physician decides to insert a pleural chest tube under nonemergent conditions. What is your responsibility as J.D.'s nurse? **[P/c/Pl/ct,ni]**
    - Provide adequate analgesia.
    - Obtain a thoracotomy tray, several size chest tubes (28 and 32), and sterile gowns and towels.
    - Set up the chest drainage system, and adjust the suction pressure.
    - Watch that sterile technique is maintained throughout the procedure.
    - Make sure the tubing connections are airtight and secured with adhesive tape or bands.
    - Position the drainage system below the patient's chest.

12. Evaluate each of the following statements about chest tube drainage systems. Place a "T" (true) or "F" (false) in the space provided. Discuss why the "false" statements are incorrect. **[E/an/S,Pl/ct,ni]**
    a. ___ It is the height of the column of water in the suction control mechanism not the setting of the suction source that actually limits the amount of suction transmitted to the pleural cavity.
    b. ___ A suction pressure of +20 cm H_2O is commonly recommended for adults.
    c. ___ Bubbling in the water seal chamber means that air is leaking from the lungs, the tubing, or the insertion site.
    d. ___ The rise and fall of the water level with the patient's respirations reflects normal pressure changes in the pleural cavity with respirations.
    e. ___ The chamber is a closed system; therefore water cannot evaporate.
    f. ___ To declot the drainage tubing, put lotion on your hands, compress the tubing, and strip long segments of the tubing before releasing.
    g. ___ You lower the bed on top of the drainage system and break it. Because you noted an air leak from the lung during your initial assessment, you may clamp the chest tube for the short time it takes to reestablish the drainage system.
    h. ___ The chest tube becomes disconnected from the drainage system. Because you noted an air leak from the lung during your initial assessment, you can submerge the chest tube 1 to 2 inches below the surface of a 250 ml bottle of sterile saline or water.
    i. ___ The collection chamber is full so you need to connect a new drainage system to the chest tube. It is appropriate to momentarily clamp the chest tube while you disconnect the old system and reconnect the new.
    j. ___ The drainage system falls over, spilling the chest drainage into the other drainage columns. The total amount of drainage can be obtained by adding the amount of drainage in each of the columns.

    <u>Answers to "False" Statements</u>
    b. Suction pressure is negative; -20 cm H_2O is common.
    e. The chest drainage system is not a closed system, and H_2O evaporates over time. Observe the H_2O level, and add sterile H_2O or NaCl, using a sterile catheter tip syringe as needed.
    f. This procedure, called chest tube stripping, is dangerous and should be avoided. Chest tube stripping can cause tissue biopsy (pieces of tissue are sucked through the holes of the chest tube); this procedure can generate up to -400 cm H_2O pressure!
    g. Clamping the chest tube in the presence of an air leak can result in a tension pneumothorax.

13. It is visiting hours. An attractive young woman approaches you at the desk and, stating she is J.D.'s wife, asks what room he is in. You know that another woman, his real wife, is in the room with him now. How are you going to handle this? **[PD/an/S,PSI/ct,ni,tc]**
    - Tell this woman he already has a visitor and ask her to wait in the visitor's lounge.
    - Go into his room, and ask his wife if she could leave for a few minutes.
    - Tell J.D. what has happened, and ask how he wants to handle this. Inform him that you refuse to get in the middle of this; this is *his* problem.
    - Notify security that you may have a potentially volatile situation.
    - Good luck and hope neither of the women is armed.

J.D. did some fast talking and managed to avoid discovery, He received aggressive antibiotic and pulmonary therapy and was discharged 5 days later.

Case Study 7: Emphysema

Difficulty: **	*Setting:* Home care
Index Words: Emphysema, obstructive sleep apnea	

C.E., a 73-year-old married man, visits his internist complaining that he becomes "so winded" with activity. C.E.'s pulse oximetry (SaO_2) registers 83% at rest. He is sent to the local hospital for a CXR and ABGs to be drawn after resting 20 minutes on room air. The next day, his physician calls C.E. and informs him that he has severe emphysema and must start on continuous oxygen therapy. The physician tells C.E. that his office will have a home health equipment company call him to make arrangements to deliver the equipment and educate him in its use. As an RN working for the company, you are assigned to make the initial home visit.

<u>Instructor Note</u>: Diagnosis of emphysema is usually made from the CXR and AGBs on room air. Insurance companies and Medicare usually pay for oxygen *only* if room air ABGs show a PaO_2 <55 mm Hg.

1. How would you prepare for the first visit? **[P/an/PI/ct,ni]**
   - Check with Medicare and C.E.'s supplemental insurance company to see what is covered; Medicare has specific contracted arrangements.
   - Call to make an appointment when both C.E. and his wife can be there.
   - Take several business cards, and be sure they have a 24-hour emergency telephone number.
   - Collect patient education materials about emphysema and the use of oxygen.
   - Pack the oxygen units, oxygen adaptors, 50 feet of oxygen tubing, several nasal cannulas, and a small in-line flow meter.

2. What issues would you address with C.E. and his wife? **[P/ap/S,PSI/ct,ni,tc]**
   - Using simple illustrations, show them what emphysema is.
   - Using simple terms, explain why C.E. needs oxygen.
   - Explain the different types of oxygen systems (compressed air, oxygen concentrator, liquid oxygen) and help them determine which system would be best for them and their lifestyle.
   - Show them the oxygen equipment and explain how to use it. Give a demonstration, then have C.E. explain everything to you and demonstrate how to use the equipment. Finally, have his wife review and demonstrate the use of the equipment.
   - Using patient education materials, review how to use oxygen safely (do's and don'ts), how to travel with oxygen, and when to seek medical treatment. Leave these materials with them, and highlight the most important information.
   - Inform them that you will visit again to reinforce the information discussed during this visit (do not overwhelm them, stick to the basics, and give C.E. a success experience).
   - Repeat instructions concerning the 24-hour emergency services available to them.

3. The next time you visit, C.E. complains about sores behind his ears. He explains, "That long oxygen tubing seems to take on a life of its own. It twists around and gets caught under doors, chairs, everything. It darn near rips the ears off my head." He asks for your help. How would you respond? **[PD/ap/PI/ct,ni,tc]**
   - Cushion the top and posterior side of the ears so the oxygen tubing doesn't rub.
   - Examine the "sores" for signs of infection and advise his wife what to look for, how to keep the area clean, and how to promote healing.
   - Show C.E. how to make a "sag line" of the oxygen tubing by tucking a loose loop of about 2 feet into his belt or pocket to protect his ears from the stress of unplanned "jerks."

   Instructor Note: Medical supply companies carry a sponge wrap. The sponge is approximately 3 inches long and has a lengthwise slit that fits over the oxygen tubing to protect the ears. The tubing must be taped in place to prevent slipping.

4. You auscultate C.E.'s breath sounds and detect the odor of Vicks Vapo Rub. When you question C.E. about the use of Vicks, he tells you that he started to apply it in and around his nose to prevent his nose from becoming dry and sore. How would you council C.E. and his wife? **[A/an/S,PI/ct,ni,tc]**
   - Remind C.E. that it is very dangerous to use vapor rubs or petroleum-based products around oxygen because O_2 is very flammable. Oxygen supports combustion and petroleum melts. All it would take is a spark to start a fire.
   - Educate him to use lanolin or water-based aloe vera moisturizing gels to keep his nasal passages moistened.

C.E. elected to use liquid oxygen because it offers more freedom and portability. It is also lighter in weight.

5. Over the next 3½ weeks, C.E. seemed to adjust well to his liquid oxygen system. However, one evening he walked to the kitchen for a snack and became increasingly short of breath. Identify 4 possible causes. **[PD/ap/S,PI/ct]**
   - The tank ran out of oxygen (liquid tanks are generally filled once a month, depending on the liter flow).
   - The oxygen flow regulator malfunctioned.
   - The tubing became disconnected from the oxygen flow regulator.
   - The tubing became kinked.

As per your instructions, C.E. removed the nasal cannula, tested the flow against his check, and felt no oxygen flowing from the catheter. He lacked the force and volume required to yell for help and was too short of breath to return to the living room to check his oxygen tank. He bent forward with his elbows on the counter top, and struggled to breathe. He became more frightened with each passing second, and his breathing seemed to become increasingly more difficult. A minute later, C.E.'s wife found him and reconnected his oxygen tubing. C.E. sat at the table for 20 minutes before he could walk back to the living room.

6. Why did C.E. assume the peculiar position at the counter top? **[A/c/PI/ct]**
   - He leaned forward. This position takes advantage of gravity; the bowels are pulled forward, thereby, allowing more room for the diaphragm to expand.
   - He placed his elbows on the table. Normally, the inspiratory muscles of the neck are responsible for lifting the first 2 ribs upward. By placing his elbows on the table, C.E. mechanically lifted the rib cage into a maximally expanded position and spared the inspiratory muscles the workload of accomplishing this task, conserving energy. This position allows maximal pulmonary expansion and minimal energy output to accomplish inspiration.

7. A week later you receive a call from C.E.'s wife. She relates the incident from the previous week and tells you that C.E. "doesn't want her out of his sight." She asks you to come to the house and "...talk some sense into him." What teaching strategies will you use with C.E. and his wife? **[P/ap/PI,PSI/ct,ni,tc]**
   - Acknowledge his feelings of fear and panic at suddenly being without oxygen.
   - Explain that fear causes the airways to dilate and makes it more difficult to get enough air in and out. (An epinephrine flush causes the bronchi to dilate, thereby increasing dead space volume.)
   - Practice pursed lip and abdominal breathing with C.E. He should practice these techniques every day so that when he has another panic attack, he can focus on one breath at a time (getting air in, then getting air out). He can relax himself enough to stop the epinephrine flush and stop the resulting bronchodilation. He can practice these breathing techniques anytime, anywhere.
   - Work out a plan whereby C.E.'s wife will check on him periodically or he can call for help.
   - Show C.E. how to check his equipment on a daily basis.
   - Have C. E. and his wife practice breathing relaxation exercises to keep him from panicking in emegencies.

8. C.E.'s wife asks you what her husband can do to help her around the house. She says, "The doctor told him to go home and take it easy. He sits in a chair all day. He won't even get up to get himself a glass of water. I've got a bad hip and this has been very hard on me." How would you address her issue? **[P/ap/PI,PSI/ct,ni,tc]**
   - Establish C.E.'s level of daily activity before he was placed on oxygen.
   - Establish which activities C.E. is experiencing particular difficulty performing.
   - Call the physician and request an occupational therapy (OT) consultation. OT can show C.E. and his wife how to accomplish tasks in the most energy-efficient way.
   - Tell him that his muscles will deteriorate if he doesn't use them. "Use it or lose it." Find out what he can reasonably accomplish.
   - Have C.E. and his wife negotiate a plan of daily activity for C.E. Function as a neutral third party.
   - Check to see if they qualify for home help.

   Instructor Note: COPD patients will experience difficulty with particular activities or under particular circumstances, such as climbing steps, inhaling fumes, anything that requires them to hold their arms over the head, bending over, and/or a humid environment (cooking and bathing).

The OT instructs the couple about energy saving ways to complete their housework. They both seem satisfied with their new division of labor. In addition, their church women's group has volunteered to help once a week with laundry, vacuuming, and other stressful tasks.

9. C.E. states, "You seem to know what you are talking about so let me ask you something. I wake up with a headache almost every morning. My wife says its because I snore so loud and don't breathe right when I sleep. Do you know anything about that?" After asking several questions you inform C.E. that it sounds like he has obstructive sleep apnea. Explain the connection between obstructive sleep apnea and morning headaches. **[A/c/PI/ct,ni,tc]**
   - When C.E. obstructs his airway, respiratory effort does not result in the movement of air. Arterial oxygen levels decline and carbon dioxide levels increase. Carbon dioxide levels cause vasodilation in the brain, and C.E. wakes up with a headache.

10. C.E. seemed impressed by your explanation. He asks if there is anything that can be done for his problem. You inform him that there is a treatment called continuous positive airway pressure (CPAP). What is CPAP and how does it work? **[A/k/PI/ct]**
   - CPAP is a method of maintaining pressure in the airways to prevent airway collapse. This enables patients to breathe while asleep.
   - CPAP entails wearing a mask over the nose or nose and mouth. The mask is connected to a machine that forces air, at a prescribed pressure, into the nose or nose and mouth.
   - Many patients are successfully treated with CPAP. Others refuse to wear the mask because of the uncomfortable feeling they experience when the air rushes through their air passages.
   - Inform C.E. that he would have to undergo testing to determine that he has obstructive sleep apnea before CPAP would be prescribed.

You comment that C.E. sounds like he has a cold. He replies, "Oh, our great-grandchildren were over to visit several days ago and they all had snotty noses. I suspect that I'll get it pretty soon. The problem is, every time I get a cold it goes straight to my lungs."

11. What information would you want to review with C.E. and his wife about the signs and symptoms of infection and when to seek treatment? **[P/ap/S,PI,HP/ct,ni,tc]**
    - Signs include an increase in quantity, color, or consistency of sputum; a cough or an increase in coughing.
    - Symptoms are fever, aching, tightness in the chest, fatigue, weakness.
    - He should seek treatment as soon as he experiences symptoms. Early intervention may prevent an upper respiratory tract infection from becoming a lower respiratory infection, and, possibly, pneumonitis.

12. Why is it important for people with lung disease to seek early intervention for infection? **[A/k/PI/ct]**
    - Invading organisms cause damage to lung tissue. People like C.E. do not have a lot of lung reserve and can suffer temporary or permanent loss of function from a pulmonary infection.

C.E. learned to manage his emphysema fairly well. His wife had her hip replaced, made a speedy recovery, and was discharged to home. She suddenly died 4 weeks later from a pulmonary embolus. C.E. was panic stricken at her loss. A psychiatric nurse practitioner was requested to work with him.

Case Study 8: Spontaneous Pneumothorax

Difficulty: **	*Setting:* Hospital ED, hospital
Index Words: Pneumothorax	

A.W., a 52-year-old woman disabled from severe emphysema, was walking at a mall when she suddenly grabbed her right side and gasped, "Oh, something just popped." A.W. told her walking companion, "I can't get any air." Her companion yelled for someone to call 911 and helped her to the nearest bench. By the time the rescue unit arrived, A.W. was stuporous and in severe respiratory distress. She was intubated, an IV of LR at KVO was started, and she was transported to the nearest ED.

On arrival to the ED, the physician auscultates muffled heart tones, no breath sounds on the R, and faint sounds on the L. A.W. is stuporous, tachycardic, and cyanotic. The paramedics inform the physician that it was difficult to ventilate A.W. A STAT portable CXR and ABGs are obtained. A.W. has a 70% pneumothorax on the R, and her ABGs on 100% oxygen are pH 7.25, $PaCO_2$ 92 mm Hg, PaO_2 32 mm Hg, HCO_3 27 mEq/L, BE +5 mEq/L, SaO_2 53%.

1. Given the diagnosis of pneumothorax, explain why the paramedic had difficulty ventilating A.W. **[PD/c/PI/ct]**
   - Air escaped from the lung into the pleural space. Eventually, enough air collected in the pleural space to cause the mediastinum to shift toward the R. The collapsed L lung, increased intrapleural pressure, and rightward shift make it difficult to ventilate A.W.

2. Interpret A.W.'s ABGs. **[A/k/PI/ct]**
   - Significant respiratory acidosis with profound hypoxemia. A.W. is near death.

3. What is the reason for A.W.'s ABG results? **[PD/ap/PI/ct]**
   - 70% of her R lung is collapsed and is not taking part in gas exchange.

4. The physician needs to insert a chest tube. What are your responsibilities as the nurse? **[P/ap/PI,PSI/ct,ni,tc]**
   - Be constantly aware of patient emotional support needs. This is a very frightening experience.
   - Prepare for immediate needle aspiration (the physician will use a 14- or 16-gauge spinal or cardiac needle)
   - Set up a chest tube drainage system, obtain size 28 and 32 chest tubes, and prepare a thoracotomy tray for a thoracostomy (chest tube insertion).
   - Monitor chest drainage.
   - Frequently assess for breath sounds.
   - Educate the patient about the procedure. Although A.W. is stuporous, you do not know what she can hear or process. Briefly tell her that her lung collapsed and that the doctor is going put a tube in her chest to get rid of the air and help her breathe.

5. As the nurse, it is your responsibility to ensure pain control. In A.W.'s case, would you administer pain medication before the chest tube insertion? **[P/ap/PI/ct]**
   - No. A.W. was stuporous on arrival to the ED. This is an emergency; you cannot take the time to obtain and administer pain medication.

6. The ED physician inserts a size 32 chest tube in the 2nd intercostal space, midclavicular line. Many chest tubes are inserted in the 6th intercostal space, midaxillary line. What factor determines where a chest tube is placed? **[PD/c/PI/ct]**
   - Air is lighter than liquid and tends to rise to the top; therefore, chest tubes inserted to remove air are placed close to the 2nd intercostal space along the midclavicular line. Fluid is heavier and tends to seek the lowest level, therefore, chest tubes inserted to remove fluids are placed at the 5th or 6th intercostal space, midaxillary line.

7. Given the information above, would you expect to observe an air leak when A.W.'s chest drainage system is in place and functioning? **[PD/c/PI/ct]**
   - Yes. If A.W. ruptured a bleb into her pleural space, inspired air would continue to escape into the pleural space and into the chest tube drainage system until the hole healed.

8. Would you expect A.W.'s lung to reexpand immediately after the chest tube insertion and initiation of underwater suction? **[PD/c/PI/ct]**
   - Not necessarily. It can take hours to days for the lungs to completely reexpand

9. The clerk tells you A.W.'s husband has just arrived; A.W. will be admitted to the hospital. How would you address this issue with her husband? **[P,I/an/PI,PSI/ct,ni,tc]**
   - Look for him in the ED waiting area, and as you walk him to his wife's room tell him that A.W. is doing much better. Inform him that one of her lungs collapsed, so the doctor put a tube in her chest to let the air out and allow the lung to expand again. Tell him that the tube will stay in her chest until the lung stays inflated on its own. That means she will have to be admitted to the hospital so she can be watched until she is OK again.
   - Accompany him into A.W.'s room and remain alert to help him into a chair or onto the floor if he experiences vertigo or a syncopal episode.
   - Explain the tubes and monitoring equipment in very simple terms (e.g., "This machine allows us to watch her heart, this one takes her blood pressure, this is the tube that lets the air out of her chest so that she can breathe better").
   - Provide tissues and tell him where the restrooms are located.
   - Ask him if he needs to use the telephone (someone may need to bring clothing, provide transportation, or stay with him to offer support).
   - Ask him if he needs anything (juice, water) to make him more comfortable.

10. You approach A.W.'s bedside and ask about what looks like two healed chest tube sites on her L chest. A.W's husband informs you that this is the third time she has had a collapsed lung. He asks if this trend will continue. How would you respond? **[PD/ap/PI,PSI/ct,ni,tc]**
    - If A.W. continues to experience spontaneous pneumothoraces in the same area of the lung, the physician may elect to "scar" the surface of the lung in that particular area. The physician instills sclerosing medication through the chest tube, and because the medication is very irritating to the lung, scar tissue forms on the outside. It is more difficult for the thick scar tissue to rupture than the thinner lung tissue. The treatment is effective, but it is also painful for the patient.

11. A.W. recovered and was discharged home 4 days later with a chest tube and Heimlich valve. The physician connected a 1-way (Heimlich) valve between the distal end of the chest tube and a drainage pouch. Discuss the purpose of this device. **[A/k/PI/ct]**
    - During inspiration, negative intrapleural pressure closes the valve and prevents air from entering the pleural space. During expiration, positive pressure opens the valve and allows air and/or fluid to drain into a plastic pouch. This valve makes it possible to discharge patients who have a residual air leak. The chest tube is removed after the air leak heals.

A.W. developed several more spontaneous pneumothoraces on the L and eventually had bleomycin instilled over the L lung to induce scarring. She said, "It felt like someone poured kerosene in and threw a lit match in after it. It was the most painful thing I ever went through."

Instructor Note: Sclerosing a lung doesn't have to feel like it is burning; it should be managed with adequate pain medication.

Case Study 9: Community-Acquired Pneumonia

Difficulty: **	*Setting:* Hospital
Index Words: Pneumonia	

C.K. is a very healthy, active 71-year-old who called his physician with complaints of chills and fever. After taking a history, the doctor instructs C.K. to go to the hospital for admission. He is given a diagnosis of R/O pneumonia. The intern is busy and asks you to complete your routine admission assessment and call her with your findings.

1. Identify the 5 most important things to include in your assessment. **[A/c/Pl/ct]**
   - Complete vital signs.
   - Auscultate lung sounds.
   - Note perfusion.
   - Question the patient about presence of pain or discomfort.
   - Determine nutritional status and fluid intake.
   - Ask about medication or drug allergies.

Your assessment findings are as follows: His VS are 154/82, 105, 32, 103°F. You auscultate crackles in the LLL anteriorly and posteriorly, his nailbeds are dusky on fingers and toes, he has cough-productive rust-colored sputum and c/o pain in his left chest when he coughs. C.K. seems to be well-nourished and adequately hydrated. He states that he "got hives" the last time he took penicillin.

2. Which of these assessment findings concern you? State your rationale. **[PD/ap/Pl/ct]**
   - C.K.'s HR, RR, and T are elevated.
   - Crackles in the LLL indicate fluid accumulation.
   - Dusky nailbeds indicate lack of oxygen uptake by the tissues.
   - The presence of rust-colored sputum indicates blood and probable infection.
   - Pain with coughing is consistent with inflammation and infection.
   - Allergy to penicillin because if he has a pulmonary infection he will be started on an antibiotic.

The intern writes the following orders: regular diet; VS with temp q2h; maintenance IV of $D_5½$ NS at 125 ml/h; cefuroxime (Zinacef) 1 g IVPB q8h; Zinacef peak and trough level with 3rd dose; 6 L O_2/nc; titrate to maintain oximeter (SaO_2) >90%; obtain sputum for culture and sensitivity (C&S) x 3; draw blood cultures x 2 sites for temp >102°F; CBC with differential, Chem 7, and urinalysis plus C&S on admission; CXR on admission and in AM.

3. Review the orders and determine what you would do first. **[E/an/Pl/ct]**
   - The patient has a fever of 103°F. Order STAT blood cultures, and try to get the first sputum specimen before beginning the antibiotic.

4. Is cefuroxime appropriate for this patient? State your rationale and indicate what action you would take? **[E/an/S,Pl/ct,ni,tc]**
   - Zinacef is an antibiotic that has proven effective against many bacteria known to cause respiratory tract infections; however, it is contraindicated for patients with severe hypersensitivity to penicillin. Before giving the drug, notify the physician of the conflict and ask if the order should be changed. The physician can order a test dose of the drug from pharmacy. If a test dose is ordered, slowly administer the cefuroxime and instruct C.K. to immediately inform you if he begins to experience anything unusual (e.g., itching, swelling, pain, rash).

5. Explain the order for the peak and trough level. How is this information used? **[A/k/Pl/ct]**
   - Trough level measures the lowest level of circulating medication; the blood level 30 minutes before administration of the next dose of medication.
   - Peak level measures the highest level of circulating medication; rate of administration and time of the blood draw depends on the drug in question.
   - Some drugs are nephrotoxic or hepatotoxic, depending on the site of metabolism. The trough and peak levels are used to adjust drug dosages to attain an effective treatment level without causing organ toxicity.

6. Is the intravenous fluid of D_5½ NS appropriate for C.K.? State your rationale. **[E/ap/S,Pl/ct]**
   - D_5½ NS and D_5¼ NS are considered "hydrating fluids." Solutions consisting of dextrose with hypotonic saline provide more water than is required for excretion of salt. C.K. has an infection and will need hydration to help the body dispose of the infectious toxins and wastes. The rate of 125 ml/h is considered maintenance of normal fluid balance.

7. What is the rationale for ordering oxygen to maintain an SaO_2 >90%? **[A/c/Pl/ct]**
   - The order means that you are to titrate the oxygen flow rate to maintain the saturation reading on C.K.'s oximeter (SaO_2) above 90%. According to the oxyhemoglobin dissociation curve, a hemoglobin saturation of 90% (SaO_2 of 90%) means that the partial pressure of oxygen in the arterial blood (PaO_2) is approximately 60 mm Hg (remember that normal PaO_2 at sea level is 80 to 100 mm Hg). Below this point on the curve, the slope becomes very steep, which means that small decreases in Hgb saturation reflect larger decreases in PaO_2 (i.e., SaO_2 of 85% reflects a PaO_2 of 50 mm Hg; SaO_2 of 80% means the PaO_2 is 44 mm Hg).

8. What is a culture and sensitivity test? **[A/k/Pl/ct]**
   - A culture is a growth of an organism on a nutrient media to specifically identify the microbe. After a microbe is isolated, its susceptibility to specific antibiotics is determined. If required, broad spectrum antibiotic therapy is prescribed until the C&S results are available and a more suitable antibiotic can be identified and prescribed.

9. Why would blood cultures be drawn if the patient spikes a fever? **[A/k/Pl/ct]**
   - According to one theory, bacteria are being shed into the bloodstream when the patient spikes a temperature. Blood cultures should be drawn STAT and before any antipyretic agent or antibiotic is given.

10. Why are blood cultures drawn from two different sites? **[A/k/Pl/ct]**
    - Blood is drawn from two different sites to increase the likelihood of culturing the offending organism. If the patient has an arterial or central venous catheter, one set of cultures may be withdrawn from the catheter after a 10 ml discard sample is withdrawn. Invasive catheters should always be suspected as a source of infection.

11. What general information can be obtained from a CXR? **[A/k/Pl/ct]**
    - Heart size.
    - Fluid accumulation (in lungs, pleural space, or around heart).
    - Congestion in large blood vessels of the chest.
    - Tumors.
    - Fractures and dislocations.
    - Placement of tubes and catheters. All invasive tubes and catheters have a radiopaque line that is visible on x-ray (e.g., central venous catheters; chest tubes; endotracheal tubes; nasogastric, duodenal, jejunostomy tubes.

12. C.K. recovers from his pneumonia and is preparing for discharge. You know that C.K. is at increased risk for contracting community-acquired pulmonary infections. Discuss 4 strategies for prevention. **[P/ap/S,Pl,HP/ct,ni,tc]**
    - Teach the importance of immunization with pneumococcal vaccine (one-time injection).
    - Teach the importance of yearly influenza vaccine. Each year the CDC predicts which 3 strains of influenza virus will infect the U.S. The vaccine is an inactivated antigen for all 3 strains.
    - Teach the importance of avoiding exposure to people with colds/flu.
    - Teach good hand-washing technique.
    - Teach him how to handle and properly dispose of secretions.
    - Teach the importance of PO fluids to thin pulmonary secretions and facilitate expectoration.

13. C.K. confides in you, "You know, my wife died a year ago and I live alone now. I've been thinking...this pneumonia stuff has been a little scary." How will you respond? **[P/an/S,PSI/ct,ni,tc]**
    - Tell him you appreciate his sharing this with you.
    - Explore whether he wants to talk more about it.
    - Inquire about his social support system. Does he have family/friends who can look in on him? Recognize that he may be experiencing such psychosocial responses as grief, fear of death, and loneliness. Ask about a psychiatric nurse specialist or social services consultation if you consider it necessary.
    - Make sure his concern is addressed in at least one concrete arrangement before he leaves the hospital.

<u>*Instructor Note*</u>: Pneumonia, etiology unknown, is properly called "pneumonitis." When "pneumonitis" is used, it should be defined according to cause, such as viral pneumonia or *Klebsiella* pneumonia.

Case Study 10: COPD with Transtracheal Oxygen

Difficulty: ** *Setting:* Outpatient clinic, hospital

Index Words: Chronic obstructive pulmonary disease, respiratory failure, pneumonia

S.M., a 67-year-old woman with severe emphysema, lives with her daughter. Six months ago, S.M. was admitted to the hospital for respiratory failure with severe hypercapnia. She received aggressive treatment with bronchodilators, mucolytics, and steroids. To improve her oxygenation, she underwent a minor surgical procedure for placement of a transtracheal (TT) catheter. She was discharged on bronchodilator and steroid therapy and continued to do well until last evening when she became profoundly short of breath and had to sit in a chair all night. This morning, the admitting nurse interviews S.M. to determine why she came to the pulmonary clinic.

1. What is hypercapnia? **[A/k/Pl/ct]**
   - Increased $PaCO_2$ levels resulting in respiratory acidosis.

2. S.M. has a TT O_2 catheter at 4 L/min. Describe the catheter and identify its function. **[A/k/Pl/ct]**
   - The TT catheter is a thin, Teflon-coated tube that is surgically placed in the trachea to deliver O_2 directly into the lungs. The catheter offers an alternative method of O_2 delivery for patients who don't like to wear a nasal cannula. Some patients are able to decrease their oxygen flow requirements using the TT O_2 catheter.

3. Identify 5 complications associated with TT O_2 therapy. **[PD/k/Pl/ct]**
   - Hypoxemia if the catheter becomes occluded.
   - Increased mucus production because "mucus balls" tend to form over the openings of the catheter and occlude the flow of oxygen. The catheter must be cleaned daily using clean technique.
   - Inflammation.
   - Bleeding.
   - Infection of the insertion site.
   - Subcutaneous emphysema (air under the skin).
   - Displacement of the catheter (flips upward into trachea/pharynx).

4. There is a possibility that S.M.'s TT catheter is occluded. What should the nurse do before removing the catheter for cleaning? **[P,I/k/Pl/ct]**
   - Provide O_2 per nasal cannula at 4 to 6 L/min before removing the TT catheter. Turbulence in the nasopharynx offers a natural resistance to air flow during inspiration. Some of the oxygen delivered by nasal cannula may remain within the nasopharynx, thus requiring an increased oxygen flow rate to deliver the same FIO_2.

The nurse cleans the catheter and removes several "mucus balls." She then completes a thorough assessment and notes the following. S.M. remains very anxious after the TT O_2 catheter is cleared. Her VS are 112/72, 114, 32, 37.0°C on 4 L/O_2 per TT catheter. She is dyspneic and uses accessory muscles of the neck and abdomen for respirations. There are scattered wheezes throughout the R lung fields and LUL, rhonchi over large airways, and breath sounds are absent from 4th intercostal space to the base on L side and greatly reduced on the R. Her skin is thin and friable, with multiple ecchymoses over both arms. She has a moderate amount of hard, dark, guaiac-positive stool.

5. Based on the assessment findings, identify 6 possible problems that S.M. may be experiencing. **[PD/ap/PI/ct]**
   - Hypoxemia (anxiety).
   - Respiratory muscle failure (fatigue of the respiratory muscles).
   - Asthma (wheezing).
   - Infection/pneumonia (rhonchi over large airways, consolidation causing absent breath sounds over LLL, and reduced breath sounds over the RLL).
   - Atelectasis (decreased/absent breath sounds).
   - GI bleeding/guaiac-positive stools (r/t steroid therapy).
   - Dehydration (stool is hard).

6. Given S.M.'s history and your knowledge of pathophysiologic processes, explain the assessment findings. **[PD/c/PI,PSI/ct]**
   - Anxiety: S.M. is anxious secondary to shortness of breath and hypoxemia.
   - Tachycardia: hypoxemia elevates the HR in an effort to increase oxygen delivery to the tissues.
   - RR of 32, SOB, dyspnea, and use of accessory muscles may be due to hypoxemia: she has bilateral wheezes as airflow passes through narrowed airways.
   - T 37.0°C is not elevated: patients with emphysema are at increased risk for pulmonary infection; however, steroid therapy suppresses the immune system and may mask signs of infection.
   - Skin is thin and blood vessels are friable as a result of steroid therapy.
   - The stool guaiac-positive: a results of steroid therapy.

The CXR reveals LLL pneumonia. S.M. is transported to the hospital and admitted to your intermediate care unit for exacerbation of COPD and pneumonia. The doctor writes the following orders: methylprednisolone (Solu-Medrol) 40 mg IV q8h; erthromycin (Erthrocin) 1g IV q6h; cefuroxine (Zinacef) 2g IV q6h; aerosol treatments using albuterol 2.5 mg (0.5 ml) in 3 ml NS alternating with acetylcysteine (Mucomyst) 5 ml of 10% concentration q4h round the clock; iodinated glycerol 60 mg PO qid; ranitidine (Zantac) 150 mg PO bid.

7. Describe why each of the medications are prescribed for S.M. **[A/ap/S,PI/ct]**
   - Solu-Medrol is a corticosteroid used to decrease the number and activity of antiinflammatory cells, inhibits bronchoconstriction, and relaxes smooth muscles (bronchioles). It has many systemic effects, so the risk/benefit ratio must be assessed.
   - Erythromycin and cefuroxine are antimicrobial agents that is effective in a variety of infections due to gram-positive and gram-negative pathogens, including multiresistant strains. Antibiotic(s) will be adjusted based upon culture results.
   - Albuterol is a bronchodilator, and Mucomyst is a mucolytic agent.
   - Iodinated glycerol is used as a mucolytic-expectorant in respiratory tract disorders such as COPD, bronchitis, emphysema, and bronchial asthma.
   - Zantac is a H_2 receptor antagonist used in the treatment of ulcer disease. This is being given because S.M. has guaiac-positive stools.

8. While you are administering the first dose of medication, S.M. states, "I don't want to be intubated again and placed on that breathing machine. I have lived with my lung disease for 30 years and I'd rather die than live on that machine." What action(s) would you take next? State your rationale. **[A/an/PSI/ni,tc]**
   - Validate her feelings.
   - Call the physician and indicate the patient's wishes. Ask him/her to come and talk to the patient about advanced directives/do not resuscitate (DNR) orders.
   - Have S.M. discuss her wishes with her daughter/family when she visits. That way there will be no misunderstanding concerning goals of medical management.

You arrange a family conference with S.M., her daughter, the physician, and yourself. After some discussion, the physician assures S.M. that medical management will focus on resolving the pneumonia and keeping her comfortable and that her wishes regarding no resuscitation efforts will be respected. The physician details the instructions in the physician orders.

9. Describe how palliative care differs from curative care. **[A/k/PI,PSI/ct]**
   - Palliative care includes measures to decrease suffering, such as administering adequate pain medication; keeping her clean; preventing skin breakdown; providing relief from anxiety, fear, and insomnia; controlling peripheral and pulmonary edema; and managing nausea and vomiting. Palliative care includes working with the daughter to determine that her needs are being met.
   - Curative care is directed toward resolving the pulmonary infection through aggressive medical treatment, which stops short of intubation and mechanical ventilation.

10. Formulate a list of 8 nursing diagnoses for S.M. **[PD/an/S,PI,PSI/ct]**
    - Ineffective airway clearance r/t pneumonia and COPD.
    - Inability to sustain spontaneous ventilation r/t pulmonary infection and COPD.
    - Impaired gas exchange r/t pneumonia and COPD.
    - Ineffective breathing pattern r/t pulmonary infection and COPD.
    - Self-care deficit r/t chronic lung disease.
    - Altered nutrition r/t infection.
    - Alteration in comfort r/t dyspnea.
    - Anxiety r/t hypoxemia.
    - Fatigue r/t increased energy requirements for breathing.
    - Spiritual distress r/t wishes to die.
    - Fear r/t dying.

11. Before leaving, the daughter stops you in the hallway and says, "I know that the doctor only gave my mother a 50% chance of survival. I realize how sick she is, but I would like to know if there is anything I can do to better her odds and make her more comfortable." How would you respond? **[E/an/S,PI,PSI/ct,ni,tc]**
    - There are several things you can do to increase your mother's chances for survival:
        - Watch that everyone washes his/her hands on entering and leaving your mother's room, including visitors, nurses, doctors, laboratory technicians, everyone.
        - Encourage your mother to cough and deep breathe.
        - Make sure that your mother keeps her oxygen on.
        - In order to breathe deeply, she has to be positioned properly in the bed. Explain when her mother needs to be "pulled up in bed."
        - You can help the nurses turn and reposition your mother.
        - Encourage your mother to drink at least 8 glasses of fluids per day.
        - Inspect all sputum that your mother coughs up (or save it for you to inspect). We need to know the quantity, color, and consistency of her sputum.
        - Limit visitors. Your mother needs several hours of uninterrupted sleep and lots of rest.
    - There are several things you can do to help your mother be more comfortable:
        - Quietly sit in the room, she will feel the comfort of having you there and yet she can sleep/rest.
        - Plan activities while she is awake so that she can have periods of uninterrupted sleep; activities such as drinking fluids, turning, cough and deep breathing, and range of motion exercises and pumping her feet up and down to promote venous return.
        - Allow your mother to talk about her life and her feelings about dying.
        - Call a minister/pastor/rabbi/bishop if she wishes to talk to a clergy.

    Instructor Note: Also, take the opportunity to ask the daughter if a family member or significant other could relieve her so that she can get adequate rest and nutrition. Explain that she has to take care of herself before she can take care of her mother. Direct other nurses to allow the daughter to be involved in her mother's care. Place a note in the Kardex and on the patient's chart.

S.M. was discharged home with a referral for hospice care. Her daughter wrote a "Thank You" note to the nurses on your floor informing you that her mother died peacefully at home 2 weeks later.

Case Study 11: Chronic Bronchitis/Lung Cancer

Difficulty: ***	*Setting:* Hospital
Index Words: Chronic bronchitis/lung cancer, respiratory failure	

The ICU nurse calls to give you the following report: "D.S. is a 56-year-old man with a PMH of chronic bronchitis. He quit smoking 12 years ago and exercises regularly. He went to see his doc c/o increasing exertional dyspnea, and a large mass was found in his R lung. Three days ago he underwent an RML and RLL lobectomy, the pathology report showed adenocarcinoma. He has no neuro deficits and his VS run 120s/70s, 110s, about 34, and he has been running a fever of 100.2°F. His heart tones are clear, he has all his pulses, and has an IV of $D_5½$ NS at 50 ml/h in his R forearm. He has a R midaxillary chest tube to PleurEvac drain, there's no air leak, and it's draining small amounts of serosanguinous fluid. He's complaining of pain at the insertion site but the site looks good, and the dressing is dry and intact. He's on 5 L O_2. He refuses pain medication. He's a real nervous guy and hasn't slept since surgery. He'll be there in about 20 minutes."

1. What additional information would you ask the nurse to provide at this time? **[A/k/PI/ct]**
   - Lung sounds and oximeter readings?
   - How he is tolerating the reduced lung volume?
   - Does he have any allergies?
   - Does he have any family that come to see him?

D.S. is transported by wheelchair past the nurses' station to a room at the far end of the hall. You enter his room for the first time to find him sitting on the edge of the bed with his left leg in bed and his right foot on the floor. You introduce yourself, tell him that you are going to be his nurse for the rest of the shift. You note that he keeps rubbing his left hand over his right chest.

2. What issues/problems can you already identify? **[PD/c/S,PI/ct]**
   - Safety issues: he is sitting on the edge of the bed and the siderails are down; he had surgery on his R chest and, if he loses his balance, he won't be able to use the R arm to help stabilize himself.
   - Pain issue: he is 3 days postop and has not received anything for pain.
   - Sleep issues: he has not slept since surgery (3 days).

3. List 4 things you would do for D.S. **[P/an/S,PI,PSI/ct,ni,tc]**
   - Raise the R siderails of the bed and explain your rationale.
   - Explain that your rooms are clustered at this end of the hallway so you can keep an eye on all your patients. This will lessen his sense of isolation.
   - Obtain his VS.
   - Tell him that you understand that his chest tube is causing pain. Ask him to describe the pain. You want to know if the pain is sharp/dull, constant/intermittent, localized/generalized, does it stay in one place or radiate someplace else, what relieves it/what makes it worse. Investigate why he has refused to take pain medication since surgery.
   - Give him the call light.

4. D.S. states, "I have a nephew who rolled his jeep and busted himself up real bad. He got hooked on those drugs, and I don't want any part of them." How would you respond to D.S.'s statement. **[P/ap/PI,PSI/ct,ni,tc]**
   - Inform D.S. that the purpose of pain is to tell you something is wrong with your body so you can seek medical attention. Beyond that, pain serves no useful purpose. Pain medication is ordered to relieve the pain so that he can move around, cough and deep breathe, and recover faster; that moving and coughing will keep fluid from accumulating in his good lung (preventing pneumonia). Inform him that patients who take pain medication recover more quickly and have fewer complications. Explain that if he waits until the pain is intense, it will take larger amounts of pain medication to relieve the pain. Tell him his body's response to pain can delay healing.
   - Explain that all of your patients take pain medication for the first 3 days after surgery; they use it to work the soreness out and after that they don't need much medication. Tell him that the two of you have to work together so that he can get better and go home. Tell D.S. that you are going to get his pain medication and ask him if he will let you administer it to him because you are going to encourage him to be more active.
   - Also tell D.S. that you will wait until his pain is relieved before removing the chest tube dressing to observe the insertion site.

5. Why is D.S. experiencing difficulty using his R arm? Given the type of surgery D.S. underwent, is this expected? **[A/c/PI/ct]**
   - Yes, it is an expected outcome of this type of surgery. The patient is placed on the L side with the R arm placed anterior and superior to the head. The standard posterolateral thoracotomy incision begins just below the R nipple in front, curves posteriorly below the tip of the scapula, and extends slightly cephalad almost to the vertebral column in back. Then all intervening muscles are divided and the long portion of the 5th rib or 4th and 5th ribs is/are dissected. Postoperatively, the patient suffers a transient nerve compression and restricted use of the arm on the affected side.

6. You administer 10 mg morphine ($MgSO_4$) IM and tell D.S. that you will return in 30 minutes; 15 minutes later he turns on his call light. When you enter the room D.S. says, "I think I'm going to throw up." What are the next 3 things you would do? **[A,P/an/S,PI/ct,ni]**
   - Turn him onto his side to reduce the risk of aspiration.
   - Grab a bath basin and place it beside his mouth (do not give patients emesis basins; it takes a great deal of concentration to confine emesis to such a small object).
   - Provide a cool washcloth to his head.
   - Ask him when he began to feel nauseated.

7. D.S. stated, "I started to feel sick a couple minutes ago. It just kept getting worse until I knew I was going to throw up." Given this information, what do you think is responsible for the sudden onset of nausea? **[PD/c/PI/ct]**
   - The morphine.

8. Would it be appropriate to give D.S. a second dose of morphine before reporting his reaction to the physician? State your rationale. **[PD/c/PI/ct,ni,tc]**
   - No, it would not be appropriate to subject D.S. to a second dose of M.S. There are many alternative medications that the physician could order.
   - Call the physician and describe your findings and observations during your initial assessment.
   - Inform him/her that D.S. has not received anything for pain since surgery.
   - Describe the patient's reaction to morphine sulfate 10 mg IM. Ask if D.S. could try Demerol.
   - Suggest that if the Demerol is more effective in achieving pain control, that D.S. be placed on a PCA pump.
   - Also request something to relieve the nausea, such as droperidoe (Inapsine) (0.25 to 0.5 ml IVP).

9. D.S.'s pain and nausea are under control an hour later. You remove the chest tube dressing and note that the area around the insertion site looks slightly inflamed, the tissue immediately around the tube looks white, and there is a small amount of purulent drainage. What action would you take next? **[P/ap/PI/ct,ni]**
   - Obtains a specimen of the drainage for C&S.
   - Cleanse the area with half-strength Betadine.
   - Apply a new Vaseline gauze around the insertion site, apply a sterile dressing, and tape the tube securely.

The next day the nurse giving you report says that D.S. has been driving her crazy all day long. She tells you that he is fine but has been paranoid and very demanding. You enter D.S.'s room to see how he is doing and to tell him you are going to be his nurse again today. You note that his head bobs up and his mouth opens, like a fish taking in water, every time he inhales. He says, "I just can't (breath) seem to (breath) get enough (breath) air."

10. Identify 6 possible problems that D.S. could have that would account for his behavior? **[PD/c/PI/ct]**
    - Pneumonia.
    - Atelectasis.
    - Bronchoconstriction (exacerbation of asthma or chronic bronchitis).
    - Pulmonary embolus.
    - Pneumothorax in the RUL, LUL, or LLL.
    - Pulmonary edema (CHF).
    - Adult respiratory distress syndrome (ARDS).
    - Splinting due to severe pain.

11. What 3 actions should you take next and give your rationale. **[I/an/S,PI/ct,ni]**
    - Obtain VS.
    - Auscultate breath sounds.
    - Note respiratory pattern.
    - Note recruitment of accessory muscles to breath.
    - Increase his oxygen (start on 100% nonrebreather mask).

D.S.'s RR is 46; you auscultate slight air movement over the large airways and no breath sounds distal to the 3rd ICS. He's sitting on the side of the bed with his arms hunched up on the overbed table. His gown is in his lap, he is diaphoretic, you note intercostal retractions with inspiration, and all muscles of the upper torso are engaged in respiration.

12. What would you do next? **[I/an/S,PI/ct,ni]**
    - Call a code. His V_T is inadequate to support life; he is creating an oxygen deficit and could have a repiratory arrest at any moment.

D.S. is successfully resuscitated and transferred to ICU. The physician returns to your floor and compliments you on your clear thinking and fast action. The nurse who gave you report comes up to you to apologize. She is relatively new and asks you to explain how you know when a patient is in the early and late stages of respiratory difficulty. She states that she wants to learn from her mistakes so she doesn't put another patient through what D.S. experienced.

13. How would you distinguish between early and late stages of respiratory failure? **[A,PD/k/PI/ct]**

    <u>Signs of Early Respiratory Failure</u>
    - Increased respiratory rate.
    - Decreased V_T.
    - Increased use of accessory muscles.
    - Sentence length begins to shorten.
    - Loss of sense of humor; energy and cognitive awareness focused on breathing.

    <u>Signs of Late Respiratory Failure</u>
    - Inability to maintain PaO_2 >50 to 60 mm Hg.
    - Increased $PaCO_2$ (acidosis pH <7.3 and somnolence without cough).
    - Respiratory rate doubles.
    - Exaggerated use of accessory muscles.
    - Sternal retractions.
    - Paradoxical respirations.
    - Clammy skin.

    <u>Instructor Note</u>: D.S. has a PMH of chronic bronchitis and has undergone a RML and RLL lobectomy; 2 of his 5 lobes have been removed. His tidal volume has been drastically reduced, and it will take approximately 6 months for his remaining lung to maximally hyperinflate in an effort to compensate for the reduced alveolar surface area. Any compromise to his respiratory system will have an exaggerated effect on him.

D.S. recovered. His CXR at 5 years showed no recurrence.

Case Study 12: Adult Respiratory Distress Syndrome

Difficulty: *** *Setting:* Hospital

Index Words: Adult respiratory distress syndrome, dysrhythmias

G.S., a 36-year-old secretary, was involved in a motor vehicle accident; a car drifted left of center and struck G.S. head on, pinning her behind the steering wheel. She was intubated immediately after extrication and flown to your trauma center. Her injuries were found to be extensive: bilateral flail chest, torn innominate artery, right hemo/pneumothorax, fractured spleen, multiple small liver lacerations, compound fractures of both legs, and probable cardiac contusion. She was taken to the OR where she received 36 units of PRCs, 20 units of platelets, 20 units cryoprecipitate, 12 units FFP, and 18 L of LR. She was admitted to the intensive care unit postop where she developed adult respiratory distress syndrome (ARDS). She has been in ICU for 6 weeks, her ARDS has almost resolved, and she is transferred to your unit. You receive the following report: Neuro: alert and oriented to person and place, she can move both of her arms and wiggle her toes on both feet; CV: heart tones are clear, VS are 138/90, 88, 26, 99.2°F, bilateral radial pulse 3+, foot pulses by Doppler only; Skin: incisions and lacerations have all healed; Respiratory: bilateral chest tubes to water suction with closed drainage, dressing are dry and intact; GI: duodenal feeding tube in place; GU: Foley catheter to down drain.

1. What additional information should you require during this report? **[A/an/S,PI,PSI/ct]**
   - Does she have an IVs?
   - Neuro: Is she oriented to time? Does she have any sensory deficits? Pupils?
   - CV: What have her vital signs been running? What is her cardiac rhythm? Any edema?
   - Skin: Does she have any staples, sutures, or open areas? Skin condition?
   - Resp: Is she on oxygen? What have SaO_2s been running? Any chest drainage? How much suction to chest drainage system? Breath sounds? Coughing? Cultured anything? Any respiratory treatments? Last CXR? Any respiratory distress?
   - GI: What type of feeding tube, solution, and rate of infusion? Any residuals? pH and guaiac? Any stools, bowel sounds?
   - GU: What has her urine output been?
   - General: What does she know and remember about the accident? Allergies and past medical history? Are there any family members, if so, any problems with them? Belongings? What medicine is she on? Pain management?

You complete your assessment on G.S. You note shortness of breath, crackles throughout all lung fields posteriorally and in both lower lobes anteriorly, and rhonchi over the large airways.

2. What is the significance of crackles and rhonchi in G.S.'s case? **[A/c/PI/ct]**
   - Crackles indicate fluid accumulation in the pulmonary tissues (parenchyma). Edematous parenchymal tissue exerts pressure on distal airways; when parenchymal pressure exceeds intraairway pressure, the airways prematurely collapse, or pop closed. Conversely, when intraairway pressure exceeds parenchymal pressure, the airways pop open. The vibrations of distal airways popping closed and open are carried to the outer chest wall and are heard as crackles.
   - Rhonchi indicate secretions in the large airways. Vibrations caused by air passing around or through the secretions are carried to the outer chest wall and is heard as rhonchi.

3. The nurse from the previous shift charted the following statement, "Crackles and rhonchi clear with vigorous coughing." Based on your knowledge of pathophysiology, determine the accuracy of this statement. **[A/ap/PI/ct]**
   - It is quite possible to clear rhonchi but physiologically impossible to clear crackles with coughing.

4. It is time to administer 40 mg furosemide (Lasix) IVP. What effect, if any, will Lasix have on G.S.'s breath sounds? **[PD/c/PI/ct]**
   - Lasix, a diuretic, will mobilize and increase excretion of excess fluids from the body. Decreased parenchymal edema may result in fewer crackles.

5. What action should you take before giving the Lasix? **[PD/c/S,PI/ct,ni]**
   - Check laboratory values; particularly Na, K, Mg, and Ca.

The 0500 laboratory values are as follows: Na 129 mEq/L, K 3.3 mEq/L, Cl 92 mEq/L, HCO_3 26 mEq/L, BUN 37 mg/dl, creatinine 2.0 mg/dl, glucose 128 mg/dl, calcium 7.1 mg/dl, ABGs on 6 L O_2/nc: pH 7.38, $PaCO_2$ 49 mm Hg, PaO_2 82 mm Hg, HCO_3 36 mEq/L, BE +2.2, SaO_2 91%

6. Keeping in mind that you are about to administer Lasix, which laboratory values concern you and why? **[A/an/PI/ct]**
   - Na, K, and calcium are low. Each of these laboratory values is likely to decrease after administering Lasix. Na levels affect blood pressure and neuromuscular reactions. K is essential for transmission of electrical impulses in cardiac and skeletal muscle. Calcium is essential for muscle contraction and blood coagulation.
   - Mg was not drawn; however, because the Na, K, and calcium are low you would want to check the Mg level.
   - The BUN and creatinine are slightly elevated; the possibility of renal impairment must always be considered in evaluating diuretic response to Lasix.

7. Given the laboratory values listed above, what action would you take before administering the Lasix and why? **[P/c/S,PI/ct,ni]**
   - Call the physician to report the abnormal laboratory values and state that no Mg level was drawn. Inform her/him that it is time to administer 40 mg Lasix IVP.

The physician prescribes the following: draw STAT Mg level, if below 1.4 mg/dl give $MgSO_4$ 3 g in 100 ml D_5W over 4h; give KCl 40 mEq in 100 ml D_5W IVPB over 4h NOW; and give CaCl 2 g in 100 ml D_5W IVPB over 3h. The laboratory is called to draw a STAT Mg level.

8. Given that KCl and CaCl are compatible, would you mix them in the same bag of D_5W? State your rationale. **[PD/c/S,PI/ct,ni]**
    - Yes, it would be permissible to mix the two medications. The KCl is prescribed to infuse over 4h and the CaCl is to infuse over 3h. However, the rationale for prescribing an infusion time is to ensure that the medication is not infused too rapidly. Frequently, the infusion rate for a KCl "flash" or "rider" is slowed due to patient complaints of intravascular pain.

9. You open G.S.'s medication drawer to draw the Lasix into a syringe. You find one 20 mg ampule. The pharmacist tells you that it will be at least an hour before he can send the drug to you. You realize it is illegal to take medication dispensed by a pharmacist for one patient and use it for another patient. What should you do? **[PD/an/PI/ct,ni]**
    - If you are unable to locate the Lasix and cannot send anyone to the pharmacy to obtain the drug, give the first 20 mg IVP, then give the second 20 mg when it is delivered. Realize that two 20-mg doses may not generate the same diuretic effect as one 40-mg dose. Compare the diuresis achieved with the two half-doses to that achieved with the single dose, and if there is a discrepancy, inform the appropriate physicians the next time a coworker pages one of them. Chart your actions and rationale!

10. While you administer the Lasix and hang the IVPB medication, G.S. says, "This is so weird. A couple times this morning I felt like my heart flipped upside down in my chest but now I feel like there's a bird flopping around in there." What are the first 2 actions you should take next? Give your rationale. **[E/an/S,PI,PSI/ct,ni]**
    - Determine if G.S. has a conducted pulse; note the rate and regularity.
    - If she has a pulse, then take her BP and determine if she is symptomatic. Monitor ABC status. If she loses her pulse, call for help and begin CPR.

11. G.S.'s pulse is 66 and irregular. Her BP is 92/70 and respirations are 26. She admits to being "a little light-headed" but denies having pain or nausea. Your coworker connects G.S. to the code cart monitor for a "quick look." You are able to distinguish normal P-QRS-T complexes but you also note approximately 22 very wide complexes per minute. The wide complexes come early and are not preceded by a P wave. What do you think has happened to G.S.? **[A,PD/an/S,PI/ct]**
    - G.S. is having premature ventricular contractions (PVCs).

12. What should your next actions be? **[P/ap/S,PI/ct,ni]**
    - Increase the oxygen concentration.
    - Hang the KCl and CaCl piggyback as quickly as possible and begin the infusion.
    - Call for a STAT portable 12-lead ECG to confirm the PVCs.
    - STAT page the physician.
    - Call for STAT ABGs.

13. What are the most likely causes of the abnormal beats? **[PD/ap/PI/ct]**
    - Low K, calcium, or Mg levels.
    - Low oxygen levels.

14. You notice that G.S. looks frightened and is laying stiff as a board. How would you respond to this situation? **[I/ap/PSI/ct,ni,tc]**
    - Put your hand on G.S.'s arm and tell her something like this: "Let me tell you what is going on. As we get older, everyone has some abnormal heart beats. It is not a problem as long as we don't have too many of them. When you told me you felt like you had a bird in your chest, I felt your pulse right away and I could tell you were having too many of those abnormal beats. Those beats are usually caused by one of two things. Either your heart muscle isn't getting enough oxygen or you don't have enough of certain minerals such as potassium, calcium, or magnesium in your blood. We are trying to determine why you are having those abnormal beats. I have already turned up your oxygen and the respiratory therapist drew your blood to see how much oxygen is in it. I have started an IV that has potassium and calcium in it, but I can't give it too fast because that could cause other problems. The lab technician drew your magnesium level about an hour ago so we'll have that result soon. I'll keep you informed as we get more information." Then ask G.S. if she has any questions and if there is anything she needs. Give her the nurse's call button, and ask her to alert you immediately if she feels any changes.

G.S.'s PVCs responded well to treatment. Unfortunately one week later, a large fat embolus lodged in G.S.'s lungs. All attempts at resuscitation failed.

Case Study 13: Status Asthmaticus

Difficulty: ***	*Setting:* Hospital
Index Words: Status asthmaticus, asthma	

F.P., a 42-year-old male RN, is admitted to the intermediate care floor for exacerbation of asthma that is unresponsive to treatment. His admission weight is 43 kg and his latest VS are 150/88, 126, 32, 102.2°F. You complete a thorough assessment and document the following. F.P. is slightly confused (Glasgow Coma Scale = 14) and very anxious. His temperature is 102.2°F but his skin is cool and clammy. He is tachycardic, dyspneic, and has a slightly productive weak cough. Wheezing is noted throughout all lung fields, and his anterior-posterior diameter is exaggerated. Bowel sounds are hypoactive, and he denies the urge to void.

1. Explain possible reasons for your assessment finding. **[PD/ap/PI/ct]**
   - Slight confusion and anxiety r/t hypoxemia.
   - Temperature elevation could stem from one of two sources: (1) the increased work of breathing will increase metabolic rate, resulting in increased heat loss and elevated temperature; and (2) infections, common in patients suffering from asthma, will activate the inflammatory response and manifest itself as fever.
   - Cool, clammy skin. Circulation is shunted from the skin to oxygenate vital organs.
   - Tachycardia. Hypoxemia stimulates tachycardia in an effort to increase oxygen delivery to the tissues.
   - Dyspnea. Narrowed airways trap air in lungs. As the PaO_2 decreases, he experiences shortness of breath and increases his respiratory rate to compensate.
   - Cough. Excessive mucus collecting in the airways renders the cilia ineffective and stimulates the cough response. However, because V_T is low, he does not have the force to expel the secretions.
   - Wheezes in all lung fields r/t airflow through narrowed airways.
   - Decreased breath sounds. Air trapping will result in decreased V_T.
   - Increased anterior-posterior chest diameter. The trapping of air within the lungs prevents the thoracic cage from returning to its resting position and results in an increased AP diameter.
   - Decreased bowel sounds due to shunting of blood away from the bowel in favor of vital organs.

You check F.P.'s laboratory values and find the following: WBC 13.5 mm^3, Hgb 17 g/dl, Hct 48%, platelets 280 mm^3, Na 147 mEq/L, K 4.9 mEq/L, Cl 109 mEq/L, CO_2 31 mEq/L, BUN 35 mg/dl, creatinine 2.0 mg/dl, glucose 134 mg/dl.

2. Which of the laboratory values listed above are abnormal? **[A/k/PI/ct]**
   - The following labs are elevated: WBC, Hgb, Hct, Na, Cl, CO_2, glucose, BUN, creatinine.

3. Relate the abnormal laboratory values to F.P.'s condition. What do the laboratory values indicate? **[E/an/S,PI/ct]**
   - These laboratory values indicate pulmonary infection and dehydration.

4. F.P.'s attending physician makes rounds on him for the first time. What information is important to convey to the doctor? **[A/c/S,Pl/ct,ni,tc]**
   - Time he arrived and his room number.
   - Assessment findings.
   - Essential history and changes since admission (brief).
   - Abnormal lab values.
   - Allergies.

The physician prescribes the following: 800 caloric mechanical soft diet; maintenance IV of NS with 30 mEq KCl/L at 125 ml/h; cefuroxime (Zinacef) 1 g IVPB q8h; albuterol 2.5 mg in 3 ml NS q4h; theophylline 260 mg IVPB over 30 minutes then aminophylline 500 mg in 500 ml D_5W to infuse at 0.5 mg/kg/h; prednisone 60 mg PO q8h; morphine sulfate 20 mg IM q3-4h prn for pain; STAT blood culture and sensitivity x 2 sites; sputum C&S; STAT CXR and ECG; acetaminophen (Tylenol) 650 mg PO for temp $>102°F$.

5. You know the patient has an elevated temperature. After reviewing the orders, what would you do first? **[P/ap/Pl/ct]**
   - Wait until the blood cultures are drawn before giving the Tylenol or starting the antibiotic.

6. You transcribe the orders listed above. Identify the orders that you should question and state your rationale. **[PD/ap/Pl/ct]**
   - Diet. This patient needs a large number of calories to support his increased metabolic rate. He needs to be encouraged to eat a high-protein high-carbohydrate diet.
   - M.S. This dosage is very high and should be questioned.
   - 30 mEq KCl to each liter of IV fluid. Because F.P.'s K was 4.9 mEq/L you would question the amount of K ordered.

7. You initiate the loading dose of aminophylline and leave the room to prepare the maintenance drip. Identify the drip rate required to infuse the ordered dose of 0.7 mg/kg/h for 12 hours, then 0.3 mg/kg/h? **[A/k/Pl/ct]**
   - F.P.'s weight is 43 kg. The solution you mixed (aminophylline 500 mg in 500 ml D_5W) contains 1 mg/ml. After the loading dose, you want to infuse the aminophylline drip at 30 ml/h for 12 hours then decrease the drip rate to 12.9 or 14 ml/h.

8. List pertinent side effects of theophylline. **[A/k/Pl/ct]**
   - Tremors.
   - N/V.
   - Cardiac dysrhythmias, cardiac arrest.
   - Tachycardia.

You enter F.P.'s room to hang the maintenance drip and find him barely responsive. His respiratory rate is 58, shallow and gasping. He exhibits an asynchronous or paradoxical respiratory pattern, you detect no breath sounds on auscultation, and he is generally cyanotic. His apical pulse is 164.

9. What actions should you take next and why? **[E/an/Pl/ct,ni]**
   - Lay the HOB flat.
   - Call for help. Have your coworker call a code.
   - Use an airway and bag valve mask device to support respirations until the code team arrives.
   - Have someone notify the physician of the patient's condition.
   - Prepare for transport to ICU.

The code team responds immediately. F.P. is intubated. The respiratory therapist begins to ventilate F.P. using a bag-valve device when the endotracheal tube (ETT) fills with thick yellow secretions. She calls for endotracheal suction.

10. Explain hyperoxygenation and why it is important to hyperoxygenate before endotracheal suctioning. **[A/c/S,Pl/ct]**
    - Hyperoxygenation is the administration of a high concentration of oxygen before removing pulmonary secretions from the lower respiratory tract. Hyperoxygenation is done to prevent hypoxemia during and after suctioning.

11. There are two methods of delivering the hyperoxygenation breaths: the ventilator or the bag-valve device. Discuss which method is the most reliable. **[A/an/Pl/ct]**
    - The ventilator method of delivering hyperoxygenation breaths has a known inspiratory volume, flow rate, inspiratory waveform, and inspiratory pressure. These factors are unknown when using the bag-valve device. Some ventilators have a preoxygenation mode that flushes the inspiratory tubing with 100% O_2; others require up to 2 minutes to flush the tubing to 100% O_2. The concentration of oxygen delivered by various bag-valve devices depends on the oxygen flow rate, size of the oxygen reservoir, ventilatory rate, one- vs two-handed compression, and bag refill time after each compression. There are many more variables to delivering O_2 by bag-valve devices than by ventilator.

12. When endotracheal suctioning (ETS) is performed, the suction regulator should not be adjusted above the maximum "low" setting. What are the consequences of having the suction regulator adjusted to a medium or high setting? **[PD/c/S,Pl/ct]**
    - Approximately 15 L/min of air are removed from the patient's lung when the suction regulator is set at maximum "low." Suction of 15 L/min x 10 seconds means that 2500 cc of air are removed from the airways if no secretions obstruct the suction catheter while the suction is applied. Because higher suction pressures remove greater quantities of air from the airway, they may be dangerous and can result in atelectasis.

13. Why are size 14 French catheters routinely used for ETS in adults? **[A/k/S,Pl/ct]**
    - Adult ETTs are sized 7.5 mm or larger. A 14 French catheter is used because the outer diameter of the suction catheter should not occlude more than half the inner diameter of the endotracheal tube. This ratio ensures that the patient can obtain adequate ventilation during endotracheal suctioning.

14. You insert the suction catheter until you feel an obstruction, withdraw the catheter 1 cm before applying suction, and begin to withdraw the suction catheter over a 10-second period. A nursing student approaches you and askes why you didn't rotate the suction catheter as you suctioned the patient. How would you respond? **[PD/c/S,PI/ct,tc]**
    - Rotation of the proximal end of the suction catheter does not result in rotation of the distal end; such rotation causes lateral movement of the distal end of the catheter. The suction catheter causes gross avulsion of the delicate tracheal tissue and promotes small areas of hemorrhage. In order to prevent unnecessary damage, the suction catheter should not be rotated. Encourage the student to obtain an ETT, pass a suction catheter through it, and rotate the suction catheter to observe the lack of rotation for her/himself.

You remove a large amount of thick, yellow secretions from F.P.'s airway and transfer him to the ICU for stabilization and further treatment. The following day he is transferred back to your unit. Because he is to be discharged tomorrow, you are interviewing him about his support systems. He appears to be agitated. Suddenly he says, "You know, I haven't told anyone, but I think I had a near-death experience the other day. I don't think I've gotten over it yet."

15. How are you going to respond? **[PD/an/PSI,HP/ct,ni,tc]**
    - Realize that this is a profound emotional experience that should be taken seriously.
    - This may be an indication that he wants to talk to you about it. Offer to listen if he wishes to share.
    - If he seems shy about discussing it with you, ask if there is someone he would like to talk to about it (e.g., priest, minister, friend, psychiatric nurse specialist, hospice nurse, specialist, social worker).
    - Offer him pen and paper and encourage him to write about his experience.
    - Ask him how he is feeling right now (important!)
    - Ask him if it was a positive or negative experience

    Instructor Note: Not all near death or "out of body" experiences are positive. Some are very frightening, such as a woman who said she "saw the fires of hell" and was terrified.

Case Study 14: The Mechanically-Ventilated Patient

Difficulty: ***	*Setting:* Home care
Index Words: Guillain-Barré syndrome	

P.R., a 31-year-old woman diagnosed with Guillain-Barré, is being cared for at home by home health care nurses because she requires 24-hour/day nursing coverage. She has been intubated and mechanically ventilated for 3 weeks and has shown no signs of improvement in respiratory muscle strength. Her ventilator settings are A/C of 12, V_T 700, FIO_2 .50, PEEP 5. Her VS are 108/64, 118, 12, 100.6°F. She is receiving enteral nutrition by nasal-duodenal tube (2800 calories/24 hours). P.R.'s three children, ages 3, 4, and 6, are staying with her sister.

1. Why is P.R.'s ventilator mode on assist/control? **[PD/c/PI/ct]**
   - P.R. must not have enough innervation to her respiratory muscles to trigger the ventilator to deliver a breath, so the machine is doing all the work.

2. P.R. is receiving lorazepam (Ativan) 1 mg slow IVP q4h to reduce her anxiety. Identify 2 factors that should be considered when choosing Ativan for P.R. **[A/k/PI/ct]**
   - Ativan is metabolized in the liver. Is her liver functioning properly?
   - What is P.R.'s level of sedation? You want her to remain alert.
   - Ativan is inexpensive.

3. Identify 9 nonpharmacologic strategies that you could use to reduce P.R.'s anxiety, increase her comfort, and reduce the need for Ativan. Be creative! **[P/ap/PI,PSI/ct,ni,tc]**
   - Observe closely for clues to overt and covert needs.
   - Develop a simple form of communication, such as a combination eye blinking/movement system.
   - Encourage communication. Allow P.R. time to communicate and provide feedback.
   - Reassure P.R. that anxiety and other negative feelings are understandable and expected.
   - Use TV and radio for reorientation.
   - Provide her (not the nurse's) favorite relaxing music.
   - Use relaxation techniques.
   - Provide back rubs.
   - Have her children tape messages/songs and play the tapes as she requests.
   - Create a special time when her children can visit.
   - Involve the family in her care.
   - Provide private time for P.R. and her husband.

4. You give P.R. a bath and note that her cheeks billow outward each time the ventilator delivers a breath. What could cause this phenomenon? **[E/an/S,PI/ct,ni]**
   - Air leak in the cuff, inflation tube, or inflation valve of the ETT.
   - The trachea could have become dilated from the constant pressure of the ETT cuff.
   - The lungs may have become increasingly stiff from pulmonary edema. When the ventilator delivers the breath, the stiff lungs resist inflation and force the air to flow around the cuff.
   - The ETT could have been pulled out (proximal to the vocal cords).

5. You try repositioning P.R., place a stopcock in the inflation valve, auscultate the lungs, check the length of the tube at the lip (the tube had not moved), and finally insert more air in the cuff before sealing the leak. Over the next 24 hours, the leak becomes worse and the ventilator's low exhaled volume alarm repeatedly sounds. What action should you take? **[I/an/S,PI/ct,ni,tc]**
   - Notify the physician of the air leak. Because the ETT has been in place for 3 weeks and P.R. shows no signs of increased inspiratory muscle strength, the physician may elect to replace the ETT or, more likely, perform a tracheostomy.

6. The physician elects to insert a No. 8 Shiley tracheostomy tube with a disposable inner cannula. P.R. becomes increasingly anxious after receiving the news. How would you prepare P.R. and her husband for the tracheostomy? **[P/an/PSI/ct,ni,tc]**
   - Show them a picture of a tracheostomy tube, and explain that placement requires a brief surgical procedure. The tract, or hole, develops in about 1 week, then the trach tube is changed monthly. Inform them that the trach tube will cause increased mucus production for the first several days, until P.R.'s body becomes use to the new tube, then secretions will decrease. The incision must be cleaned at least q4h until the secretions subside, then q8-12h. Like any incision, you have to use sterile technique and observe for signs of infection.
   - Once P.R. is able to breathe on her own, the tube is removed, the stoma is covered with a dressing, and the hole takes about 3 days to heal. P.R. will have a slight scar at the base of her neck where the tube was inserted.

7. P.R. undergoes the tracheostomy procedure without complications. When you return in the morning and assess the new tracheostomy you note that the trach tape looks tight. You are unable to insert 1 finger between P.R.'s neck and the trach tape. Discuss whether or not this is problematic. **[PD/c/PI/ct]**
   - Yes. If the trach tape is tied too tightly, the tracheostomy flange completely covers and compresses the stoma. This could result in infection of the incision or the leakage of air into the surrounding subcutaneous tissues.

8. What should your next actions be? **[I/ap/S,PI/ct,ni]**
   - Ordinarily, the trach tapes are not changed for 48 hours after tracheostomy; however, it is required in this case. Immediately perform trach care, observe the incision, palpate the surrounding tissues, and tie the trach tapes loose enough to allow 1 finger to fit under the tapes.
   - Document the findings and notify the physician.
   - Complete an incident report, and write a note to inform the previous nurse about the incident.

9. You note that the tissue surrounding the incision is edematous. As you palpate the area, your fingers sink into the skin and you auscultate a popping sound through your stethoscope. Is this to be expected? **[PD/c/PI/ct]**
   - No. P.R. has subcutaneous emphysema around the incision.

10. Based on your decision in question 9, what action should you take? **[I/ap/PI/ct,ni]**
    - Instruct P.R. that a small amount of air has leaked into the tissue around the incision, that you have loosened the trach tape, and that the air will be reabsorbed in a day or so. In the mean time, keep P.R.'s head of the bed elevated to allow the air to escape from the trach incision.

11. That afternoon, a powerful storm causes a power failure. What should you do? **[I/ap/S,PI,PSI/ct,ni,tc]**
    - Get the resuscitation bag, connect it to the portable oxygen tank, and manually ventilate P.R.
    - Reassure her that she is going to be OK and that someone will stay with her until the power is restored.

12. Within minutes of the power failure, the rescue unit arrives at the door. How did they know you needed assistance? **[A/k/PI/ct]**
    - The local rescue unit should be notified, before the patient's discharge, about every ventilator-dependent person residing within their service area. In case of power failure, the unit personnel check on those residents.

13. You evaluate P.R.'s activity tolerance and note that she desaturates when turned to her R side. You auscultate tubular breath sounds in the entire R lung posteriorally. Based on your knowledge of pathophysiology, explain the probable cause of the desaturation. **[PD/an/PI/ct]**
    - Normally, pulmonary tissue carries vibrations from the airways to the anterior chest wall. Because parenchymal tissue is not dense, the vibrations are weak and barely audible with deep inspiration. However, when the parenchyma becomes edematous with large amounts of fluid (as occurs during infection), the pulmonary tissue augments the vibration of inspiratory air waves through the chest wall, which result in the auscultation of tubular breath sounds. In addition, it becomes increasingly more difficult for gases to diffuse through the thickened membranes; thus, when oxygen demands increase, as with increased activity, the body is unable to meet the increased demand and the blood becomes desaturated.

You notify the physician of the change in P.R.'s breath sounds. The paramedic unit transports P.R. to the hospital where she is readmitted for recurring pneumonia.

14. P.R.'s husband arrived shortly after the paramedics transported P.R. to the hospital. He collapses into the nearest chair, tears begin to roll down his cheeks, and he says, "It has been almost a month now. Are you sure she will recover?" How would you respond? **[I/ap/PSI/ni,tc]**
    - Assure him that P.R. will recover. Reinforce that the recovery time varies from person to person but most people with Guillain-Barré syndrome recover in weeks to months with little to no residual lung impairment.
    - Validate his feelings of frustration and disappointment. Tell him that it has been hard on him, that both he and P.R. have been through a tremendous ordeal. Reassure him that it will end.
    - Ask him if he has anyone to talk to such as family or a support group.

P.R. underwent aggressive antibiotic therapy and was discharged to home 5 days later. P.R. progressed slowly. It took 4 months for her to recover, but recovery was complete.

Case Study 15: Emphysema

Difficulty: ***	*Setting:* Hospital
Index Words: Emphysema	

D.Z., a 65-year-old man, is admitted to a medical floor for exacerbation of his emphysema (COPD). He has a PMH of HTN, which has been well controlled by enalopril (Vasotec) for the last 6 years. He presents as a thin, poorly nourished man who is experiencing difficulty breathing. He complains of coughing spells that are productive of thick yellow sputum. D.Z. seems irritable and anxious when he tells you that he has been a 2-pack a day smoker for 38 years. He complains that he sleeps poorly and lately feels very tired most of the time. His VS are 162/84, 124, 36, 102°F, SaO_2 88%. His admitting diagnosis is chronic emphysema with an acute exacerbation; etiology to be determined. His admitting orders are as follows: diet as tolerated; out of bed with assistance; O_2 at 2 L/NC; maintenance IV of D_5W at 50 ml/h; sputum C&S x 3; ABGs in AM; CBC, Chem 7, and theophylline level on admission; CXR in AM; prednisone 40 mg PO tid; cefuroxime (Zinacef) 1 g IVPB q8h; theophylline (Theo-Dur) 300 mg PO bid; albuterol aerosolized 2.5 mg (0.5 ml) in 3 ml NS q6h; enalapril (Vasotec) 10 mg PO q AM.

1. Explain the pathophysiology of emphysema. **[A/k/PI/ct]**
   - Emphysema results when the membranes between alveoli are destroyed and larger alveolar spaces are created. These alveolar membranes contain pulmonary capillaries and elastic fibers. The function of the elastic fibers are to hold open the small airways during expiration. Thus, destruction of alveolar membranes results in premature closure of the small airways and air trapping during expiration.

2. Are D.Z.'s VS and SaO_2 appropriate? If not, explain why. **[A/c/PI/ct]**
   - His SBP should be $\leq$140 mm Hg.
   - HR is tachycardic (124).
   - RR fast (36) due to hypoxemia.
   - Temp is elevated and may indicate an inflammation/infection.
   - Oximeter is low (88%) because of poor diffusion of oxygen across alveolar membrane.
   - Hypoxemia has contributed to anxiety, and anxiety is making the hypoxemia worse.

3. Identify 3 nursing measures that you could try to improve oxygenation. **[P/ap/PI,PSI/ct,ni]**
   - Positioning: sit patient in a chair that has arm rests; elevating his arms lifts the rib cage and allows more lung expansion.
   - Diaphragmatic breathing: encourages the patient to think about coordinating breathing to provide maximum lung expansion.
   - Pursed-lip breathing: may increase pressure throughout the airways and allow airways to stay open longer; more air may be expelled.
   - Anxiety: can increase the patient's sense of dyspnea; try controlled relaxation breathing exercises and/or biofeedback.

4. Explain the main purpose of the following classes of drugs: antibiotics, bronchodilators, and corticosteroids. **[A/k/PI/ct]**
   - Antibiotics kill or suppress the growth of microorganisms.
   - Bronchodilators reduce airway resistance.
   - Corticosteroids inhibit the number and activity of antiinflammatory cells, inhibit bronchoconstriction, and relax smooth muscles (bronchioles).

5. What are the 2 most common side effects of bronchodilators? **[A/k/PI/ct]**
   - Tremors.
   - Tachycardia.

6. You deliver D.Z.'s dietary tray and he comments how hungry he is. As you leave the room he is rapidly consuming the mashed potatoes. When you pick up the tray you notice that he hasn't touched anything else. When you question him he states, "I don't understand it. I can be so hungry, but when I start to eat I have trouble breathing and I have to stop." Explain this phenomenon based on your knowledge of the breakdown of carbohydrates (CHO). **[PD/c/PI/ct]**
   - Carbohydrates (CHO) break down into CO_2, which is eliminated by the respiratory system; increased CO_2 levels stimulate the respiratory system to increase respirations. The respiratory system is already taxed and is unable to meet the increased workload of the CHO load. The patient experiences shortness of breath and becomes anorectic.

7. Identify 3 strategies that might improve his caloric intake. **[P/ap/PI/ct,ni]**
   - Provide small, frequent meals.
   - Provide supplemental higher-fat foods.
   - Arrange for the family to bring the patient's favorite foods (try to avoid high carbohydrates and high sodium).
   - Include D.Z.'s wife in the discussion because problems with appetite often persist after discharge from the hospital.

8. Identify 3 expected outcomes of D.Z.'s treatment. **[P/an/PI/ct]**
   - Subjective reports of absence of dyspnea at rest and minimal dyspnea on exertion.
   - A decrease in respiratory rate and an increase in depth of respirations.
   - Return to prehospital ABGs.
   - Improved appetite

9. You answer D.Z.'s call light and he asks for a carton of milk. You remind him that milk causes an increased production of thick mucus. He replies, "Yes, but you told me that I had to have lots of protein." How should you respond? **[E/ap/PI/ct,ni,tc]**
   - Yes, a high protein, moderate fat, and moderate-CHO diet is very important to people who have lung disease. But, milk and milk products can cause thick mucus production in many patients, thereby, making it more difficult to breathe.

10. You notice a box of dark chocolate on D.Z.'s overbed table. He tells you that he wakes at night and eats 4 to 5 pieces of chocolate. Several of your COPD patients have identified a craving for chocolate in the past. What is the basis for this craving? **[A/c/PI/ct]**
    - Chocolate contains theobromine which acts to relax smooth muscles, including those of the bronchioles. Milk chocolate contains 5 mg theobromine per ounce, cocoa 5 to 10 mg/oz, and dark chocolate 35 mg/oz.

11. What would you do to address dietary and nutritional teaching needs with D.Z. and his wife? **[P/c/PI/ct,ni]**
    - Request that a registered dietitian (RD) consult with C.K. and his wife concerning the specific needs and requirements of the COPD patient. The RD can help them individualize his dietary plan.

12. List 6 educational topics that you need to explore with D.Z. **[P/ap/S,PI,PSI/ct,ni,tc]**
    - Infection control.
    - Activity and exercise.
    - Medication regimen including importance of keeping a current list of medications and allergies with him.
    - Fluid requirements.
    - When to seek medical attention.
    - Home oxygen therapy.
    - Pulmonary hygiene.

D.Z.'s wife approaches you in the hallway and says, "I don't know what to do. My husband used to be so active before he retired 6 months ago. Since then he's lost 35 pounds. He is afraid to take a bath and it takes him hours to dress—that's if he dresses at all. He has gone downhill so fast that it scares me. He's afraid to do anything for himself; he wants me within calling distance at all times. I have to keep working. His medical bills are draining all our savings, and I have to be able to support myself when he's gone. You know, sometimes I go to work just to get away from the house and his constant demands. He calls me several times a day asking me to come home, but I can't go home and I don't want to. I just don't know what to do."

13. How would you respond to her? **[E/an/PI,PSI,HP/ct,ni,tc]**
    - Reassure her that her experiences and feelings are typical of those expressed by many spouses of patients with COPD. Inform her about the Better Breathers Club (BBC) of the local chapter of The American Lung Association; that the BBC offers education and social support for COPD patients and their families and significant others. Tell her that she needs to be able to vent her feelings and get advice from people who are in her same situation. Reinforce that it is something she has to do for herself.
    - Wish her well. Spouses experience considerable suffering in living with someone with COPD. They are often left embittered, emotionally exhausted, and financial drained.

CHAPTER 3. MUSCULOSKELETAL DISORDERS

Case Study 1: Osteoporosis

Difficulty: *	*Setting:* Outpatient clinic
Index Words: Osteoporosis	

M.B. is a 55-year-old woman presenting to the clinic complaining of episodes of feeling "hot and sweaty" during the day and waking up at night soaked with perspiration. Because her sleep is so disrupted, she is tired all day and is having trouble concentrating at work. She says that the episodes are becoming unbearable and is seeking treatment for them.

1. You suspect she is premenopausal. You obtain her prior medical and surgical history and her current medication regimen. List 3 questions that would be important to ask in exploring the possibility of menopause being related to her symptoms. **[A/k/Pl/ct]**
   - Did her mother or sisters experience a natural menopause (not a surgically or medically induced menopause)? At what age?
   - How often are her menstrual periods at this time and how would she describe them?
   - Does she experience other symptoms, such as fatigue, depression, crying spells, difficulty thinking or concentrating, dizziness or fainting spells, irritability, painful vaginal intercourse, mild stress incontinence, dry skin, and cardiac palpitations.

2. You are concerned with the possible development of osteoporosis in M.B. List at least 8 questions you would ask to determine her risk for development of osteoporosis. **[A/k/Pl/ct]**
   - Does she smoke? (This is a very powerful risk factor!)
   - Does she drink?
   - What is her weight for height?
   - How often and how vigorously does she exercise, and what type of exercise does she do?
   - What is her typical diet with emphasis on quantifying intake of dairy products, fruits, green vegetables, and fat.
   - What is her intake of carbonated beverages?
   - Does she currently take estrogen replacement, phenytoin (Dilantin), calcium supplements, or aluminum antacids? Does she take supplemental vitamin D?
   - Does she have a history of glucocorticoid intake?
   - Does she currently experience joint or back pain?
   - Does she have a family history of osteoporosis?

   Instructor Note: Because vitamin D is essential to calcium metabolism in the body, calcium supplement without additional vitamin D, especially in northern climates, may be of little value. Also, beware the "classic" high-risk profile of the "slender, white female smoker."

3. She is not currently taking estrogen replacement therapy. What 3 questions would be important to ask M.B. to determine if there are any contraindications or precautions to this therapy for her? **[A/k/PI/ct,tc]**
   - Does she have a history (personal or family) of uterine or breast cancer and when was her last mammogram?
   - Does she have a history of cerebrovascular disease, thrombophlebitis, or pulmonary embolism?
   - Does she have a history of liver, gallbladder, renal, or pancreatic disease?
   - Does she or a first degree relative have IDDM?

4. M.B. says that she does have frequent "backaches." Spinal films are ordered. Later you receive a report stating that the films appear normal with no significant findings. What would be an appropriate explanation of these findings? **[PD/c/PI/tc]**
   - There is usually a loss of at least 30% to 50% of bone mass before radiolucency is seen on x-ray identifying osteoporosis. Dual beam photometry is a much more useful diagnostic test for osteoporosis. Low back pain is frequently an early symptom of osteoporosis. It also is a symptom of poor muscle strength in the back and postural muscles.

5. What would be appropriate supportive measures for M.B. to relieve the noninjury-related low back pain in the absence of fracture? **[P/k/S,PI,HP/ct]**
   - Hyperextension exercises to strengthen paravertebral muscles.
   - Avoid heavy lifting and falls.
   - Consistent exercise specific for her age and condition.
   - Proper body mechanics.
   - Heat application prn for discomfort, with cold applied to acute injuries.
   - NSAIDs.
   - Refer her to a physical therapist for evaluation for orthotics (prescribed shoe inserts to correct weight distribution on feet).

6. M.B. reports that she does not like milk or milk products and rarely includes them in her diet. How can M.B. increase her calcium intake at this time? **[P/an/HP/ct,tc]**
   - Include seafood and green vegetables in her diet.
   - Decrease her fat intake and phosphorus intake (diet soda).
   - Try to get adequate exposure to sunshine and take products that are supplemented with vitamin D. Caution M.B. to wear sunscreen.
   - Take a calcium supplement, such as calcium carbonate or calcium gluconate, in divided doses and with meals to increase absorption.

7. M.B.'s physician told her that her blood calcium was normal. "If I have enough calcium in my blood, I couldn't have osteoporosis, could I?" she asks you. How will you respond and why? **[A/k/PI/ct,tc]**
   - You will explain that blood calcium is not a good diagnostic test for osteoporosis. People can have large calcium losses from bone and still have normal blood levels.

8. M.B. says she rarely exercises. What advice should be given concerning exercise? **[P/k/HP/ct,tc]**
   - Exercise regularly to decrease calcium loss from bones. Emphasize movement and weight-bearing.
   - Start slowly and increase very gradually. Walking is excellent. Bicycling, stationary cycling, and low-impact aerobic movement/dancing are also effective. Avoid jogging because it adds pressure to weight-bearing joints.

9. M.S. states she still is not certain she has a well-balanced diet with sufficient calcium and vitamin D. What would you suggest to her? **[P/ap/PI,PSI,HP/ct,ni,tc]**
   - Refer her to a registered dietician for dietary analysis and recommendations.
   - Use a quality nutritional analysis computer program.

Case Study 2: Low Back Strain

Difficulty: *	*Setting:* Hospital ED, home
Index Words: Low back strain, rehabilitation	

J.C. is a 41-year-old man who comes to the ED C/O acute low back pain. He states that he did some heavy lifting yesterday, went to bed with a mild backache, and awoke this morning with terrible back pain. He admits to having had several episodes of similar back pain each year over the last 10 years. In the past, the pain has been treated by diazepam, codeine, and several weeks of bed rest. J.C. has a PMH of duodenal ulcer and takes Prilosec for symptom relief. He is 6 ft tall, weighs 265 lb, and has a prominent "pot belly." The ED admitting clerk calls J.C.'s insurance company to authorize payment for treatment at your facility. J.C.'s HMO has identified him as a consumer of "high cost care" with poor prior outcome. The ED is authorized to perform emergency treatment only and the case manager will make a home visit within 24 hours to devise a treatment plan. The ED physician diagnoses muscular strain of the lower back and orders the following: cyclobenzaprene (Flexeril) 10 mg QID, Feldene 20 mg QD; bed rest for 2 days then gradually increase activity; ice packs to the lower back 30 minutes out of every hour.

You are a case manager (RN) working for Grubabuck HMO and make the initial visit to J.C.'s residence. His wife lets you in and you find J.C. lying on the sofa with his knees flexed and watching videos.

1. What questions would be appropriate to ask J.C. in evaluating the extent of his back pain and injury? **[A/c/PI/ct]**
   - Obtain a clear chronologic narrative of problem onset, setting, manifestation, and treatment. Principal symptoms should be described.
   - Location: Where does it hurt? (Etc.)
   - Quality: What does it feel like?
   - Quantity or severity: How bad is it?
   - Timing (onset, duration, frequency): When does it happen or when is it worse?
   - Setting: Where are they when it happens or under what conditions is it worse?
   - Factors that aggravate or relieve the pain: What makes it feel better? What makes it worse?
   - Associated manifestations: Is there anything else they feel with it?
   - The meaning of the symptom to the patient and the impact on his/her life.

2. What observable characteristic does J.C. have that makes him highly susceptible to low back injury and chronic pain? **[A/c/S,PI/ct]**
   - His "pot belly" puts undue strain on his lower back muscles.

3. Why do you think that cyclobenzaprine was prescribed instead of diazepam? **[I/c/S,PI,PSI/ct,ni]**
   - Cyclobenzaprine is a centrally acting skeletal muscle relaxant.
   - Diazepam is a schedule IV drug because of the risk of abuse. It is a sedative hypnotic, anticonvulsant, and muscle relaxant.

4. What does J.C. need to know concerning Feldene considering his PMH? **[P/c/PI/ct,ni,tc]**
   - Feldene can precipitate peptic ulceration and GI bleeding as with other NSAIDS. J.C. should be instructed to take Feldene with food and if he should experience abdominal pain or other GI discomfort, he should contact his physician before continuing with the medication.

You determine that J.C. needs an interdisciplinary approach to treatment and rehabilitation for his chronic back problem. Your goal is to minimize J.C.'s long-term health care costs by rehabilitating his back, helping him reduce his weight to reduce stress on his back, and treating his current injury. You coordinate referrals for J.C. to see four health care experts on your team.

5. You refer J.C. to a physiatrist. What is a physiatrist, and what can a physiatrist do to help J.C.? **[PD/k/S,PI,HP/ct]**
   - A physiatrist specializes in injury prevention and medical rehabilitation. Physiatrists have an M.D. or D.O. and have specialty training in their field.

6. What expert would work with J.C. to help him lose weight? What are her/his credentials? **[PD/k/S,PI,PSI,HP/ct]**
   - A dietician would be the health care expert to help J.C. in weight loss through healthy eating patterns. A dietician has a bachelor's degree or higher and is designated as an R.D. (registered dietician) in most states.

7. What kind of expert will work with J.C. using exercise and various treatment modalities to restore his back muscles? **[PD/k/S,PI,HP/ct]**
   - A physical therapist requires a bachelor's or master's degree and is designated as a P.T. or an R.P.T. They use massage, therapeutic exercise, heat, and cold, as well as other modalities to treat a wide variety of problems and injuries. They also specialize in injury prevention.

8. What kind of expert will work with J.C. on body mechanics and strengthening him for occupational- and home-related work? **[PD/k/S,PI,PSI,HP/ct]**
   - An occupational therapist requires a bachelor's or master's degree and is designated as an O.T. or O.T.R. They specialize in optimizing performance of activities of daily living, occupational, and daily role-related activity. They also can help patients with energy-saving techniques.

9. A physical therapist teaches J.C. maintenance exercises he can do on his own to promote back health. What 3 common exercises would be included? **[I/k/S,PI,HP/ct]**
   - Knee-to-chest: Lie on back with knees bent at 90% angle and feet flat on the floor. Clasp hands behind one knee at a time and gently pull toward chest. Alternate knees. Repeat.
   - Partial sit-ups: Lie on back with knees flexed and feet flat on the floor, with arms extended beside knees. Inhale deeply. Tuck chin and exhale while slowly lifting shoulders from the floor. Hold position for count of 5 while continuing to exhale and inhale while slowly returning to resting position. Repeat.
   - Pelvic tilt: Lie on back with knees flexed and feet flat on the floor. Inhale deeply. Exhale slowly as you tighten buttocks and abdomen, pressing back into floor. Hold for count of 5 while exhaling and relax.

Case Study 3: Ankle Sprain

Difficulty: *	*Setting:* Hospital ED
Index Words: Trauma, sprained ankle, substance abuse	

D.M., a 25-year-old man, hops into the ED complaining of right ankle pain. He states that he was playing basketball and stepped on another player's foot, inverting his ankle. You note swelling over the lateral malleolus down to the area of the 4th and 5th metatarsal, and pedal pulses are 3+ bilaterally. His VS are 124/76, 82, 18. He has no allergies and takes no medication. He states he has no prior surgeries or medical problems.

1. When assessing D.M.'s injured ankle, what should be evaluated? **[S/k/PI/ct]**
   - Pulses, pain, paresthesia, paralysis, pallor.

2. What should initial nursing management of the ankle involve that would prevent further swelling and injury to the ankle? **[I/ap/PI/ni]**
   - The ankle should be immobilized with the leg elevated above the patient's heart. Ice bags should be applied to the ankle, and elastic wrap should be used to apply mild compression.

3. You note there is significant swelling over the 4th and 5th metatarsal. How would you further evaluate this finding? **[A/ap/PI/ct]**
   - Apply pressure over the area to assess for pain. If pain is present, x-ray films should include the ankle as well as the foot. Inversion injuries commonly result in fracture of the 5th metatarsal.

X-rays are negative for fracture and a third degree sprain is diagnosed. The physician orders an ankle splint with elastic wrap and crutches with instructions. The physician instructs D.M. not to bear weight on his ankle for 2 days.

4. Describe the technique for applying an elastic wrap. Give the rationale. **[I/c/S,PI/ct]**
   - The elastic wrapping should begin distally to prevent milking of venous blood flow and extravascular fluid downward. The wrap should be unrolled with very little tension and should be smooth and without wrinkles. A figure-8 wrap should be used at the ankle joint. Capillary refill should be checked after application.

5. When instructing D.M. to use crutches, his weight should rest on what part of his body while the crutch is bearing the weight? Explain why. **[I/c/S,PI/ni,tc]**
   - His hands, wrists, and arms. The axillary area should never be used to support the weight; this can result in nerve damage. The top of the crutches should be 2 fingerwidths below the axilla. Arms should be kept straight with hands on the grips.

6. You are to instruct D.M. on application of cold and heat, activity, and care of the ankle. What would be appropriate instructions in these areas? **[I/k/S,PI/ni,tc]**
   - Do not bear weight on the affected ankle for 48 hours. Use crutches for walking.
   - Remain on bed rest as much as possible with affected ankle elevated on pillows (above the heart) for 48 hours.
   - Apply an ice bag to the ankle for 20 minutes out of every hour while awake.

7. D.M. is given a prescription for acetominophen/hydrocodone (Lortab) for pain. What instructions concerning this medication should you give him on discharge? **[I/c/S,PI/ct,ni,tc]**
   - D.M. should not combine this drug with other medications without checking with a pharmacist first. Lortab should never be taken with alcohol. He should not drive or operate heavy machinery after taking the medication. Patients with a history of heavy alcohol consumption should be warned against using medications containing acetaminophen.

8. Four days later D.M. hobbles into the ED and sheepishly informs you that he "did it again, only this time it was touch football." He states that the pain pills worked so well he thought it would be OK. You detect the odor of beer on his breath. What are you going to do? **[A,I/c,an/S,PI,PSI/ct,ni]**
   - Elevate, ice, and assess the ankle.
   - Raise the siderails, instruct him not to climb out of bed, and provide a call button.
   - Obtain VS and assess neurologic status (assess his level of ETOH-related impairment).
   - Ask D.M. how much beer he has ingested, how long ago, how many pain pills he took, and when he took them.
   - Inform the physician of his recent visit to the ED, prescribed medication, and current problem.

9. You remove his sock and find a large hematoma forming on the lateral aspect of the ankle. You inquire about D.M.'s pain perception. He states, "It doesn't feel too bad now but I sure saw stars when it popped." What is the significance of his statement? **[PD/c/S,PI,PSI/ct]**
   - His ankle is probably fractured.
   - He has ingested a significant quantity of beer; enough to dull his sensory perception.

Case Study 4: Rheumatoid Arthritis with Hip Arthroplasty

Difficulty: *	*Setting:* Hospital
Index Words: Arthroplasty, infection, rheumatoid arthritis	

S.P. is admitted to the orthopedic ward. She has fallen at home and has sustained an intracapsular fracture of the hip at the femoral neck. The following history is obtained from her. She is a 75-year-old widow with 3 children living nearby. Her father died of cancer at 62 years of age; mother died of CHF at 79 years of age. Ht 5'3", wt 118 lb. She has a 50 pack/year smoking history and denies alcohol use. She had severe rheumatoid arthritis with UGI bleed in 1993 and CAD with CABG 9 months ago. Since that time she has engaged in "very mild exercises at home." VS are 128/60, 98, 14, 37.2°C. Medications: nizatidine (Axid) 150 mg bid, prednisone (Deltasone) 5 mg PO qd, and methotrexate (Amethopterin) 2.5 mg/weekly.

1. List 4 risk factors for hip fractures. **[PD/k/PI/ct]**
   - Age; high-risk for fall.
   - Decreased estrogen (menopause).
   - Smoking.
   - Lack of exercise.
   - Corticosteroid therapy.
   - Antimetabolite therapy.

2. Place a check (✓) mark next to each of the responses in #1 that represent S.P.'s risk factors. **[PD/c/PI/ct]**
   - All of them are applicable.

S.P. is taken to surgery for a total hip replacement. Because of the intracapsular location of the fracture, the surgeon chooses to perform an arthroplasty rather than internal fixation.

3. List 4 critical potential postoperative problems for S.P., and explain why you think each is important. **[P/c/S,PI/ct]**
   - Potential for bleeding.
   - Potential for atelectasis .
   - Potential for pneumonitis.
   - Potential for DVT.
   - Potential for embolism.

4. How would you monitor for excessive postoperative blood loss? **[P/c/S,PI/ct,ni]**
   - Monitor amount of drainage in drainage system (100-150 ml/h is excessive and should be reported) or on dressing.
   - Observe vital signs q 15 min X 4, q 30 min X 4, q 1 hour X 4, then q 4 hours.
   - Minotor Hct levels.

5. There are 2 main goals for maintaining proper alignment of S.P.'s operative leg. What are they, and how are they achieved? **[P/k/S,Pl/ct,ni]**
   - Abduction of the hip should be maintained by using pillows or an abduction bolt between S.P.'s legs.
   - Extreme flexion of the hip is avoided by elevating the head of the bed no more than 60 degrees.

6. Postoperative wound infection is a concern for S.P. Describe what you would do to monitor S.P. for wound infection. **[I/c/S,Pl/ct,ni]**
   - Monitor vital signs at least every 4 hours.
   - Monitor amount and character of drainage from incision.
   - Monitor for indicators of joint infection, such as warmth, edema, decreased range of motion, fever, and purulent drainage.
   - Monitor nutritional status.
   - Monitor hematocrit/hemoglobin, white blood count, and differential.

7. Taking S.P's rheumatoid arthritis into consideration, what interventions should be implemented to prevent complications secondary to immobility? **[I/k/S,Pl/ct,ni]**
   - Active range of motion exercises in nonsurgical joints to prevent stiffness and pain.
   - Use TED hose or sequential compression devices on legs and/or feet.
   - Reposition and provide skin care every 2 hours. Monitor for development of pressure sores.
   - Deep breathe and cough. Monitor breath sounds, O_2 saturation, and secretions.

8. What predisposing factor, identified in S.P.'s medical history, places her at risk for infection, bleeding, and anemia? **[PD/c/S,Pl/ct]**
   - She has been taking methotrexate, which may cause leukopenia, thrombocytopenia, or anemia.

9. Explain 4 techniques you will teach her to help her protect herself from infection r/t medication-induced immune suppression. **[I/c/S,Pl,HP/ct,ni,tc]**
   - Effective hand washing.
   - Identifying and avoiding people with communicable diseases.
   - Avoid uncooked foods.
   - How to identify prodromal signs of infection and promptly seek medical intervention.
   - Use dishwasher with hot water to wash dishes to prevent contamination.

Case Study 5: Fractured Tibia Fibula with Osteomyelitis

Difficulty: *	*Setting:* Hospital
Index Words: Trauma	

H.K. is a 26-year-old man who tried to light a cigarette while driving and lost control of his jeep. The jeep flipped and landed on the passenger side. H.K. was transported to the ED with a deformed, edematous R lower leg and a deep puncture wound approximately 5 cm long over the deformity. Blood continues to ooze from the wound.

1. What further assessment should the nurse make of the leg injury and what precautions should she take in making this assessment? **[A,P/c,ap,Pl/ct]**
   - The 5 Ps should be assessed: pain, pulses, pallor, paralysis, and paresthesia. However, when an open fracture is suspected or when obvious displacement of bone is present, the limb should be immobilized and the patient should not be asked to demonstrate mobility. Toes or fingers can be wiggled when fractured arms or legs are being assessed.

2. What would be the most appropriate method for controlling bleeding at this wound site? **[P,Ic/Pl/ct,ni]**
   - A heavy dressing of gauze sponges applied over the site with light pressure should be sufficient. Oozing will usually subside or diminish considerably with heavy dressing and a little time.

3. What is the best way to immobilize the leg injury before surgery? **[P/K/Pl/ct]**
   - A posterior splint made of metal, plaster, or plastic (whatever is available) padded with soft roll then wrapped with gauze will allow for swelling of the extremity, bleeding of the wound, and further assessment and management of the injury.

H.K. is taken to surgery for internal fixation of the tibia and fibula fractures. He returns with a full leg cast.

4. Describe nursing assessment of a patient with a long leg cast involving trauma and surgery. **[P,I/c/Pl/ct,ni]**
   - The 5 P's should be assessed, paying special attention to capillary refill, temperature, color, movement, and sensation of toes.
   - Assess tightness of cast at edges because continued swelling may result in tightening of cast and compartment syndrome.
   - Assess for increasing or excessive pain because these may indicate infection or ischemia.
   - Assess drainage on cast by drawing a line around edges of drainage at regular intervals.
   - Assess odor of cast. Foul odor of cast may indicate infection.

5. In assessing H.K.'s cast on the third day postop, you notice a strong foul odor. Drainage on the cast is extending and H.K. is complaining of pain more often and seems considerably more uncomfortable. VS are 123/78, 102, 18, 39°C. What is your analysis of these findings? **[PD/an/Pl/ct]**
   - H.K. exhibits symptoms of infection and is a likely candidate for a posttraumatic osteomyelitis. Findings must be reported to the physician so further treatment can be initiated.

H.K. returns to surgery. The wound over H.K.'s fracture site has become necrotic with purulent drainage. The wound is debrided and cultured then a posterior splint is applied. H.K. returns to his room with orders for wet to moist dressing changes. The physician suspects osteomyelitis and orders ampicillin (Unasyn), nafcillin (Unipen), and gentamycin (Gentak).

6. As you continue to assess H.K. over the following days, what evidence will you look for that antibiotics are effectively treating the infection? **[P/k/Pl/ct,ni]**
   - WBCs will decrease on lab work.
   - Patient temperature will be within normal limits.
   - Wound will show signs of healing and purulent drainage will cease.
   - Pain in leg will decrease.

7. What should H.K. be taught concerning the care of his cast? **[P,1/ap/Pl/ct,ni,tc]**
   - Do not put powders, especially those containing corn starch, or lotions inside the cast. The corn provides food for bacterial growth, and lotions can macerate the skin.
   - If he perspires under the cast, blow cool air into the end of the cast using a hair dryer.
   - If it itches under the cast, *do not* insert objects between the cast and skin to scratch.
   - Immediately report numbness, tingling, burning, pallor, cyanosis, change in temperature, tenderness, drainage, and unusual or severe pain.

Case Study 6: Fractured Hip with Postoperative Complication

Difficulty: **	*Setting:* Hospital
Index Words: Fracture, pulmonary embolus	

M.M., a 76-year-old retired schoolteacher, underwent ORIF of his R femur. He has been on bed rest for the first 2 days postoperatively. 0600 VS were 132/84, 80 reg, 18 unlabored, and 37.2°C. He is AA&Ox3 (awake, alert, and oriented). No adventitious heart sounds. Breath sounds are clear but diminished in the bases bilaterally. Bowel sounds are active in all 4 quadrants, and he is taking sips of clear liquids. An IV of D_5½ NS is infusing TKO in his L hand and should be saline locked in the AM if he is able to maintain adequate PO fluid intake. His lab work shows Hct 34%, Hgb 11.3 mg/dl, K 4.1 mEq/L, PTT 44 seconds. Pain is controlled with neperidine (Demerol) 25 mg and promethazine (Phenergan) 25 mg IM q3h. He is also taking Nitropatch, heparin 5000 units SQ bid, and docusate sodium.

At 2330 on the second postoperative day, you answer M.M.'s call light and find him lying in bed breathing rapidly and rubbing his R chest. He complains of R-sided chest pain and appears to be restless.

1. What are you going to do? **[PD/an/PI/ct,ni]**
   - Take VS.
   - Rapidly assess heart, lungs, and neurologic status.
   - If readily available, obtain pulse oximeter reading.

He is slightly hypotensive, tachycardic, tachypneic, restless, and slightly confused. The pulse oximeter reads 86%, so you start him on 3-6 L O_2/nc. You identify faint crackles in the posterior bases bilaterally; they were clear this AM.

2. You contact the physician. What information is important to report? **[P,I/an/PI/ct,ni,tc]**
   - Identify yourself, the patient, the diagnosis, attending physician, and postop status. Give a quick summary of M.M.'s progress since surgery.
   - Tell how M.M. turned the call light on (indicates cognitive awareness) and c/o pain in his R chest.
   - He was slightly hypotensive, tachycardic, tachypneic, restless, and slightly confused.
   - He has crackles in posterior bases; his lungs were clear this AM.
   - You started him on O_2, because his SaO_2 reading was 86%.

3. The physician orders ABGs on room air, continuous pulse oximetry, STAT CXR, and STAT 12-lead ECG. What information will the physician gain from each of the above? **[A/c/PI/ct]**
   - ABGs: oxygenation status.
   - Pulse oximetry: monitor oxygenation trends.
   - CXR: determine fluid status in lungs.
   - ECG: determine rate, rhythm, and ischemia.

4. Why would the physician order a blood gas on room air as opposed to with supplemental O_2? **[A/c/PI/ct]**
   - The physician wants to evaluate his pulmonary status. An A-a gradient is best obtained on room air or 100% O_2. This will help determine the need for a V/Q (ventilation/perfusion) scan. Simply remove M.M. from oxygen for 20 minutes and obtain ABGs.

The ABGs return as follows: pH 7.55, $PaCO_2$ 24 mm Hg, HCO_3 24 mEq/L, and PaO_2 56 mm Hg at sea level. SaO_2 is 86% on room air. Chest x-ray shows a small R infiltrate. VS are 150/92, 110, 28, 37.2°C.

5. What is your interpretation of the ABGs, and what do you think the physician will order next? **[PD/c/PI/ct]**
   - ABGs show an acute respiratory alkalosis with hypoxemia. The physician will probably order a V/Q scan and PTT. If the scan shows a probable pulmonary emboli, a heparin infusion will be initiated.

6. The V/Q is performed, and the interpretation reads "strongly suggestive of a pulmonary embolus." What are the most likely sources of the embolus? **[PD/k/PI/ct]**
   - Deep vein thromboembolism from immobility.
   - Fatty embolism from femoral fracture.

7. Based on the latest PTT of 40 seconds, the physician orders a heparin bolus of 5000 units IV followed by an infusion of 1200 units/hour. The PTT 4 hours later is >120 seconds. Based on these results, what action would you take? **[I/ap/PI/ct,ni]**
   - The physician should be notified and the infusion should be stopped or reduced with follow-up PTT. PTT should be 2 to 2½ times the control value.

8. The next day, the physician's orders read, "Coumadin 2.5 mg, PT in AM, DC heparin." What is wrong with these orders? **[A/ap/S,PI/ct]**
   - It will take 3 days for warfarin (Coumadin) to have an effect. Heparin should be continued until the PT levels are within a therapeutic range on warfarin, then the heparin should be DC'd. A PT should not be drawn until after 3 days of warfarin therapy; this will save M.M. some money.

9. Thrombolytics, such as streptokinase and urokinase, have been beneficial in the treatment of pulmonary embolus. Why would this medication be contraindicated in M.M.'s case? **[A/ap/S,PI/ct]**
   - M.M. has had surgery within the past 10 days, placing him at risk for hemorrhage if thrombolytics are used.

10. List 3 priority nursing diagnoses for M.M. related to his present status. **[PD/an/S,PI/ct]**
    - Impaired gas exchange r/t pulmonary embolism and V/Q mismatch.
    - Ineffective breathing pattern r/t hypoxemia and pain.
    - Tisk for inadequate tissue perfusion r/t hemorrhage secondary to anticoagulant therapy.
    - Risk for infection related to surgery, immobility, and ineffective breathing pattern.

11. Several days later, you hear M.M. requesting his son to bring in a "decent razor" because he is tired of the stubble left by the unit's shaver. How would you address this issue? **[I/ap/S,PI/ct,ni,tc]**
    - Get their attention, and ask if anyone has told him about why he is supposed to use a shaver instead of a razor.
    - Inform both of them that M.M. is taking a blood thinner and is not permitted to use a straight razor because of the risk of bleeding.

Case Study 7: Finger Amputation

Difficulty: **	*Setting:* Hospital ED
Index Words: Trauma, amputation	

You are working in the ED when a 27-year-old man runs through the door with a blood-soaked towel over his left hand. D.W., a machinist, states he caught his hand in an automatic shear and cut off his left index finger. His coworker has the finger wrapped in a paper towel. You grab a pair of gloves while you direct D.W. to lay on a stretcher where you remove the towel and apply firm pressure to the stump with sterile sponges. A coworker takes his VS and announces 196/122, 144, 22. To distract him, you gather information about his PMH, allergies, and tetanus status. He has a history of depression for which he takes Prozac and is allergic to Darvocet. He has no significant medical history other than depression.

1. What is your first nursing priority in dealing with D.W.'s amputated finger? **[P/a/S,Pl/ct]**
   - Control the bleeding of the amputated finger.

2. D.W.'s finger is bleeding profusely. Would you apply a tourniquet to the finger or not, and why? **[I/ap/S,Pl/ct,ni]**
   - You would not apply a tourniquet because this would compromise circulation to the tip of the amputated digit. Direct pressure around the tip of the digit with sterile sponges would be the best way to control the bleeding.

3. An x-ray of the index finger reveals an amputation of the proximal DIP joint. The fracture has left a jagged protruding bone that can be seen from the distal tip. After controlling the bleeding, what would be the appropriate management? **[P/an/Pl/ct]**
   - Handle the finger with sterile technique, and prepare for immediate intravenous administration of antibiotics.

4. What would be suitable treatment of the amputated appendage? **[P/ap/Pl/ni]**
   - Wrap the finger in sterile sponges soaked with sterile normal saline. Place the wrapped finger in a plastic bag and place the plastic bag on top of ice. D.W. and the appendage will be evaluated for replantation.

5. D.W. has not had a tetanus shot in the last 10 years. You have run out of adult TD and you only have pediatric DPT available. Would it be suitable to give the pediatric DPT? **[P/c/S,Pl,HP/ct]**
   - A pediatric DPT contains pertussis vaccination which could serve as an antigen in an adult (adults may have anaphylaxis). Obtain the proper vaccination from the pharmacy, or have the medication delivered to surgery or postop unit for administration. D.W. has 72 hours to obtain the tetanus toxoid. Stress the importance of obtaining an injection of tetanus toxoid.

6. What factors influence the success of the reattached digit? **[A/k/Pl/ct]**
   - Finding the digit.
   - Keeping the digit cool to decrease the metabolism within the digit. Be careful not to freeze the tissue.
   - Timing is important. Get the patient to surgery as soon as possible.
   - The condition of the amputated digit.
   - Thorough cleansing of the wound.
   - Prophylactic antibiotics to prevent infection.

7. List 3 nursing diagnoses for D.W. **[PD/an/Pl,PSI/ct]**
   - Risk for infection d/t to open fracture.
   - Body image disturbance r/t traumatic amputation.
   - Acute pain r/t amputation.
   - Impaired tissue integrity r/t traumatic amputation.

8. You repeat his VS and record the following: 118/86, 78, 18. Do you find the VS changes to be reassuring or distressing and why? **[A/an/Pl/ct]**
   - This change is a positive change. He was extremely anxious on arrival and his VS reflected his anxiety as hypertension.
   - If D.W. were becoming shocky, he would be exhibiting such signs and/or symptoms as pallor, tachycardia, increased respiratory rate, and diaphoresis.

9. The OR calls for D.M. Before he leaves you need to start an IV. What type of solution would you hang and why? **[I/ap/S,Pl/ct,ni]**
   - 0.9 NS with blood tubing in case D.M. requires blood during surgery.

10. Why would it be important to further question D.M. about his allergy to Darvocet? **[PD,P/c/Pl/ct]**
    - To determine the extent of a reaction (GI complaints to sudden death).
    - This will help determine future pain management.

Case Study 8: Fractured Mandible and Leg

Difficulty: **	*Setting:* Hospital ED and hospital, rehabilitation center
Index Words: Fracture, trauma	

B.G. is struck by a vehicle while riding his motorcycle and is transported to your ED by ambulance. He is found to have a fractured mandible and multiple fractures of the R tibia and fibula.

1. When a patient comes in with facial trauma such as B.G.s, what two other injuries should you assume exist until ruled out? Explain. **[A/c/S,Pl/ct]**
   - Cervical spine injury and head injury.
   - Because they are not obvious, they can be overlooked and can result in long-term injury or death.

B.G. is taken to the operating room for intermaxillary fixation (wiring of the jaw) and pinning of the fractured tibia and fibula.

2. B.C. returns from surgery with his jaws wired together. What nursing diagnosis or patient problem statement express your primary concern for B.G. postoperatively? **[PD/k/S/ct]**
   - Risk for airway obstruction r/t vomiting with wired jaws.
   - Potential for aspiration of vomitus.
   - If B.G. were to vomit, he will have difficulty expelling the contents of his mouth, and his airway may become blocked.

3. What precautions will you take to ensure a patent airway in B.G. if he begins vomiting while his jaws are wired? **[I/k/S,Pl/ct,ni]**
   - Wire cutters should be kept taped to the head of the bed (visible at all times), and suction equipment (wall suction or suction machine, suction canister, tubing, and tonsilar suction or Yankauer) should be set up at all times. The head of his bed should be elevated to decrease swelling and the likelihood of aspiration. B.G. will likely have a NG tube in place postoperatively, and this should be kept patent and connected to suction to prevent vomiting.

4. If B.G. begins vomiting with his jaws wired, what actions should you take? **[I/c/S,Pl/ct,ni]**
   - Immediately turn B.G. on his side or maintain a sitting position. Suction equipment should be used to suction his mouth as much as possible. The nurse should not hesitate to cut the wires connecting the top teeth and the bottom teeth if unable to clear the airway adequately.

B.C. is transferred to a rehabilitation facility for treatment of his leg injury.

5. His jaw remains wired. What instructions should you give him concerning oral care and safety? **[I/c/S,PI,HP/ct,ni,tc]**
   - Leave a set of wire cutters taped to the head of his bed.
   - He must carry a second set of wire cutters with him at all times.
   - If he vomits, he should lean forward and "blow" food out of his mouth.
   - Mouth care is very important. Some facilities use diluted peroxide or a special mouth rinse for oral care. Teeth should be kept clean with soft toothbrush and WaterPik.

6. During his stay at the rehabilitation facility, what nutritional teaching does B.G. need to prepare him for discharge? **[P,I/c/S,PI/ct,ni,tc]**
   - B.G. should drink high-calorie, high-protein liquids with liquid vitamin supplements or a commercial liquid supplement (instant breakfast-type mixes can be much more cost-effective than commercial preparations).
   - He can expect to lose approximately 10 pounds, but excessive weight loss should be reported to his physician.
   - Do ***not*** try to force solid or semisolid food between the wires!

B.G. has daily dressing changes, antibiotics, and physical therapy; wound debridement is prn.

7. Two weeks after B.G.'s accident, you enter his room to do his afternoon shift assessment. The shades are drawn, he is sitting in the corner with his face to the wall, and you have been told he refused to go to physical therapy this afternoon. He answers your questions in flat, monosyllabic tones. When you ask him what is wrong, he explodes in anger, even more frustrated because his wired jaw keeps him from being able to talk well. What are you going to do? **[A,PD,I/an/PSI/ct,ni,tc]**
   - There are medical emergencies and emotional emergencies. This is an emotional emergency and requires effective crisis management techniques. It is common for people like B.G. who have been "cooped up" and debilitated for more than a few days to "hit bottom." This is a time they become discouraged and overwhelmed by the continuing loss of control and pain or other symptoms. You are very busy but you recognize the importance of acknowledging B.G.'s distress.
     - Sit down. It signals B.C. that you will focus on him without distraction, and it conveys dignity and worth.
     - Express your concern. Ask him to talk to you, to tell you what's going on with him. Some people have trouble articulating their feelings or experiences. Two "permission" statements that can help nurses are:
     - "I've never been through this myself, so I don't know exactly how you feel, but I can imagine it's really (tough/hard/painful/discouraging/frustrating, etc.). Help me understand what you're going through right now...."; and
     - "A lot of folks who go through things like you're going through tell me how (scary/discouraged/frustrated/hopeless/tired of hurting, etc.) they feel. Have *you* had any feelings like that?"
     - Acknowledge the validity of his feelings.
     - Offer to negotiate issues of control. Little changes can make a big difference to someone who is discouraged and miserable.
     - Follow up on your promises and plan.

8. B.G. tells you, "I got a good look at my leg today when the bandage was off...It looks really ugly. I wanted to throw up." What are you going to say? **[I/ap/PSI/ct,tc]**
   - Acknowledge that it takes a long time for wounds like his to heel.
   - The reason he is here is so his leg has the best possible chance for healing.
   - It might look ugly to you for awhile, but we're letting it heal from the inside out. You need to know that you always will have a scar. But we're most concerned that you have a healthy leg.

B.G. was discharged to home but returned to the rehabilitation facility for physical therapy and continued wound management for 3 months. Several months later you see B.G. at the grocery store. You call his name, he waves and walks toward you. You notice that he walks with a slight limp. He tells you that his leg healed but he has pain in his knee when he walks or hikes any distance.

9. What could be causing pain in B.G.'s R knee (remember that his R foreleg had originally been injured)? **[PD/an/PI/ct]**
   - B.G. may be experiencing pain caused by gait changes as a result of his injury.

10. You suggest B.G. ask his physician about a prescription for a foot evaluation and orthotics. What are orthotics and what purpose do they serve? **[PD/c/PI/ct]**
    - B.G. will be referred to a sports medicine center, orthopedist, podiatrist, or physical therapist to have his gait and foot evaluated. Orthotics are mechanical inserts that are placed inside the shoes to correct defects in musculoskeletal structure and function. This will contribute to a normalized gait and relief of the stressed joint that is being "punished" by the attempt to compensate for gait changes.

Case Study 9: Traction for Fractured Femur

Difficulty: **	*Setting:* Hospital
Index Words: Trauma, fracture	

J.F., a 67-year-old woman, was involved in an auto accident and is life-flighted to your facility. She sustained a ruptured spleen, fractured pelvis, and compound fractures of the L femur. On admission she underwent a splenectomy (5 days ago). Her pelvis was stabilized with an external fixator device 3 days ago, and yesterday her L femur was stabilized using balanced suspension with skeletal traction. She has a Thomas ring with Pearson attachment on her L leg. She has 20 lb of skeletal traction and 5 lb applied to the balanced suspension (her L femur is elevated off the bed at approximately 45 degrees, the foreleg is parallel to the bed and lies in a sling that the nurse adjusts on the frame, and the foot hangs freely). This morning S.G. was transferred to your orthopedic unit for specialized care. You are the nurse assigned to care for J.F. on the night shift.

1. You enter J.F.'s room for the first time. What aspects of the traction would you want to inspect? **[A/k/S,Pl/ct,ni]**
   - Inspect body alignment. Does the traction maintain the leg in proper alignment with the rest of the body (not at an angle).
   - Inspect the weights to make sure they hang freely and are well off the floor.
   - Inspect all knots to make sure they are secure and away from the pulleys.
   - Inspect the ropes to make sure they move freely in the pulleys and are not frayed.
   - Inspect all pulleys to make sure they are tightly attached to the support bars.
   - Inspect the position of the sling that supports the lower leg. Make sure the Achilles tendon does not support the weight of the entire lower leg.
   - Inspect the skin around the skeletal pin. Make sure it is not in contact with the frame.
   - Inspect the skeletal pin through the L femur. Make sure it is not in contact with the frame.

2. When inspecting the skeletal pin sites, you note that the skin is reddened for an inch around the pin on both the medial and lateral L leg. What does this finding indicate, and what action would you take? **[I/an/S,Pl/ct,ni]**
   - Slight redness would be expected, but redness that extends for a 1-inch radius from the pin indicates infection.
   - Perform pin care according to physician preference or institutional policy. Use sterile technique.
   - Obtain wound cultures as needed.
   - Check WBC results; note trends and look for increase.
   - Monitor VS.

3. You find J.F.'s body in the lower 75% of the bed, her L upper leg is at an exaggerated angle (>45 degrees), the knot at the end of the bed is caught in the pulley, and the 20-lb weight is dangling just above the floor. What are you going to do? **[I/ap/S,PI/ni]**
   - Get lots of help to lift J.F. to the head of the bed.
   - Have one person pull up slightly on the 20 lb-traction weight, and another person lift up slightly on the 5-lb suspension weight so that the group can move J.F. toward the head of the bed.
   - Have both people gradually release their weights at the same time and observe the L upper leg return to a 45 degree angle.
   - You must recheck the traction mechanics after each position change.

4. When you lift J.F., you notice that her sheets are wet. Because you have lots of help in the room, you decide to change J.F.'s linen. How would you accomplish this task? **[I/ap/S,PI/ct/ni]**
   - First determine why the sheets are wet. If the bed is wet with perspiration, J.F. will need to have a bath blanket placed beneath her torso. If she spilled water in the bed, then the bed can be made with the same quantity and type of linen as you remove from the bed.
   - Obtain all the linen that will be needed, and arrange it in the order that it will be required to change the bed quickly.
   - Lift J.F. vertically while two people quickly strip then remake the bed from the top down.
   - Lower J.F. onto the bed.
   - Everyone gently and simultaneously pull on the sheets to ensure a wrinkle-free surface beneath J.F.

   Instructor Note: Tell the students about a bed roll. A bed roll is made by laying linen on a clean, unoccupied bed and rolling it from the bottom to the top. Once the patient is lifted, two people quickly strip the bed then drape the bottom sheet over the top of the mattress and roll the linen toward the bottom of the bed. This method is very fast and spares the backs of your co-workers.

5. J.F. tells you that she feels like she needs to have a bowel movement but it is too painful to sit on the bedpan. How would you respond? **[I/ap/PI/ct,ni,tc]**
   - Show J.F. a fracture pan and tell her that the flat end fits under her buttock and is not as uncomfortable as the larger pans.
   - Place her on the fracture pan and provide privacy.
   - Make sure she has her call light, and instruct her to turn it on when she is finished.

6. J.F. expels a few small, hard, round pieces of stool. What could be done to promote normal elimination? **[I/c/S,PI/ct,ni]**
   - Institute a bowel regimen (stool softeners, roughage, increase fluid intake, etc).
   - Carefully document each bowel movement.

   Instructor Note: Some facilities provide a chocolate cake that is guaranteed to get results. The recipe calls for prunes to be added. Patients say it is very moist, tastes good, and it works!

You ask J.F. if she is ready for her bath, and she responds positively. You let her bathe the parts she can reach and engage her in a conversation as you attend to the rest of her body. While performing peri care you notice that the folds of skin around her peri area are reddened and excoriated.

7. Given that J.F. has been on antibiotics for the last 5 days, what is the likely cause of the problem, and what needs to be done to encourage healing? **[P/ap/PI/ct]**
   - The most likely cause would be *Candida*.
   - Wash the area with soap and water. Dry thoroughly and allow maximal exposure to the air. Separate opposing skin surfaces by placing a clean, dry wash cloth or gauze pad between the skin surfaces.
   - Institute skin care protocol or inform the physician and follow prescribed treatment.

8. You ask J.F. what she is doing to exercise while she is confined to bed. She looks surprised and states that she isn't doing anything. What activities can J.F. engage in while on bed rest? **[P/ap/PI,HP/ct,ni]**
   - She can pump her right ankle to facilitate circulation in her right leg.
   - Obtain a trapeze and teach J.F. how to use it to lift her upper body off the bed and reposition herself.
   - Obtain a physical therapy consult if not already ordered. PT has elastic bands that can be tied to the siderails to offer resistance to upper extremities, handgrip devices that can be squeezed, putty, etc.

9. You realize that maintaining skin integrity is a challenge in J.F.'s case. What measures will you take to prevent skin breakdown? **[P/k/PI/ct,ni]**
   - Institute pressure point monitoring.
   - Pad any skin that comes into contact with the traction.
   - Frequently reposition J.F.
   - Encourage her to use the trapeze bar to frequently reposition herself.
   - Massage skin over bony prominences.

10. Although J.F. is recovering nicely, she is becoming increasingly withdrawn. You enter her room and find her crying. She tells you that she is all alone here, that she misses her family terribly. You know that her son is flying into town tomorrow but will only be able to stay a few days. What can be done so that J.F. benefits from her family support system? **[P/ap/PSI/ct]**
    - Call the son and have him bring pictures of the grandchildren for J.F.
    - Have the grandchildren tape record messages and send them to J.F.
    - Arrange for uninterrupted time for phone calls.
    - Ask children to draw pictures for grandma's room and tape the pictures to the crossbar over J.F.'s bed (don't just hang them on the wall).
    - Ask J.F. about her children and grandchildren.

Case Study 10: Fractured Hip in Emergency Department

Difficulty: ***	*Setting:* Hospital ED
Index Words: Fracture, compartment syndrome, hypovolemia, hypertension	

You are working in the ED when M.C., an 82-year-old widow, arrives by ambulance. Because M.C. had not answered her phone since noon yesterday, her daughter went to her home to check on her. She found M.C. lying on the kitchen floor, incontinent of urine and stool, and complaining of pain in her R hip. Her daughter reports a PMH of hypertension, angina, and osteoporosis. M.C. takes propanolol (Inderal), nitropatch, indapamide (Lozol), and Premarin daily. The daughter reports that her mother is normally very alert and lives independently. Upon examination, you see an elderly woman, approximately 100 lb, holding her right thigh. You note shortening of the right leg with external rotation and a large amount of swelling at the proximal thigh and right hip. M.C. is oriented to person only and is confused about place and time. M.C.'s VS are 90/65, 120, 24, 36.4° C; her SaO_2 is 89%. Preliminary diagnosis is fracture of the right hip.

1. In view of M.C. history of hypertension and the fact that she has been without her medications for at least 24 hours, explain her current VS. **[PD/c/PI/ct]**
   - She should be hypertensive by this time. However, several factors may have contributed to her low BP, high pulse, high respirations.
     - She may not have had fluid intake for 24 hours, leading to a significant net fluid loss.
     - Her current injury may have contributed to significant compartmentalized intravascular fluid loss.
     - She has lost fluid through urinary and bowel incontinence as well as insensible loss (respiratory).

     This net hypovolemia, characterized by decreased intravascular volume, results in a low BP.
   - In order to compensate for decreased circulating blood volume, the HR increases to try to maintain an adequate cardiac output. The loss of RBCs into the thigh compartment contributes to generalized hypoxemia; respiratory drive increases in an attempt to maintain oxygenation.

2. Based on her history and your initial assessment, what 3 priority interventions should be initiated? **[I,E/an/S,PI/ct,ni]**
   - Titrate administration of O_2/nc to keep SaO_2 above 90%.
   - Start an IV of LR and administer a fluid challenge (administer 200 ml over 5 minutes, evaluate vital signs, then administer another 200 ml over 5 minutes). Then continue to administer IV fluids to support vital signs and urine output.
   - Monitor lung sounds and vital signs for fluid overload because of her history of angina and risk of CHF.

3. M.C.'s daughter states, "Mother is always so clear and alert. I have never seen her act so confused. What's wrong with her?" What are 3 possible causes for M.C.'s disorientation that should be considered and evaluated? **[PD/an/Pl/ct]**
   - Hypovolemia with associated electrolyte imbalances and hypoxemia.
   - Head injury at time of fall.
   - Cerebrovascular accident or cardiac dysrhythmias before the fall, resulting in loss of balance or temporary loss of consciousness.

X-ray films confirmed the diagnosis of intertrochanteric femoral fracture. Knowing that M.C. is going to be admitted, you draw admission labs and call for an orthopedic consult.

4. What laboratory and diagnostic studies would be ordered to evaluate M.C.'s condition, and what critical information will each give you? **[A/an/Pl/ct]**
   - CBC will evaluate blood loss.
   - Chem 8. The Na, K, Cl, CO_2, Ca, and glucose will be used to evaluate electrolyte status. The BUN and creatinine will be used to calculate the BUN/creatinine ratio which is used to evaluate renal function.
   - Urinalysis will assess for presence of hemoglobinuria related to trauma or myoglobinuria related to rhabdomyolysis. Rhabdomyolysis results from prolonged pressure on muscular tissue with damage to cells. Release of myoglobin into vascular system may result in damage to renal tubules that become occluded with myoglobin.
   - Type and crossmatch for 4 units of PRBCs (packed red blood cells) to replace blood loss.
   - PT and PTT to evaluate presence of bleeding disorders.
   - Electrocardiogram is necessary because M.C. is especially at risk for myocardial ischemia, infarction, and presence of dysrhythmias.
   - CXR for admission.

5. What are the 5 Ps that should be guide the assessment of M.C.'s right leg before and after surgery? **[P/k/S,Pl/ct]**
   - Pulses, pallor, pain, paresthesia, paralysis.

6. In evaluating M.C.'s pulses, you find her posterior tibial pulse and dorsalis pedis pulse to be weaker on her right foot than on her left. What would be a possible cause of this finding? **[PD/ap/S,Pl/ct]**
   - This is probably caused by compartment syndrome in which vascular supply is compressed by excessive swelling. This is an emergency condition. Hypovolemia may be a contributing factor if the blood pressure remains low.

7. In planning further care for M.C., list 4 potential complications for which M.C. should be monitored. **[P/ap/Pl/ct]**
   - Risk of fat emboli is high in the presence of long bone fracture.
   - Venous thromboembolism may occur as a result of immobility.
   - Compartment syndrome may occur because of an excessive amount of swelling into tissue that compresses the vasculature and nervous tissue.
   - Hemorrhage into muscle may result in significant blood loss and shock.
   - M.C.'s history places her at higher risk for developing CHF, CVA, or MI.

8. M.C. keeps asking about "Peaches." No one seems to be paying attention. You ask her what she means. She says Peaches is her little dog and she's worried about who is taking care of her. How will you answer? **[I/an/PSI,HP/ni,tc]**
   - You are aware of the significant role pets play in the lives of many elderly. You tell her you will find out and let her know. You ask the daughter to come back to be with her mother and tell the daughter she is asking about Peaches. Ask the daughter to talk to her mother about the anticipated care for her dog. This social support and validating her concerns can contribute toward cognitive stabilization.

M.C. is placed in Buck's traction and sent to the orthopedic unit until an open reduction and internal fixation (ORIF) can be scheduled. M.C.'s cardiovascular, pulmonary, and renal status will be closely monitored.

Case Study 11: Above-the-Knee Amputation

Difficulty: *** *Setting:* Hospital

Index Words: Insulin-dependent diabetes mellitus, above-the-knee amputation, hyperbaric therapy

E.B., a 69-year-old man with insulin-dependent diabetes mellitus (IDDM), is admitted to a large, regional medical center with severe pain in his R foot and lower leg. The foot and lower leg is cool and without pulses (absent by Doppler). Arteriogram demonstrates severe atherosclerosis of the right popliteal artery with complete obstruction of blood flow. Despite attempts at endarterectomy and intravascular urokinase over several days, the foot and lower leg become necrotic. Finally the decision is made to perform an AKA (above the knee amputation) on E.B.'s R leg. E.B. is recently widowed and has a son and daughter who live nearby. In preparation for E.B.s surgery, the surgeons wish to spare as much viable tissue as possible. Hence, an order is written for E.B. to undergo 5 days of hyperbaric therapy for 20 minutes bid.

1. What is the purpose of hyperbaric therapy, and what purpose does it serve in a patient like E.B.? **[PD/c/PI/ct]**
   - It optimizes the viability of hypoxic tissue beds by the process of hyperoxygenation. It can rejuvenate cells that are borderline, but cannot restore cells that are already dead. Hyperbaric oxygenation therapy is the process of administering oxygen to a patient enclosed in a chamber at a pressure greater than sea-level pressure.

As you are preparing E.B. for surgery, he is quiet and withdrawn. He follows instructions quietly and slowly without asking questions. His son and daughter are at his bedside and they also are very quiet. Finally, E.B. says, "I don't want to go like your mother did. She lingered on and had so much pain. I don't want them to bring me back."

2. You look at his chart and find no advanced directives. What is your responsibility? **[P/c/PSI,HP/ct,ni,tc]**
   - On admission, all patients must be informed about advanced directives and are given the opportunity to state their wishes in writing at this time.
   - Tell him you overheard his conversation. You can find no advanced directives in his chart. Without them, the medical personnel have no alternative but to fully resuscitate if it becomes necessary.
   - Ask him if he wishes to state advanced directives (his specific wishes). Notify the approporiate hospital representative to talk to E.B., and obtain written instructions to ensure his wishes are carried out.
   - Notify the physician that he needs to clarify with this patient what he does and does not want done. Physicians often are not aware of the existence of advanced directives or patient's stated wishes.

3. What is your assessment of E.B.'s behavior at this time? **[PD/an/PSI,ct]**
   - E.B. is most likely in the initial phase of anticipatory grief, which involves numbness, shock, and denial. These responses may have a variety of manifestations. E.B.'s manifestations of this phase seem to involve blunted affect, passive behavior, social withdrawal, and immobility.

4. What are some appropriate nursing interventions and responses to E.B.'s anticipatory grief? **[P,I/ap/PSI/tc]**
   - Demonstrate acceptance and support of E.B. during whatever phase of grief he may be in.
   - Provide simple explanations and instructions because E.B. may have difficulty concentrating and understanding at this time.
   - Identify and validate E.B.'s feelings.
   - Help him identify his resources at this time. His son and daughter are present and supportive.
   - Reassure E.B. that every effort will be made to meet his needs, and assistance will be provided during his recovery and rehabilitation.

E.B. returns from surgery with the right stump dressed with gauze and an elastic wrap. The dressing is dry and intact, without drainage. He is drowsy with the following VS: 142/80, 96, 14, 36.6°C. He has a maintenance IV of D_5.9 NS infusing at 125 ml/h in his right forearm.

5. The surgeon has written to keep E.B.s stump elevated on pillows for 48 hours; after that, have him lay in prone position for 15 minutes qid. In teaching E.B. about his care, how would you explain the rationale for these orders? **[P/an/S,PSI/ct,tc]**
   - Elevation of the stump will decrease swelling and promote healing at the end of the stump.
   - Lying prone will prevent the development of hip contractures.

6. In reviewing E.B.'s medical history, what factor may affect the condition of E.B.'s stump and ultimate rehabilitation potential? **[PD/an/PI,HP/ct]**
   - Diabetes and atherosclerosis may decrease the ability of the stump to heal. Prosthesis may not be possible for a diabetic who has problems with a healing stump.

You have just returned from a 2-day workshop on guidelines for the care of surgical patients with IDDM. You notice that E.B.'s blood glucose has been running between 130 to 180. The sliding scale insulin intervention does not begin until a blood glucose of 200 is reported. You recognize that patients with blood glucoses exceeding 140 suffer from impaired wound healing.

7. Identify 4 interventions that would facilitate timely healing of E.B.s stump. **[P/ac/PI/ct,ni,tc]**
   - You ask the surgeon for a Certified Diabetes Educator consult to help regulate E.B.'s blood glucose.
   - Request more frequent glucose monitoring.
   - Sliding scale insulin interventions should begin at 150.
   - Enlist the family's cooperation in not bringing in outside food.
   - Request a physical therapy consult for activity to simulate more normal daily caloric expenditure.

8. What should the postoperative assessment of E.B.'s stump dressing include? **[A/k/S,Pl/ct,ni]**
   - Amount of drainage should be monitored closely to detect presence of hemorrhage.
   - Character of drainage should be monitored for presence of purulent drainage and possible infection.
   - Presence of excessive edema may impair healing.
   - Dressings initially should be snug but not constrictive to prevent edema.

9. On the evening of the first post-op day, E.B. becomes more awake and begins to complain of pain. He states, "My leg is really hurting, are you sure it's gone?" How would you respond to E.B.'s question? **[I/c/PSI/tc]**
   - Phantom pain will usually mimic the pain that existed before removal of the limb. It is most common immediately following the amputation and will eventually subside. (There is controversy concerning telling a patient about phantom pain before surgery. Some feel a preoperative warning will help patients identify and report it; others feel anticipation may precipitate the pain.)

E.B. will be discharged to his daughter's home with a wheelchair and crutches. He will be evaluated for a prosthesis and begin training when his stump is ready.

10. What instructions should be given E.B.'s daughter concerning safety around the home at this time? **[I/c/S/tc]**
    - Remove throw rugs.
    - Examine carpeting or linoleum for holes or uneven surfaces that may contribute to falls.
    - Make sure the shoe he is wearing fits well and does not have lose or torn soles. Watch for wear on the shoe and replace it as needed.
    - Because of the loss of weight on one side of E.B.'s body, he will loose his balance easily at first. Assist him as much as needed to maintain balance, especially on stairs.
    - He should only use a wheelchair designed for amputees because the loss of weight in front may cause a regular wheelchair to tip backward.

Case Study 12: Hand Injury

Difficulty: ***	*Setting:* Hospital ED, short-stay surgery
Index Words: Trauma	

J.T. has injured his hand at work and is accompanied to the ED by a co-worker. You examine his hand and find a piece of a drill bit sticking out of the skin between the 3rd and 4th knuckle of his left hand. There is another puncture site about an inch below and toward the center of the hand. Bleeding is minimal. J.T. is 41 years old, has no significant medical history, and NKDA (no known drug allergies). He states the accident occurred when a mill at work malfunctioned and knocked his hand onto a rack of drill bits. His last tetanus booster was 3 years ago. It is your job to provide the initial care for J.T.'s injury.

1. You examine J.T.'s hand. What should you include in your initial assessment and why? **[A/c/Pl/ct]**
   - Control of bleeding.
   - Assess blood supply to each digit. Document capillary refill, color, and temperature. Swelling in a digit can quickly compromise circulation.
   - Assess sensory perception (sharp/dull) of each digit, palm, and back of hand to identify nerve damage.
   - Assess motor function (flexion and extension) of each digit to determine injury to tendons and ligaments.

   Instructor Note: A Doppler can be used to confirm the arterial flow to each digit. The surgeon will find this very helpful.

You record that J.T.'s fingers are warm with capillary refill <2 seconds. Sensory perception is intact. He is able to flex and extend the distal joints but not the proximal joints of the 3rd and 4th fingers.

2. You notice J.T.'s wedding band and promptly ask him to remove it. Why is this important? **[A/c/S,Pl/ct]**
   - The wedding band needs to be removed as quickly as possible before there is further swelling of the finger. Rings can compromise circulation to an edematous digit.

   Instructor Note: Have the secretary contact his wife and inform her that J.T. injured his hand at work and is in the ED of your hospital. Ask if she can come to the hospital.

3. J.T. asks you why he can't just pull the bit out and go home. How should you respond to his question? **[P/ap/S,Pl/tc]**
   - Tell J.T. that you never remove an impaled object; removing the object may cause further damage and possibly precipitate extensive bleeding.

4. What common diagnostic test will identify fractures and the location of metal fragments in J.T.'s hand? **[P/c/Pl/ct]**
   - An x-ray of the hand will tell the physician if there are any fractures, the number and location of metal fragments, and the position of the drill bit in J.T.'s hand.

The drill bit is impaled ½ inch below the surface of the skin, and there are no fractures. Because the hand contains so many blood vessels, nerves, ligaments and tendons, the ED physician decides to consult a surgical hand specialist. The surgeon suspects tendon damage and decides to operate immediately.

5. What do you need to do to prepare J.T. for immediate surgery? **[I/ap/S,Pl/ct,ni]**
   - Make sure that someone has contacted J.T.'s wife and informed her that he is going to require surgery.
   - Make sure that J.T.'s signed surgical consent form is on the chart.
   - Answer any and all questions that J.T. may ask.
   - Help J.T. remove all clothing and put on a hospital gown.
   - Collect all J.T.'s valuables; they should be given to his wife or locked in the hospital safe.
   - J.T. should have a CBC, Chem 7, PT/PTT, and UA done. Make sure that all laboratory results are posted on the chart.
   - Have J.T. empty his bladder.
   - Start an IV as prescribed.
   - Ask J.T. when he last ate, and inform the anesthesiologist.

   Instructor Note: The nurse should accompany the surgeon to J.T.'s bedside, listen to the explanation of the surgery, and witness J.T. signing the surgical consent form. Ask J.T. to explain, in his own words, what is going to be done to his hand. Ask him to explain, using his own words, the risks involved in this surgery. This method ensures informed consent.

6. You record that J.T. has had no food since 8:00 PM yesterday and drank "some water" this AM. Based on this information, do you anticipate problems during surgery and why? **[P/k/S,Pl/ct]**
   - No problems are anticipated. If J.T. had eaten today, it would have been necessary to insert a nasogastric tube and empty his stomach.

   Instructor Note: Because J.T. drank water, the anesthesiologist may choose to give metoclopramide (Reglan) IV to facilitate natural emptying of J.T.'s stomach before surgery.

7. Should J.T. be given a tetanus booster before he goes to surgery? **[A/k/Pl/ct]**
   - No. J.T. has a nontetanus-prone wound and has had a booster within the past 10 years.

The surgeon repairs two partially severed tendons and wraps the hand in a very large, padded dressing. The distal ½ inch of each digit protrudes from the bulky dressing.

8. While in the short-stay recovery area, J.T. asks the nurse why his fingers look yellowish-brown. How should she respond to his question? **[A/k/Pl/tc]**
   - The coloring comes from an iodine soap that was used to scrub his hand before surgery. He should be reassured that the coloring can be wiped off.

The surgeon tells J.T. that he had to repair tendons in his 3rd and 4th fingers and instructs J.T. that he is not to work. He gives J.T. prescriptions for an antibiotic and an antiinflammatory agent. He instructs J.T. to make an appointment to see him in the surgery clinic in 2 days.

9. What instructions should the nurse in the short-stay area discuss with J.T. and his wife give before releasing J.T.? **[I/an/S,PI/ni,tc]**
   - Call and make the appointment in the surgery clinic for J.T. Record this information on a card and give it to the wife.
   - Keep his hand elevated and apply ice for the next 48 hours.
   - Explain that if he experiences any numbness, tingling, or burning sensation; if his fingers turn dusky; or if he experiences a lot of pain during the night he should go to the ED.
   - Explain that someone should check on him every 2 hours during the night. Check the color of his fingers; give him medication if it is due; ask him about numbness, tingling, or burning; and apply fresh ice.
   - Explain the purpose of each medication, how to take it, and what side effects to look for.
   - Stress that the more swelling he has, the more pain he will experience.

10. J.T. says, "How in the world is the ice supposed to keep my hand cold with this big bandage on it?" How will the nurse reply? **[PD/ap/S,PI/tc]**
    - Your hand isn't supposed to be cold, it should be kept cool.
    - Enough of the cold will get through the dressing if J.T. keeps ice on the dressing at all times.
    - The ice, elevation, compression of the dressing, and the medication will all help to keep the swelling down.

11. J.T. says, "I'll be able to keep my hand up when I'm awake but what about when I go to sleep?" What suggestion can the nurse make to help J.T. comply with the instructions? **[PD/ap/S,PI/ct]**
    - Suggest that J.T. sleep alone tonight so he can spread out over the bed.
    - When he goes to bed, put pillows under and all around his arm so that it won't slide down and begin to swell.
    - Tell J.T. to expect to wake up several times during the first night. Explain that many patients complain that they just can't get comfortable that first night but assure him that it gets better.

J.T.'s recovery was uncomplicated, and he regained the full use of his hand.

Case Study 13: Post-polio Syndrome

Difficulty: ***	*Setting:* Out-patient clinic
Index Words: Post-polio syndrome, pain	

Instructor Note: There is, regrettably, little information about post-polio syndrome in the nursing literature. The post-polio phenomenon only began to be recognized in the early 1980s. Students may have to engage in a "scavenger hunt," and exercise creativity to find information. This case can make an excellent group project on helping individuals adapt to chronic degenerative processes.

Dr. C., a 53-year-old nursing professor, comes to your chronic fatigue clinic for evaluation of long-term fatigue, weakness, and pain which have become increasingly disruptive to her life-style. Over the years, she sought medical advice about her fatigue but received vague and often conflicting advice such as "get more exercise," "get more rest," "lost weight," "eat better," "exercise more and lose weight," and "pull yourself together." Despite treatment for "depression," the fatigue remains unrelenting. Nothing seems to help. She confides in you that she is so discouraged and tired of dragging through each day that she has thought of suicide but it violates her belief system.

1. You ask her to describe her symptoms. What questions will you ask about her fatigue, weakness, and pain? **[A/k/PI,PSI/ct]**
   - These questions provide a guide for investigating symptom phenomena:
     - Location: Where does she feel it (fatigue, weakness, pain)?
     - Quality: What does it feel like?
     - Quantity or severity: How bad is it?
     - Timing (onset, duration, frequency): When does it happen or when is it worse?
     - Setting: Where is she when it happens or under what conditions is it worse?
     - Factors that aggravate or relieve: What makes it feel better? What makes it worse?
     - Associated manifestations: Is there anything else she feels with it?
     - The meaning of the symptom to her and what is its impact on her life (Bates, 1991).

Dr. C. describes her fatigue as daily, unrelenting, and worse in the evening. The overall fatigue, together with muscular weakness ("feels rubbery") and "nervelike" pain, is aggravated by activity and long days. She experiences nausea when extremely fatigued. She has difficulty negotiating inclines and stairs. Although rest makes her feel better, she feels guilty about "taking the time." She says she rarely attends social events, is having trouble doing her housekeeping and has had to give up doing yardwork. She tells you she worries a great deal about her future and whether she'll be able to work until retirement.

You take a detailed history in preparation for a physical and psychosocial evaluation. At age 17, she developed polio. She described this experience as sudden onset (over a 6-hour period) with fatigue, high fever (104.8°F) with shaking chills, weakness and aching all over. The next day, she dragged her feet, experienced constipation, became anorexic, had chills, indescribable muscle aches, and constant pain. The asymmetrical muscular weakness affected all her extremities, especially her legs. This was followed by over 6 months of hospitalization featuring the Sr. Kenny method of treatment. The moist, hot packs helped relieve the extreme neuromuscular pain. Together with gentle exercise (swimming pool), they helped prevent contractures. "It was that experience that motivated me to become a nurse," she said and smiled. "It has always been a point of pride that I worked so hard and overcame such a vicious disease." Based on her history and your experience with other patients, you suspect her fatigue, weakness and pain are manifestations of post-polio syndrome (PPS).

2. What comments did she make (above) indicating that her functional status (ability to function on a daily basis) is currently compromised (list 5)? **[PD/c/PI,PSI/ct]**
   - Decreased attendance at social events.
   - Decreased ability to do housework.
   - Inability to do yard work.
   - Trouble with occupation activity.
   - Difficulty with mobility (inclines and stairs).

3. What questions do you need to ask to gain an understanding of her support systems? **[A/c/S,PI,PSI/ct,tc]**
   - Social support: What kind of family and significant other relationships does she have?
   - Financial support: What kind of disability insurance, retirement, medical insurance, financial security, and income does she have?
   - Disability support: What kind of problems is she having at work? What kind of supportive help would facilitate her occupational performance (this is important for documenting Americans with Disabilities Act requests for "special accommodations").
   - Physical support: What specific kinds of problems is she having in terms of her energy levels and strength? What kind of changes in her environment (home, housekeeping, transportation, etc.) would help her?

4. Dr. C. admitted she is used to "pushing herself even when it hurts." Then she asks if you think an exercise program would be good for her. How would you respond? **[I/k/PI,HP/ct,ni,tc]**
   - Tell her that exercise is a good idea for most people, but post-polio syndrome presents special problems. Explain that when the muscles are overused and stressed, there is thought to be long-term, irreversible loss in muscle functioning. When she pushes herself so hard, she probably is damaging her muscles. She would do better to learn to pace herself and limit unnecessary activity to preserve her muscle function as much as possible. Too *little* as well as too *much* activity results in deterioration of muscle function.

Instructor Note: A pedometer could be used to help her monitor her activity so she doesn't over tax herself. The pedometer can help her identify when pain and weakness set in; she needs to stop just short of that point. For instance, if 1 ½ miles per day results in pain, monitor herself and stop at 1 ¼ miles. If she pushes herself too far, particularly for several days in a row, inflammation sets in. Look for edema to occur. Advise her not to push past the point of fatigue.

5. Dr. C. undergoes some diagnostic tests to confirm the diagnosis of post-polio syndrome. What type of tests might be used for muscle evaluation? **[A/k/PI/ct]**
    - Muscle strength testing using dynamometers or isokinetic dynamometers to gain absolute measurements of strength of specific muscle groups.
    - Electromyography is an electrophysiologic study to determine the electrical activity of specific muscles.

The diagnosis of post-polio syndrome (PPS) as a source of Dr. C.'s fatigue, weakness, and pain is confirmed by the physiatrist. Dr. C. is surprised that she had never heard of PPS and that none of the other physicians had ever suggested it to her. She expresses interest in learning more about her diagnosis.

6. What resources could you refer her to for further information? **[I/k/PI,PSI,HP/ct,ni,tc]**
    - The medical center library may have research-based information.
    - The Easter Seal Foundation is an excellent source of professional education, group support, and consumer education on PPS. Give Dr. C. their local telephone number.
    - Local PPS support groups can be an exceptional source of emotional and social support, especially in view of the lack of knowledge on the part of many health care professionals.

7. On a follow-up visit, you work with Dr. C. on ways to adapt her lifestyle to her limitations. List several prosthetic devices that may help control her fatigue, weakness, and pain, and prevent further loss in muscular functioning. **[P/c/PI,HP,ct,ni,tc]**
    - Wheelchair.
    - Crutches.
    - Electric scooter.
    - Braces.

    Instructor Note: Insurance will often pay as much as 80% of the cost for prosthetic devices that have been prescribed by a physician.

8. What other suggestions could you make to help her adapt to her limitation? **[P/c/PI,PSI/ct,ni,tc]**
    - Help with her housework.
    - Handicapped parking sticker or license plate.
    - Have a family member or significant other help her objectively evaluate her activity (very important).

9. On her next visit, Dr. C. tells you she was "shocked" at the idea of thinking of herself as "handicapped." She states, sadly, "I thought I had beat this years ago, but now my old enemy has come back to haunt me." How do you explain her comments? **[PD/an/PSI/ct,ni]**
   - Shock and grieving are common human responses to profound threats to health. Each person processes these threats differently as they adapt to a new lifestyle with altered expectations.

   Instructor Note: It is important to see these responses as a step in growth and development. To deny people this processing of pain and suffering is to insult the human spirit. These responses are *not* to be confused with depression.

Although this case featured someone whose poliomyelitis generally affected the lower body, others experience polio over their whole body, even affecting arm movement and breathing. Many individuals with PPS also develop trouble breathing and swallowing, so a history of polio should always be a question asked on geriatric assessments.

CHAPTER 4. GASTROINTESTINAL DISORDERS

Case Study 1: Partial Gastrectomy

Difficulty: *	*Setting:* Hospital, home care
Index Words: Gastrointestinal hemorrhage, partial gastrectomy	

The charge nurse on your surgical floor notifies you that your next admission will be H.C., a 70-year-old woman who has an active gastrointestinal (GI) bleed and has just been informed that she has adenocarcinoma of the lung. Her VS are 130/80, 80, 18, 37.2°C. When H.C. arrives on the floor, no family members are present, she has slightly pink coloring, and denies pain although she does appear anxious. Her PMH (past medical history) includes PUD (peptic ulcer disease) with reflux esophagitis, COPD (chronic obstructive pulmonary disease), hypothyroidism, and "fluid retention." PSH (past surgical history) includes TAH (total abdominal hysterectomy) and appendectomy (1965), benign R breast biopsy (1994), and laparoscopic Nissen fundoplication (1994). Her regular medications include nizatidine (Axid) 150 mg bid, $FeSO_4$ 325 mg qd, potassium chloride (K-Dur) 20 mEq bid, hydrochlorothiazide (HCTZ) 15 mg qd, levothyroxine (Synthroid) 0.1 mg qd, salmeterol (Serevent) 2 puffs bid, and theophylline (Slo-Bid) 200 mg PO tid.

H.C.'s admission orders brought up from the ED include the following: admit to GI unit; Dx (diagnosis) of gastric ulcer, adenocarcinoma of the lung, longstanding COPD; VS q4h; NPO (nothing by mouth); IV D_5 NS with 20 mEq KCl/L at 125 ml/h; I&O; CBC with differential; electrolytes, Chem 20, PT/PTT in AM; UA (urinalysis) on admission; O_2 at 4 L/nc prn to keep SaO_2 >92%; fa,ptodome (Pepcid) 20 mg IV at 12h; no NSAIDs, ASA; Guaiac all stools; call MD when husband arrives.

1. Which orders would require some clarification? Why? **[PD/c/S,PI/ct]**
   - The admitting diagnosis does not address the active GI bleed.
   - IV of D_5 NS at 125 ml/h: a COPD patient may not be able to tolerate the high sodium content and rapid infusion rate.
   - Does the physician want any admitting laboratory studies performed?
   - Maintaining an SaO_2 of >92% is contraindicated for a COPD patient.

You put in a call to the physician for clarification of orders. In the meantime, you proceed with the admission process.

2. What are the major components of the nursing assessment you will perform on H.C.? **[A/k/PI,PSI/ct,tc]**
   - A thorough history (including PMH and family history [Hx]) and medication allergies.
   - A complete physical assessment including VS.
   - Obtain background on patient's support system and a psychosocial history.
   - Identify her current emotional status and address any questions.

Throughout the assessment, H.C. appears to be SOB. Her sentences are getting shorter with pauses for breathing between. You ask H.C. to stand on the bedside scale. As she stands, she suddenly sits back on the bed c/o dizziness and nausea.

3. H.C. had been admitted for a GI bleed. Reviewing the data above, list possible indicators of gastrointestinal hemorrhage. **[A/an/S,Pl/ct,ni]**
   - Hypotension, tachycardia.
   - Bloody emesis.
   - Occult blood in the stools (guaiac test).
   - Decreasing hematocrit and hemoglobin (H&H).
   - Increasing abdominal girth.
   - Vertigo and nausea.
   - Dyspnea.

The physician finally calls to clarify H.C.'s orders: draw STAT H&H, change IV to D_5½ NS at 100 ml/h, titrate O_2 to maintain $SaO_2 > 86\%$, and give furosemide (Lasix) 10 mg IVP (IV push) if K > 3.8 mEq/L. The lab work returns: Hgb 10 g/dl, Hct 30%, K 3.4 mEq/L.

4. Based on these laboratory findings, what are you going to do? **[E/ap/S,Pl/ct,ni]**
   - Call the physician with the results; you will probably need to administer K before giving the Lasix.

Dr. B. arrives and discusses the options with Mr. and Mrs.C. It was decided to go ahead with partial gastrectomy to remove the ulcer. The pulmonary consultant indicates that H.C.'s adenocarcinoma has metastasized to adjacent tissues to the extent that H.C. is not a candidate for lung resection. Radiation is planned to begin as soon as possible following this GI surgery.

5. What preop care would you expect to give? **[P/k/S,Pl,PSI/ct]**
   - Complete preop teaching about anticipated postop status: NGT (nasogastric tube) and sore throat; continued NPO orders; pain management; importance of turning, coughing and deep breathing; early ambulation.
   - Enemas until clear.
   - Maintain NPO status—oral care.
   - Discuss sources of anxiety including final directives, family issues, etc.
   - Complete preop checklist.
   - Check the latest preop lab results. Are the H&H and K WNL (within normal limits)? If not, is the surgeon aware?
   - Hibiclens showers (not always done).

6. In view of H.C.'s history, which part of your preop teaching do you think will be most necessary for H.C. and why? **[PD/c/Pl/ct]**
   - It is important for H.C. to understand that there will be a lot of pain due to the high incision and that this can compromise her respiratory status. It is imperative that she understand how to use pain medication to enable her to cough and deep breathe to prevent atelectasis.

7. H.C. returns to the floor after surgery. She has had a large wedge resection of her stomach with a partial selective vagotomy and a pyloroplasty. She is quite lethargic with stable VS. Her EBL (estimated blood loss) during surgery was minimal (100 ml). She has an NGT in place to intermittent LWS (low wall suction). What should you know about NGT postoperative management? Be sure to include drainage and emergency issues. **[P,I/c/S,PI/ct,ni]**
   - The tape and tube at the nares should be checked regularly for sign of ischemia.
   - The NGT drainage probably will be slightly bloody the first 6 to 12 hours after surgery.
   - The physician should be notified immediately if you find bright red drainage, excessive drainage, or excess bloody drainage.
   - Do *not* irrigate or reposition the NGT (the sutures are very delicate and can easily be broken).
   - Use wrist restraints if necessary to prevent H.C. from pulling out the NGT (especially in the initial postop period, when she may be confused from the anesthetic).

8. If H.C.'s NGT is pulled partially out, what is the best action? Why? **[I/c/S,PI/ct,ni]**
   - Tape NGT into its current position and notify MD for further directions. Nurses do not reposition NGT in patients with gastric surgery because of the possibility of suture line disruption; this can contribute to hemorrhage.

9. The second day postop, H.C. still has an NGT and a pulse oximeter. Where might you expect H.C. to have some skin breakdown? **[PD/c/PI/ct]**
   - With an NGT there is always a risk of skin irritation and breakdown where the tube exits the nares.
   - The O_2 nasal cannula may lead to breakdown around the ears.
   - The finger probe can cause breakdown at the base of the fingernail.
   - If H.C. is not moving around and getting up to ambulate fairly often, she is at risk for breakdown over bony prominences such as the coccyx, elbows, heels, or hip areas.

10. How can the nurse best prevent skin breakdown? **[P,I/ap/S/PI/ct,ni]**
   - Monitor the nares around the NGT and position the tubing to prevent pressure on the nares.
   - Most respiratory therapy departments have sponge pads that fit over the nasal cannula tubing to cushion behind the ears.
   - The pulse oximeter finger probe should be moved frequently to prevent skin breakdown; change the probe every time you turn or change the patient's position.
   - H.C. needs to be turned q2h if she is not turning herself. Dangling her the night of surgery and ambulating her the first day postop is the best treatment for skin and lungs alike.

H.C. has no postop complications and is discharged to her home with her husband on the 5th POD (postop day).

11. What warning signs would you teach the patient to call her surgeon for? **[P,I/ap/S,PI/ct,ni,tc]**
    - She should call his office about any questions she has and ask to speak to the registered nurse or physician. (Many offices have technicians or office help who answer to "nurse" so patients must be sure to ask for the *registered nurse*.) She must call him for any increased redness in or around the wound, increased pain, any increase of temperature over 101 °F, any drainage from the wound including clear drainage, any swelling of the wound, or any separation of the wound edges. Be sure she has a thermometer at home and knows how to use it.

12. H.C. is preparing for discharge when she turns on her call light. As you enter the room, she says, "I'm leaking." You examine her incision and note that her surgical wound has opened slightly (dehiscence). What action would you take? **[I/ap/s,PI,PSI/ct,ni,tc]**
    - Have H.C. lay in bed with the HOB raised to take pressure off the abdominal cavity.
    - Cover the wound with NS-soaked gauze and sterile towel.
    - Give her the call light, instruct her not to get out of bed, and tell her you are going to call her doctor.
    - Call H.C.'s physician and explain what happened.

After examining H.C., the physician instructs you to dress the wound with a wet-to-moist dressing. You contact the home health nurses for follow-up care for H.C., and she is discharged to home.

13. In addition to dressing changes, what related services might the home health nurses provide for H.C. and her husband? **[PD/c/PI/ct]**
    - Photograph the wound once a week.
    - Assess wound healing process.
    - Culture the wound prn.
    - Teach H.C.'s husband how to irrigate and pack the wound.
    - Teach H.C.'s husband about her medications.

Three weeks later, H.C. was discharged from home care and started her radiation treatments.

Case Study 2: Hepatocellular Carcinoma

Difficulty: *	*Setting:* Hospital
Index Words: Hepatocellular carcinoma, cancer	

C.E., a 54-year-old woman, is being admitted to your unit with a tentative diagnosis of liver tumor. She has experienced increasing fatigue, anorexia, and a steady weight loss of 18 kg over the last 3 months. Her current weight is 52 kg; she is 5'6" tall. She bruised easily, has mild to moderate jaundice, experiences a "heavy fullness" in the midepigastric area, and c/o a persistent dull ache in the epigastric area that radiates to her back. She describes the pain as constant but not severe and reports that the fullness never goes away, not even when she hasn't eaten for a long time. As an afterthought she adds, "Its strange that I have lost weight and yet my skirts are too tight at the waist." Current VS are 102/60, 84, 28, 38.0°C. The abnormal laboratory results are WBC 12 mm^3, K 3.4 mEq/L, protein 4.8 g/dl, albumin 2.9 g/dl, total bilirubin 2.5 mg/dl, Alk phos 215 U/L, GGT 665 U/L, LDH 225 U/L, AST 130 U/L, ALT 168 U/L, AFP 9.5 mg/ml.

1. Which labs indicate possible liver tumor? **[A,PD/c/PI/ct]**
   - Prot, Alb, T-bili, Alk phos, GGT, LDH, AST, ALT, AFP.

2. Which of the above labs relate(s) to hepatocellular carcinoma? **[PD/c/PI/ct]**
   - Alpha-fetoprotein (AFP).

3. How would you assess C.E. to evaluate her fluid and electrolyte status? **[A/k/PI/ct]**
   - Note skin turgor.
   - Moistness of mucous membranes.
   - Edema in extremities.
   - Monitor increase in abdominal girth.
   - I&O.
   - Any abnormal fluid losses (i.e., vomiting, diarrhea, bleeding).
   - Daily weights.
   - Tremors, profound muscle weakness, lethargy, dizziness, syncope.
   - Lab values (i.e., serum electrolytes, Hgb and Hct, BUN and creatinine).
   - Nervous system changes including changes in level of consciousness.

4. What is the significance of assessing abdominal girth? How would you do this? **[A/k/Pl/ct]**
   - In the presence of liver disease, a measurable increase in abdominal girth is indicative of ascites. Ascites is fluid that is accumulating within the peritoneal cavity—this type of fluid loss is called "3rd spacing." A lack of colloidal osmotic pressure has allowed fluid to seep out of the vasculature into potential spaces such as the peritoneal cavity. Ascites develops as the liver fails and loses its ability to produce the albumin that retains water in the vasculature. To measure the girth, measure the circumference of the abdomen at its widest point when the patient is lying supine. Mark both sides of the abdomen with ink so later measurements are taken at the same place. You may need to secure 2 paper tape measures together to adequately reach around the patient. Leave the tape measure where it can be readily found at the bedside. Record measurements. And remember to record the *total* of the tapes if more than 1 tape is used.

5. Based on the information above, you would want to complete a respiratory and a neurologic assessment. Why are these 2 systems important? **[A/c/Pl/ct]**
   - The hepatic mass may compress the diaphragm, inhibit lung expansion during inspiration, and result in frequent, shallow respirations.
   - The nervous system is affected by the buildup of toxins in the blood due to a failing liver. Increased toxins are manifest by impaired cognitive functioning and memory problems, peripheral sensory deficits, and lack of coordination.

6. What diagnostic tests might be used to determine if C.E. has a liver tumor? **[PD/K/Pl/ct]**
   - Abdominal ultrasonography.
   - Abdominal CT scan.
   - Arteriogram.
   - Liver biopsy is required for a definitive diagnosis. The diagnosis of cancer is determined by the pathologist's report).
   - Laboratory tests are presence of alpha-fetoprotein (AFP, a tumor-marker) and hepatitis B surface antigens. Sometimes, these patients are at risk for hepatitis B, but tests are often negative for it.

7. C.E. is to go for an MRI. What will you do to prepare her for this test? **[P/c/Pl/ct,ni]**
   - Remove all metal from C.E., ask her about metal implants, inform patient that she will be in a long tube (a mild sedative such as versed can be given if patient has a problem with claustrophobia), and tell her that she receives *no* radiation in this test.

8. The radiologist informs the physician that C.E.'s MRI shows many lesions in the R lobe of the liver. The physician comes to the floor to biopsy C.E.'s liver. How will you assist during the biopsy? **[P/PA/Pl,PSI/ct,ni,tc]**
   - Explain the procedure to C.E.; be sure she understands how important it is to hold still and hold her breath on command. Practice this with the patient. Stay with her, hold her hand, and talk to her during the biopsy. These procedures can be very painful. Be assertive with the physician about the issue of premedication, and allow sufficient time for the medication to take effect.

9. What can be done to minimize bleeding from the biopsy? **[P,I/k/PI/ct,ni]**
   - Hold pressure on the site by turning patient onto her R side to lie with a folded bath blanket under the costal margin for several hours after the biopsy.
   - Bed rest for 24 hours after the biopsy.
   - Vital signs should be checked every half hour for several hours then every hour for up to 24 hours.
   - Vitamin K (1-5 mg IV x 1), then check the patient in 24h and after the biopsy. Another name for vitamin K is phytonadione (Aquamephyton); it is used to increase coagulation.

10. The oncologist, C.E., and her husband discuss risks and options for treatment. List 4 general types of treatments used for solid tumors. **[P/c/PI/ct]**
    - Surgery.
    - Biotherapy.
    - Chemotherapy.
    - Radiotherapy.
    - Treatment often consists of a combination of these treatment types, including multiple drug agents.

C.E. decides to have surgery. She has a difficult time waking up after surgery so she is sent to ICU overnight. Her doctor tells you, "We basically opened her up and closed her—the liver was a mass of tumors and the intestines were also heavily involved. The frozen specimens were malignant. The tumor had invaded the major blood vessels so we couldn't resect anything. Her prognosis is less than 6 months."

11. How will you approach C.E. when you readmit her to the unit later that day? **[P/ap/PSI/ct,ni,tc]**
    - Be supportive.
    - Focus on her controlling her physical discomfort.
    - Ask C.E. and her husband, "What is your understanding of what the doctor has told you?" The patient, under the influence of anesthesia, usually does not remember the postop discussion with the physician or their diagnosis. The spouse may be suffering from shock and may not know how to discuss the diagnosis with his wife, or they may not have remembered or understood much of what the physician said.
    - Suggest that they make a list of questions to ask the doctor.
    - Make every effort to be present when the doctor does come to discuss these items with the patient. You can later clarify things the patient and her family may not understand. You can also act as a patient advocate if the patient appears reluctant to ask questions during this and subsequent discussions.
    - Try to answer their questions honestly and completely. The general rule is to leave the initial discussion of the diagnosis and prognosis to the doctor.

You are present when C.E. and her husband discuss the surgical findings with the physician. Both C.E. and her husband are stunned—"You couldn't take it out?!!!" Solemnly the surgeon shakes his head and says he is sorry but there is nothing he can do. He turns and leaves the room. You ask if they'd like to be alone for a while and quietly leave.

12. When you return to care for C.E., you are rebuffed by an angry woman. "Just leave me alone! I don't need your help! What use is all this anyway?!!" How would you interpret C.E.'s response? **[PD/c/PSI/ct]**
    - This angry outburst is not personally directed at you, the nurse. C.E. is caught up in her anger at her prognosis—a normal response. She is beginning to cope with her reality.
    - Make sure she has tissues and tell her that you will leave the room for now but that you will return later to see if she feels like talking.
    - See that she and her husband are referred to an oncologist who is skilled at symptom management; pain, fatigue, dyspnea, and thirst are the most distressing symptoms in individuals with terminal illnesses.

    Instructor Note: Not all people go through the various stages of death and dying in the same order or at the same rate. Some people don't go through the process at all; others cheerfully remain in denial the entire time. It is important to respect others' "coping" styles and not to judge according to our expectations and standards. After all, it is their life.

Before C.E. leaves the hospital, you introduce C.E. and her husband to the idea of hospice care. Tell them that C.E. will require home health nurses when she goes home but eventually she will deteriorate and may want hospice nurses to support them both. Give them the hospice card and write the name of a contact person on it.

Instructor Note: The ONS (Oncology Nursing Society) is a large nursing organization that consists of nurses committed to the care of cancer patients in a wide variety of settings. Nurses who have passed the ONS-sponsored special cancer specialist examination have the letters OCN (Oncology Certified Nurse) after their names. This organization has well-developed and high-quality resources for nurses interested in improving their care of people with cancer.

For more information: call 1-412-921-7373or write to 501 Holiday Drive, Pittsburgh, PA 15220.

Case Study 3: Acute Diverticulitis

Difficulty: *	*Setting:* Outpatient clinic
Index Words: Diverticulitis	

T.H., a 57-year-old stockbroker, has come to the gastroenterologist for treatment of recurrent mild to severe cramping in his abdomen and blood-streaked stool. You are the RN doing his initial work-up. Your findings include a mildly obese (male-pattern obesity) man who demonstrates moderate guarding of his abdomen with both direct and rebound tenderness, especially in the LLQ. His VS are 168/98, 110, 24, 38.0°C, and he is slightly diaphoretic. T.H. reports that he has periodic constipation. He has had previous episodes of abdominal cramping but this time the pain is getting worse. He has NKDA (no known drug allergies.

PMH: T.H. has a "sedentary job with lots of emotional moments," has smoked a pack a day for 30 years, and had "2 or 3 mixed drinks in the evening" until 2 months ago. "I haven't had anything to drink in 60 days." He denies regular exercise—"Just no time." His diet consists mostly of "white bread, meat, potatoes, and ice cream with fruit and nuts over it." Denies hx of cardiac or pulmonary problems and no personal hx of cancer, although his father and older brother died of colon cancer. He takes no "regular" medications and denies the use of any other drugs.

1. Identify 4 general health risk problems T.H. exhibits. **[A/c/PI/ct]**
   - Male-pattern obesity.
   - 30-year history of smoking.
   - Probable recent abuse of alcohol (ETOH).
   - Low-fiber foods.
   - No regular exercise.
   - Stressful job.

2. Identify a key factor in his family history that may have profound implications for his health and present state of mind? **[A/c/PI,PSI/ct]**
   - Marked family history of colon cancer; now he has blood in his stool.

3. Identify 3 key findings on his physical exam, and indicate their significance. **[PD/c/PI/ct]**
   - Sporadic crampy abdominal pain: this type of pain is often triggered by muscle spasms of the colon and is acute and persistent; pain may arise from a number of sources, including irritable bowel syndrome, diverticulitis, and appendicitis but when found in the LLQ and combined with a low-grade fever is classic for diverticulitis.
   - Guarding of the abdomen with rebound tenderness: these involuntary findings are usually linked to irritation or inflammation of the peritoneum.
   - Constipation with associated blood streaks on the outside of the feces: if the evacuation of the constipated stool required significant straining, the blood could come from hemorrhoids, malignant polyps, or bleeding diverticula.

Based on physical exam and history, the physician diagnoses T.H. as having acute diverticulitis and discusses an outpatient treatment plan with him.

4. What is diverticulitis? What are the consequences of untreated diverticulitis? **[PD/k/PI/ct]**
   - It is an inflammatory or infectious condition in and around the colon that develops when weak areas of the intestinal wall protrude and create little outpouches called diverticula. Bits of feces caught in the diverticula can block the small neck of the diverticulum or can attract other debris to form a fecalith. The fecalith exerts excess pressure on the relatively thin walls of the pouch, causing inflammation and constriction of the blood supply to that area. If the diverticula perforate and intervention is not initiated promptly, the patient will eventually show signs and symptoms of localized infection and eventually peritonitis.

5. While the patient is experiencing the severe crampy pain of acute diverticulitis, what nursing interventions would you perform to help him feel more comfortable? **[P,I/ap/PI/ct,ni,tc]**
   - Instruct T.H. to "rest the bowel" during an acute attack of diverticulitis: including bed rest, clear liquids only, warm baths or packs to the abdomen; these measures are helpful in mild to moderate diverticulitis.

6. What is the rationale for ordering bed rest? **[PD/k/PI/ct]**
   - Bed rest helps decrease intestinal spasm and pain; anticholinergics (e.g., propantheline [Pro-Banthine]) may also be prescribed to decrease spasms.

7. What classes of medications would be prescribed for someone hospitalized for acute diverticulitis? **[PD/k/S,PI/ct]**
   - Antibiotics.
   - Analgesics.
   - Anticholinergics (e.g, propantheline bromide).
   - Bulk-forming laxatives.
   - Stool softeners.

Metronidazole (Flagyl) or clindamycin (Cleocin) are antibiotics that are used in conjunction with a broad-spectrum penicillin, cephalosporin, or aminoglycoside to treat diverticulitis. T.H. is being sent home with prescriptions for Flagyl 500 mg PO q6h and amoxicillin (Augmentin) 500 mg PO q8h.

8. Given his history, what questions *must* you ask T.H. before he takes the initial dose of Flagyl? State your rationale. **[PD/k/S,PI,PSI/ct,ni,tc]**
   - You should ask T.H. if he is drinking *any* alcohol or taking Antabuse. Explain that Flagyl, when taken with alcohol or disulfiram (Antabuse), can induce an acute psychosis or a profound disulfiram reaction.

9. What is a disulfiram reaction? **[PS/k/PI/ct]**
   - When disulfiram interferes with the metabolic breakdown of alcohol, the resulting accumulation of acetaldehyde results in a profound systemic reaction. Without this enzyme, even a sip or two of alcohol will remain in the blood at an unacceptably high level of acetaldehyde, a potent poison to the system. This level of acetaldehyde is manifested by facial flushing, pounding headache, sweating, slurred speech, abdominal cramps, profound nausea, vomiting, tachycardia, fever, palpitations, marked drop in blood pressure, dyspnea, and a sense of chest constriction. This may begin as early as 10 minutes after alcohol (or Flagyl) is taken and can last up to 24 hours.

10. Aside from warning T.H. about the interactions just described, what instructions should you give him regarding his Flagyl prescription? **[PD/k/PI/ct]**
    - Take immediately before, with, or after meals to prevent GI distress.
    - Take the medication without interrupting the schedule or skipping doses. If a dose is missed, take it as soon as possible unless close to the next dose; do not double the dose.
    - His urine may turn reddish-brown; this is the effect of the medication and is benign.
    - He may develop a yeast (*Candida*) infection. Report any furry tongue, stomatitis, glossitis, color changes of the tongue, or proctitis at once.

11. What information would you want to know before starting T.H. on ampicillin? **[PD/k/PI/ct]**
    - Has he ever taken penicillin or any cephalosporins such as Keflex? If so, did he have a reaction? If so, describe the reaction.

12. What are the signs or symptoms of an allergic reaction? **[PD/k/PI/ct]**
    - The allergic reaction may be anything from a rash or hives to full-blown anaphylactic reaction. In the more serious reactions, the patient will develop periorbital edema and edema within the mouth and throat; often the patient first notices that his tongue is getting thicker and speech is not clear.

13. What will you do if the patient indicates a history of an allergic reaction to PCN? **[PD/c/PI/ct]**
    - First, clarify the allergic reaction.
    - Hold the drug until notifying the physician.
    - It is easier to change the prescription to another antibiotic.

14. In order to prevent future episodes of constipation, what dietary changes would you discuss with T.H.? **[PD/c/PI,HP/ct]**
    - After the acute phase has resolved:
      - Keep fluid intake to at least 8 to 10 cups/day.
      - Consume soft foods that are high in digestible fiber, such as wheat bran, whole grain breads and cereals, peas, carrots, lettuce, peaches, plums, seedless grapes.
      - *Do not eat* foods that do not completely digest or could get caught in the diverticula, such as cucumbers, celery, tomatoes, corn, popcorn, strawberries, raspberries, figs, nuts, and seeds (particularly sesame and caraway).

15. What measures can T.H. take to avoid recurrent acute diverticulitis? **[PD/c/PI,HP/ct]**
    - Avoid constipation.
    - Maintain high fluid intake.
    - Avoid straining with defecation.
    - Use bran or perhaps bulk-forming agents to soften stool, increase mass, and decrease intraluminal pressures due to straining.
    - Weight loss to decrease pressure on the abdominal contents.
    - Regular moderate activity.

T.H. returns for a check-up 14 days later, all signs and symptoms of diverticulitis gone. He is working on his lifestyle changes and reports he is walking 30 min qd. Only 10% to 25% of patients with diverticulitis require any surgery (usually a colectomy). Those who do often suffer recurrent uncontrollable diverticulitis.

Case Study 4: Ruptured Spleen

Difficulty: *	*Setting:* Outpatient clinic; hospital ED
Index Words: Ruptured spleen, trauma, orthostatic hypotension	

A healthy 14-year-old boy, R.K., is admitted to an outpatient clinic. About 4 hours ago, he had been rollerblading and fell while jumping some obstacles. His left arm was caught under him as he fell. He had some "sharp" pain in the LUQ immediately after the fall. This pain eased off gradually but is coming back now. His mother brought him to the clinic because he fainted every time he tried to stand up. He c/o nausea and has vomited twice. R.K. appears somewhat pale and slightly diaphoretic. He denies being SOB (short of breath) or dizzy when lying down. VS are 104/52 (supine), 92, 24, afebrile.

1. What are R.K.'s key symptoms? **[A/c/Pl/ct]**
   - LUQ pain.
   - Orthostatic hypotension.
   - Nausea and vomiting (N/V).
   - Pallor, diaphoresis.

2. What organs lie in the LUQ (left upper quadrant)? **[A/k/Pl/ct]**
   - Stomach.
   - Pancreas (tail).
   - Spleen.
   - Small bowel.
   - Large bowel.

3. What are the nurse's assessment priorities? (list in order of priority). **[A/c/S,Pl/ct,ni]**
   - ABCs.
   - VS.
   - Ask about medication allergies.
   - Listen to lungs bilaterally A&P.
   - Examine abdomen visually, auscultate, then gently manually palpate.
   - Assess for abdominal spasms.
   - Assess for point or rebound tenderness.

4. The clinic is not equipped to care for R.K. What should they do next? **[I/ap/Pl/ct,ni,tc]**
   - Call 911 to have R.K. transported (ambulance or air) to nearest large ED.

5. While the nurses are waiting for the transport unit, what interventions would they initiate? **[I/an/S,Pl/ct,ni]**
   - Draw a STAT Hct/Hgb.
   - Start 18-gauge IV of LR (lactated Ringer's) at 125 ml/h.
   - Inform the Emergency Department (ED) of R.K.'s condition.

6. R.K. is sent by ambulance to your ED, which is 5 miles away. You are the RN receiving R.K.. What do you do *first*? **[I/ap/Pl/ct,ni,tc]**
   - ABCs include taking VS.
   - Identify yourself, ask patient how he feels, tell him what you are doing and why.

7. R.K. does not have SOB, dizziness, or N/V while lying down. Given the circumstances of the accident, what is the significance of this statement? **[PD/c/PI/ct]**
   - Absence of these symptoms makes it unlikely that R.K. has pneumothorax or head injury.

8. R.K.'s CT scan reveals a ruptured spleen; he needs immediate surgery. What additional information do you need to obtain before he goes to the OR? **[PD/k/PI/ct]**
   - You need a parent for parental consent because he is a minor.
   - Past medical and surgical history.
   - Current medications.
   - Medication allergies.
   - Last time he ate.

   Instructor Note: If death is imminent, surgery will proceed without these.

9. What is the greatest danger of a splenic rupture? **[PD/k/PI/ct]**
   - Internal hemorrhage that could be fatal.

10. Before surgery, which labs should be drawn? **[I/c/PI/ct]**
    - CBC with diff, type and cross (T&C) for blood, Chem 7, amylase.
    - An amylase is drawn because the pancreas is in the same location as the spleen; if R.K. fell hard enough to rupture his spleen, he also may have damaged his pancreas.

R.K. is taken to OR and undergoes an exploratory laparotomy and splenorrhaphy. Estimated blood loss (EBL) is 1600 ml, most of which was infused by means of the Cell Saver.

11. What is a splenorrhaphy, and why should this be done instead of a splenectomy? **[PD/c/PI/ct]**
    - Splenorrhaphy is the suturing of a splenic wound; the spleen provides several major functions of the immune system; total loss of this organ is often associated with overwhelming postsplenectomy infection (OPSI); it is current practice to preserve as much of the spleen as possible.

12. R.K. is 14 and he heals rapidly. He is discharged on the 5th postop day after having his sutures removed. What factors may have favored his wound healing? **[A/ap/PI/ct]**
    - His age.
    - Good nutritional status.
    - Normal oxygenation.
    - Lack of preexisting medical conditions.
    - Good wound care.

Case Study 5: Choledocholithotomy

Difficulty: **	*Setting:* Hospital
Index Words: Choledocholithotomy	

T.B., a 60-year-old retiree, is admitted to your unit from the ED. Upon arrival you note that he is trembling and nearly doubled-over with severe abdominal pain. T.B. states that he has severe RUQ (right upper quadrant) pain that radiates to his back, and he is more comfortable walking bent forward than lying in bed. He admits to having had several similar bouts of abdominal pain in the last month but "none as bad as this." He feels slightly nauseated but has experienced N/V during previous episodes. T.B. experienced an acute onset after eating fish and chips at a fast food restaurant. His daughter insisted on taking him to the hospital.

Assessment findings are an AA&Ox3 man of medium build who MAEW (moves all extremities well). Moves restlessly and continually, c/o of notable fatigue. Breath sounds clear throughout, anterior and posterior. Heart sounds clear without adventitious sounds, heart rate regular, all pulses 3+ bilat. Bowel sounds audible x 4 quadrants, abdominal guarding noted with exquisite tenderness to light palpation over R side, especially RUQ. Has sharp inspiratory arrest with palpation of the RUQ. Reports light-colored stools x 1 wk. Voids medium amber urine per urinal without difficulty. Skin and sclera slightly jaundiced. Admit VS are 164/100, 132, 26, 37.46, 36°C.

1. What structures are located in the RUQ of the abdomen? **[A/k/Pl/ct]**
   - Liver, gallbladder, head of the pancreas, duodenum, right kidney, colon.

2. Which of the above organs are palpable in the RUQ? **[A/k/Pl/ct]**
   - Liver: in some people.
   - Colon: if it contains stool.

Abdominal ultrasound demonstrates several retained stones in the common bile duct. T.B. is admitted to your floor and is scheduled for an open cholecystectomy in the AM.

3. Given T.B.'s diagnosis, what laboratory values would be important to evaluate? **[PD/ap/Pl/ct]**
   - CBC, direct and indirect bilirubin, PT/PTT, ALT (alanine aminotransferase), AST (aspartate aminotransferase), ALP (alkaline phosphatase), amylase, UA (urinalysis).

4. List 4 preop preparations that need to be done. **[PD/c/Pl/ct]**
   - Preop labs need to be drawn.
   - Preop antibiotics need to be ordered.
   - Bowel prep: enema, clear liquids this evening, NPO after midnight.
   - Preop teaching: what cholecystectomy entails, postop pain and pain management, need for vigorous postop pulmonary toilet.

5. T.B. is medicated with meperidine (Demerol) 100 mg IM for pain. He reports that, on a scale of 1 to 10, his pain has decreased from 10 to 4 in 1 hour. Why is Demerol preferred to morphine sulphate? What else could be done for T.B.'s pain? **[P/ap/PI,PSI/ct,ni,tc]**
   - Demerol is not as likely to cause spasms of the Sphincter of Oddi as morphine sulfate is; such spasms could contribute to increased pain in the biliary tree.
   - Other pain treatments would include supportive positioning while in bed, antiemetic medication if nausea becomes a problem. Preopteaching might also decrease the patient's anxiety and, thus, his perceived pain. Careful maintenance of the IV site will enhance your ability to medicate this patient efficiently.

6. What data charted in the assessment are consistent with common bile duct obstruction? **[A/c/PI/ct]**
   - Jaundice, light colored stools, medium amber urine.

7. At 2330, T.B. spikes a temperature to 38.6°C (tympanic). He is started on a broad spectrum antibiotic: Imipenem/cilastatin (Primaxin) 500 mg IV q6h. What, if anything, needs to be done before the antibiotic is begun? **[PD/ap/S,PI/ct,ni]**
   - Check medication allergies, check IV site, call physician and ask if culture and sensitivity (C&S) of blood, sputum, and/or urine needs to be collected before starting ATB (antibiotic therapy) therapy.

8. T.B. undergoes a cholecystectomy. Why is a T-tube drain installed during surgery? **[PD/k/PI/ct]**
   - The T-tube prevents the CBD (common bile duct) from scarring closed postop.

The first day after surgery, the drainage should have a small amount of bloody drainage. This soon changes to dark green (bile-colored) drainage. Initially the T-tube drains approximately 500 ml per day then gradually decreases. The second day postop, you enter T.B.'s room to complete your shift assessment. You note a small amount of bile drainage on his gown and moderate amount on the abdominal dressing. When you remove the tape to change the dressing, you note that T.B.'s skin is blistered and reddened.

9. In order to protect the blistered area from further damage, you apply a hydrocolloid dressing, such as DuoDERM, HydraPad, Restore, or Ultec to the damaged skin. What are the benefits of this type of dressing? **[PD/k/PI/ct]**
   - The hydrocolloid dressing creates a moist environment, provides a barrier to external bacteria, protects from reinjury, fosters autolytic debridement, is waterproof, and reduces pain.

10. What measures can be taken to prevent healthy tissue around a wound like this from damage or breakdown? **[P,I/k/PI/ct,ni]**
    - Wash the area with soap and water and allow to thoroughly dry, apply a protective skin barrier to the healthy tissue, then apply Montgomery straps. Montgomery straps eliminate the need for repeatedly stripping tape off the skin for dressing changes.

11. T.B. recovers uneventfully and will be discharged with his T-tube still in place. What does he need to know about this drain? **[I/ap/S,PI/ni,tc]**
    - Know how to empty T-tube bag, the importance of keeping the bag below the level of the T-tube insertion site, and how to avoid tension on the drainage bag by securely fastening it to trousers or undershirt.
    - T-tube may need to remain in place anywhere from 6 weeks to 6 months depending on healing of the CBD, so T.B. needs to understand how to maintain his activity with a continuously draining system.
    - How to clean the insertion site (daily showering is usually adequate), apply a dry sterile dressing every day, and protect his skin from drainage using zinc oxide or a karaya gel patch.
    - How to monitor for infection (redness, warmth, swelling, unusual drainage at the insertion site), obstruction (recurrence of RUQ pain, N/V, light colored stools, brown urine, or jaundiced sclera/skin), and T-tube dislodgement (sudden decrease in drainage or obvious shift in the tube).

12. What other discharge teaching does he need? **[A,P/c/PI/ct,ni,tc]**
    - Time, date, and location of his follow-up appointment.
    - Telephone number/answering service of physician in case of emergency.
    - Importance of immediately reporting signs and symptoms of complications: infection (redness, swelling, warmth, drainage) and fever.
    - Onset of or increase in pain.
    - Purpose of medications/treatments.
    - Importance of taking medications as prescribed.

Case Study 6: Appendicitis

Difficulty: **	*Setting:* Hospital
Index Words: Appendicitis, substance abuse	

W.T., a 22-year-old white man, presented to the ED with a complaint of "bad" abdominal pain. The generalized abdominal pain started 24 hours ago but seemed to "ease up" after he vomited. Several hours later the pain returned but had shifted to the RLQ and has remained there. The pain is steadily getting worse. W.T. reports marked nausea and "dry heaves," and he has no appetite. He has also had diarrhea for the last day. VS are 124/76, 92, 16, 38.8°C. W.T. works in a bar, has no health insurance, and his history is positive for tobacco ("1½ packs a day"), ETOH ("6-pack of beer a day"), and marijuana ("couple of hits a day"). He is allergic to PCN ("I itched all over").

1. What organs are located in the RLQ? **[A/k/PI/ct]**
   - Large bowel, small bowel, appendix, right ureter, right spermatic cord.

2. In what order will the ED nurse examine this patient's abdomen? **[A/c/PI/ct,ni]**
   - Observe, auscultate x 4 quads, then gently palpate abdomen beginning anywhere but the most painful quadrant. Palpate RLQ last.

3. Next, the patient's abdomen is checked for rebound tenderness. How is this done and what does it indicate? **[I/c/PI/ct]**
   - Rebound tenderness is elicited when the examiner presses steadily into the abdomen and then suddenly releases pressure. The patient is asked if pain is felt more on application or on the *release* of pressure. Also ask where pain is felt. Pain on release of pressure is called rebound tenderness and may indicate localized or generalized peritoneal inflammation. Location of the pain elsewhere than where palpated may present the real source of the problem.

You note no masses and localized rebound tenderness in the RLQ. W.T.'s lab work returns: WBC 15.5 mm^3, Hgb 14.6 g/dl, Hct 43.8%, platelets 280 mm^3; the UA is unremarkable.

4. One of these labs is markedly abnormal and when combined with the physical findings, is usually indicative of a specific diagnosis. Identify the abnormal lab value, the assessment findings, and probable diagnosis. **[A,PD/an/PI/ct]**
   - Elevated WBC correlated with RLQ, fever, rebound tenderness, nausea and vomiting, and diarrhea is usually indicative of acute appendicitis. You might suspect right-sided diverticulitis in an older person.

W.T. is sent to the OR for an open exploratory laparotomy for probable acute appendicitis. He underwent an appendectomy for a purulent but unruptured appendix and is admitted to your unit at 2330. His VS are stable and his orders include: D_5½ NS with 20 mEq KCl/L at 100 ml/h; cefoxitin (Mefoxin) 2 g IV q8h x 2 doses; diet as tolerated; up ad lib; meperidine (Demerol) 50 mg IM q4h prn for pain; when tolerating PO fluid, change pain medication to Tylenol #3 1-2 PO q4h prn for pain; droperidol (Inapsine) ¼ to ½ ml IV q6h prn.

5. Which of the above orders need to be clarified before a dose is given? Explain. **[PD/c/S,PI/ct,ni]**
   - Demerol: When did W.T. last receive pain medication? This will be recorded on the OR sheet record.
   - Inapsine: The physician did not give an indication for Inapsine use; this drug is an antiemetic.
   - Cefoxitin: This drug is not contraindicated for patients with hypersensitivity to penicillins; the cross-reactivity between PCN and cephalopsporins is 5% to 7%.

6. Just how will you determine the seriousness of W.T.'s allergic reaction to PCN? **[P/ap/S,PI/ct,ni,tc]**
   - Ask the patient what kind of a reaction he had when he took penicillin. Also ask if he has ever taken any other kinds of antibiotics. See if the following names mean anything to him: cephalosporins such as Ceclor, Keflex, Ancef, Kefzol, Mandole, and did he have a reaction them?

7. What type of reaction is considered an allergic reaction? **[PD/k/PI/ct]**
   - Any manifestations of the inflammatory response such as rash, hives, pruritus, laryngeal edema, or wheezing or crowing respirations. Any of these can signal onset of an anaphylactic reaction.

   Instructor Note: Patients who experience side effects or other types of reactions to medication often report being "allergic" to that medication. The most commonly listed GI side effects are abdominal cramping, nausea and vomiting, and diarrhea.

8. During the morning report you are told that W.T. has had an uneventful night; his VS are stable, and his IV of D_5½ NS at 100 ml/h is infusing on time. He received his second and final dose of prophylactic cefoxitin and he had no signs of allergic reaction. He will probably be discharged this AM. What questions do you want to ask the night nurse before she leaves? **[PS/ap/PI/ct]**
   - Has he had pain medication? How much? When?
   - How are his bowel sounds? Has he passed flatus?
   - How did he tolerate clear liquids?
   - What has his urine output been?

9. Indeed, W.T. appears stable and discharge orders are written the afternoon after surgery. What key issues need to be addressed in his discharge teaching? **[PD/ap/S,PI/ct,ni,tc]**
   - Patient teaching issues to be addressed in every recovering abdominal surgery patient include: (1) signs and symptoms of infection, (2) limit weight lifting to no more than 10 pounds for 6 weeks, (3) nature of and directions for medications to be taken at home, (4) who and what number to call in an emergency, (5) recommended activity progression, and (6) date and time of the follow-up visit.

Many inherent individual factors will affect the scope and direction of patient teaching. Consider W.T.'s background; he works in a bar, his history is positive for tobacco, ETOH, and Marijuana. These factors should not be glossed over. To address them would ensure the best chance of a full recovery.

10. Outline patient teaching on pain that would address these issues. **[P/ap/S,Pl/ct,ni,tc]**
    - Tylenol #3 is an analgesic (pain killer). Tylenol #3 may affect motor control, so W.T. should avoid driving a vehicle, operating machinery, avoid using knives, or clipping his toenails. If he drives and is picked up by the police, he may be cited with DUI (driving under the influence). He should not drink when taking Tylenol #3.
    - Tylenol #3 can be constipating. Be sure to call the MD if no BM in 4 days. May want to take stool softener until 1st BM. Since he is a young man, he may never have been constipated and may not take this seriously.

11. There are several additional areas for teaching that are not addressed above. Can you think what they might be? **[I/ap/S,Pl/ct,ni,tc]**
    - The patient smokes: need to emphasize that clean lungs and good respiratory toilet will oxygenate tissues better and allow his wound to heal faster.
    - W.T. is going home the day after surgery: who will be staying with him or helping him for the first few days?
    - W.T. drinks alcohol daily: if he continues, he may run into trouble with stopping. This needs to be explored. You may need to discuss withdrawal with him. A 6-pack per day is a considerable ETOH intake on a regular basis and can contribute to nutritional deficiencies that may affect healing.
    - W.T. smokes mariajuana. He needs to be referred to a substance abuse program.

Case Study 7: Small Bowel Obstruction

Difficulty: **	*Setting:* Hospital
Index Words: Bowel obstruction, electrolyte imbalance	

While you are working as a nurse on a GI/GU floor, you receive a call from your affiliate outpatient clinic notifying you of a direct admission, ETA (estimated time of arrival) 60 minutes. She gives you the following information: A.G. is an 87-year-old woman with a 3-day history of intermittent abdominal pain, abdominal bloating, and N/Vs. A.G. moved from Italy to join her grandson and his family only 2 months ago and she speaks very little English. All information was obtained through her grandson. PMH: colectomy for colon cancer 6 years ago, ventral hernia repair 2 years ago. No hx of CAD, DM, or pulmonary disease. She takes only ibuprofen occasionally for mild arthritis. Allergies include sulfa drugs and meperidine. A.G.'s tentative diagnosis is small bowel obstruction (SBO) secondary to adhesions. A.G. is being admitted to your floor for diagnostic work-up. Her VS are stable, she has an IV of D_5½ NS with 20 mEq KCl at 100 ml/h, and 3 L O_2/nc.

1. Based on the nurse's report, what signs of bowel obstruction did A.G. present? **[A/k/Pl/ct]**
   - A.G. has had abdominal pain with bloating/distention for 3 days. These are 2 of the primary symptoms of intestinal obstruction.

2. Are there other signs or symptoms that you should observe for while A.G. is in your care? **[A/k/Pl/ct]**
   - Other signs and symptoms include nausea and vomiting, hypoactive or hyperactive bowel sounds, and constipation. Any signs of dehydration will also support the diagnosis of bowel obstruction.

3. A.G. and her grandson arrive on your unit. You admit A.G. to her room and introduce yourself as her nurse. As her grandson interprets for her, she pats your hand. You know that you need to complete a physical examination and take a history. What will you do first? **[P,I/c/Pl/ct,ni]**
   - First, establish rapport. Her patting your hand may be a cue. You may take her hand when you talk to her and address her, don't look at the interpreter.
   - Watch A.G.'s condition. If she appears weak, you may have to wait to get a detailed history when she can think more clearly. Cover the basics in your assessment first in case you have to wait until later for more detail.
   - If she looks as if she can tolerate both, get both.

4. The grandson, an attorney, tells you elderly Italian women are extremely modest and may not answer questions completely. How might you gather information in this case? **[P/c/Pl/ct]**
   - Divide information into critical information and "nice-to-know" information; address the former first.

4. What key questions must you ask this patient while you have the use of an interpreter? **[A/ap/Pl/ct,tc]**
   - Time/date of her last bowel movement, time of her last urination, color and amount of stool and urine, when did she last eat, clarify allergies again. Any hx of cardiac or pulmonary problems?
   - Ask about medication allergies.
   - Double-check medications. Remember, U.S. brand names you are familiar with will be considerably different from drug names used elsewhere. Patients rarely are familiar with generic names. In addition, the drugs often appear differently (e.g., color, size, shape).
   - Ask detailed questions about her pain using the acronym COLDERRA: Characteristics, Onset, Location, Duration, Exacerbation, Radiation, Relief, Associated signs/symptoms.

   Instructor Note: In using interpreters, try for an adult family member. If no family member is present, access your facility's social services resources for interpreters and check with your patient's reference group or church. Look at the patient, not the interpreter. Keep your sentences short and simple—it's easier on the interpreter. When doing a physical assessment, an interpreter can stand behind the curtain or with his/her back to you to preserve the patient's privacy. Don't let the interpreter "escape" until and unless you have a language chart of significant words in both languages. Also, be sure to get her/his telephone number for necessary communication.

5. How would the description of A.G.'s pain differ if she has a small vs. large bowel obstruction? **[A/ap/Pl/ct]**
   - Small bowel pain would have a rapid onset of intermittent, colicky, crampy pain that is relieved by vomiting.
   - Large bowel pain is described as persistent, crampy pain that develops more gradually.

6. With some difficulty, you insert an NGT into A.G. and connect it to intermittent LWS. How will you check for placement of the NGT? **[PD/c/S,Pl/ct,ni]**
   - Several different methods exist to check placement. A combination of 2 may be best.
   - X-ray confirmation is the most reliable way to determine NGT placement.
   - Aspirate and check the pH of the gastric contents; theoretically, if the pH is less than 3, the NGT is in the stomach. However, research has shown this thinking to be faulty. Most gastric pH are <8, nasointestinal pHs tends to read >4, and pulmonary pH ranges from 6 to 9. Of course the pH will be affected by antacids. (*Nursing Research, 42*(6), 324-331.)
   - Another method is widely taught to nursing students. Briskly inject 10 to 20 cc of air into the NGT as you listen in the epigastric area of the abdomen for a rush of air or gurgling. This method has been associated with the greatest incidence of error. Air injected into NGTs placed in the lungs or duodenum is audible in the gastric area.

   Instructor Note: Do not use the old technique where one places the end of the tube in a glass of water to observe for bubbles because this may allow the patient to aspirate if the tube is misplaced, or air escaping from the stomach can be misleading.

7. List in order, the structures through which the NGT must pass as it is inserted. **[A/k/PI/ct]**
   - Nares, nasal septum, nasopharnyx, pharyngeal area, past the epiglottis, esophagus, cardiac sphincter, and into the stomach.

8. What comfort measures are important for A.G. while she has an NGT? **[P,I/c/PI/ct,ni]**
   - Properly tape the tube so that it does not pull on the nares or cause ulceration.
   - Pin the tube to her gown at such an angle that the tube does not apply pressure on the nares.
   - Regularly observe and cleanse the nares.
   - Provide good oral care.
   - Obtain prescription for Cetacaine spray or lozenges if A.G. "complains" of a sore throat (use your communication chart—be sure you have a "pain" set of words).
   - Help A.G. turn in bed to avoid traction on the tube.

9. You note that A.G.'s NGT has not drained in the last 3 hours. What can you do to facilitate drainage? **[P,I/ap/ct,ni]**
   - Check the connections to make sure the tube is connected to the suction source.
   - Have A.G. change position (turn) to see if this allows the tube to drain more freely.
   - Check for placement by gently irrigating A.G.'s NGT with 20 cc of air; if that doesn't work, irrigate with 20 ml NS (if not contraindicated).
   - Finally, change the position of the NGT and retape.

10. The NGT suddenly drains 575 ml, then it slows down to about 250 ml/2h. Is this an expected amount? **[PD/c/PI/ct]**
    - The typical NGT output is roughly 1500 ml/24 hours, but the GI tract actually produces more than 8000 ml/24 hours. Given that A.G. probably has an obstruction, 250 ml/2 hours is a smaller amount than one might expect. The actual amount of drainage from the gut will vary depending on exactly where the obstruction is located.

11. You enter A.G.'s room to initiate your shift assessment. A.G. has been hospitalized 3, days and her abdomen seems to be more distended than yesterday. How would you determine if A.G.'s abdominal distention has changed? **[A/ap/S,PI/ct,ni]**
    - Measure A.G.'s abdominal girth (measured at the widest point in her abdomen) and compare the number with those taken on previous shifts. Abdominal girth and bowel sounds need to be part of the official chart as well as available at the bedside.

After 3 days of NGT suction, A.G.'s symptoms are unrelieved. She reports continued nausea, crampy, and sometimes very strong abdominal pain; her hand grips are weaker; and she seems to be increasingly lethargic. You look up her latest laboratory values and compare them to the admission data. Her Na has changed from 136 to 132 mEq/L, K has changed from 3.7 to 2.8 mEq/L, Cl from 108 to 97 mEq/L, CO_2 25 to 31 mEq/L, BUN from 19 to 31 mg/dl, creatinine from 1 to 1.4 mg/dl, glucose 126 to 79 mg/dl, albumin from 3.0 to 2.1 g/dl, and protein from 6.8 to 4.9 g/dl.

12. Which lab values are of concern to you? Why? **[PD/ap/S,PI/ct]**
    - The electrolyte of greatest concern is the K level: A.G. is likely losing K through her NG drainage. A K of 2.8 mEq/L is life-threatening, and A.G. is at risk to developing cardiac dysrhythmias.
    - The protein and albumin are low and indicate progressive malnutrition or poor liver function: without them, A.G.'s colloidal oncotic pressure is decreased and fluids leak from the cardiovascular space to the interstitial spaces. Mobilization of fluids out of the cardiovascular space can result in hypotension and shock; proteins are essential for healing.
    - The BUN and creatinine are elevated: could indicate acute renal failure, dehydration, or increased protein catabolism due to malnutrition. Because A.G. has not been started on TPN (total parenteral nutrition), her body could be catabolizing protein for energy.
    - The Na, Cl, and glucose are decreased: A.G. could be loosing Na and Cl through the NG drainage. Glucose could be decreased due to starvation; she is not taking in the daily calories required for energy production.
    - Na, K, Cl, and CO_2 changes may arise from NGT drainage losses resulting in metabolic alkalosis; ask about mg levels.

13. What measures do you anticipate to correct each of the imbalances described in question #12? **[P/c/PI/ct]**
    - KCl (potassium chloride) will be diluted and given intravenously as a separate infusion, called a "rider" or "flash," similar to a piggyback. Because the rate must be very carefully controlled, these riders are always infused by IV pumps. The actual rate will depend on the patient care setting and patient condition. Without telemetry, the rate of KCl infusion may not be greater than 10 mEq/h.
    - Albumin levels can be increased by giving albumin IVPB; 25 g of NSA (normal serum albumin) provides the same osmolality as 2 units of fresh frozen plasma (FFP); 100 ml of 25% NSA provides the same plasma protein as 500 ml of plasma (2 units of whole blood). Albumin expands plasma volume, maintains cardiac output, and mobilizes fluids from the interstitial space to the intravascular space.
    - Na and Cl could be increased by changing the concentration of the maintenance IV as tolerated by the patient (e.g., D_5 NS)
    - All the abnormalities could be regulated by giving total parenteral nutrition (TPN).

In view of A.G.'s continued slow deterioration, the surgeon meets with the patient and her family and they agree to surgery. The surgeon releases an 18-inch section of proximal ileum that has been constricted by adhesions. Several areas looked ischemic, so these were excised, and an end-to-end anastomosis was done. A.G. tolerated the procedure well and recovered rapidly from the anesthesia in the postanesthesia care unit (PACU). Once on the unit, her recovery was slow but steady. A.G. went home in the care of her grandson and his wife on the 7th postop day. Discharge plans included walking several times per day in the house, importance of cough and deep breathing (C&DB) and use of the incentive spirometer (IS) q2h, and observing the wound for signs and symptoms of infection.

Case Study 8: Hepatitis A

Difficulty: **	*Setting:* Outpatient clinic
Index Words: Hepatitis A	

P.M., a 24-year-old house painter, has been too ill to work for the last 3 days when he arrives at your outpatient clinic. He seems an alert but acutely ill young man of average build, with a deep tan over exposed areas of skin. He reports headaches, severe myalgia, a low-grade fever, cough, anorexia, and nausea and vomiting, especially after eating any fatty food. P.M. describes vague abdominal pain that started about the same time as the other problems. PMH: no health problems, nonsmoker, drinks a "few" beers each evening to relax. Assessment: VS are 128/84, 88, 26, 38.1 °C; alert and oriented x 3, MAEW (moves all extremities well) except for aching pain in his muscles; very slight scleral jaundice present; heart tones clear and without adventitious sounds; breath sounds clear throughout A&P; abdomen soft and palpable without distinct masses. You note moderate hepatomegaly; liver edge is easily palpated and tender to palpation. P.M. mentions that his urine has been getting darker over the last 2 days.

P.M. is presenting with the key signs of hepatitis. Lab work is sent for identification of his precise problem. Results: Na 140 mEq/L, K 3.9 mEq/L, Cl 102 mEq/L, CO_2 26 mEq/L, BUN 10 mg/dl, creatinine, 1.0 mg/dl, platelets 86 mm^3, direct bilirubin 1.6 mg/dl, total bilirubin 2.3 mg/dl, albumin 3.8 g/dl, total protein 6.2 g/dl, ALT (SGPT) 66 U/L, AST (SGOT) 52 U/L, LDH 205 U/L, ALP 176 U/L, PT 12 s, PTT 32 s, urine urobilinogen 1.6 E U/L, albuminuria 160 mg/dl, bilirubinuria +, +IgM-class anti-HAV.

1. Which key diagnostic tests will determine exactly what type of hepatitis is present? **[A/k/Pl/ct]**
   - Testing is done for the presence of or specific ratio of serologic markers (specific antibodies): anti-HAV, IgM, IgG for hepatitis A; HBsAg for hepatitis B; and HCV for hepatitis C.
   - The immunoglobulin against hepatitis A virus (IgM-class anti-HAV) will occur during the first week of clinical disease and last approximately 8 weeks. This is an excellent test for acute hepatitis A infection.

2. A Chemistry 20 panel was drawn. Which of the labs listed above specifically indicates liver disease? **[A/k/Pl/ct]**
   - ALT (alanine aminotransferase, also known as SGPT) is specific for hepatocellular disease such as hepatitis, cirrhosis, liver tumor, hepatotoxic drugs, or cholestasis.

   Instructor Note: The laboratory batteries, such as the Chem 7 and Chem 20, do not always feature the same drugs from laboratory to laboratory. Warn students to check exactly what is included in these when they start working at a new site.

3. List 8 or more drugs that can cause increased ALT levels. **[A/k/Pl/ct]**
   - Acetaminophen, ampicillin, carbamazepine, cephalosporins, clofibrate, codeine, indomethacin, isoniazid (INH), methotrexate, methyldopa, nafcillin, oral contraceptives, phenothiazines, phenytoin, procainamide, propranolol, quinidine, salicylates, tetracyclines, and verapamil.

   Instructor Note: Refer to most laboratory and diagnostic test textbooks.

4. Considering that the basic pathology of hepatitis involves inflammation, degeneration, and regeneration of the hepatocyte, what type of diet will you strongly encourage P.M. to follow? **[PD/k/Pl/ct]**
   - Normal hepatic diet is adequate protein (approx. 70 to 100 g/d), high CHO (300 to 400 g/d), and moderate fat (approx. 80 to 150 g/d). In the case of simple hepatitis, there appears to be no scientific basis for the "old thinking" that urged fat restriction.

5. Differentiate between hepatitis A, B, and C on the basis of the mode of transmission and prevention. **[A/k/Pl/ct]**
   - Hepatitis A: mainly fecal-oral transmission; prevention includes good handwashing.
   - Hepatitis B: mainly blood-body fluids through broken mucous membranes or sexual contacts; prevention include vaccine for high-risk population, and avoid sharing needles.
   - Hepatitis C: mainly parenteral transfusions; prevention includes avoiding needless transfusion.

6. Name 3 major activities that can be done in a community to prevent the spread of hepatitis (any/all types)? **[P,I/c/HP/ct,tc]**
   - Screen all donated blood.
   - Avoid use of commercially obtained blood.
   - Avoid all unnecessary blood transfusions.
   - Use of vaccines as available (HBV now).
   - Vaccinate populations at high risk, including health care, day care, and food services workers; educate this group about handwashing and use of gloves.
   - Vaccinate postexposure when appropriate.

7. In P.M.'s case, the IgM-class anti-HAV antibody is positive. This indicates that P.M. is infected with hepatitis A and is in the acute or early convalescent period of the disease. Is this disease contagious? What precaution would you take? **[P,I/c/S,Pl/ct,ni,tc]**
   - Hepatitis A *is* contagious through the fecal-oral route; however, by the time jaundice has developed, the virus is no longer being shed by the fecal route. Despite this, universal precautions are important with the hospitalized patient. Teaching thorough and timely handwashing is a main method of prevention.

8. Pruritus is usually associated with jaundice. What will you do to ease this problem for P.M.? **[P,I/ap/S,PI/ct,ni,tc]**
   - Provide light loose covers and clothing.
   - Maintain cool room temperatures with a dehumidifier if possible.
   - Place cool compresses on itchy areas.
   - Apply soothing emollients such as oatmeal, baking soda, cornstarch in warm bath water.
   - Use only mild soap.
   - Dry skin thoroughly after bathing by patting, not rubbing.
   - Avoid bathing so frequently that dry skin forms.
   - Teach P.M. relaxation techniques.
   - Use distraction (e.g., videos, TV, music, sports discussions).
   - Give P.M. soft cloth to gently rub itchy areas.
   - Warn him not to use fingernails to scratch.
   - Show him how to wash his hands.
   - Use of topical corticosteroids or antihistamines may help. These require an order in hospital but can be bought over the counter (OTC) outside the hospital.

9. How would you explain to P.M. the likely progression of his disease? **[PD/AP/PI,PSI/ct,ni,tc]**
   - Begin by explaining that the clinical course of viral hepatitis can be variable; typically will pass through 3 phases, and that P.M. is probably near the end of phase 1.
   - Phase 1, or prodromal phase: onset may be abrupt with hepatitis A and more gradual with other types of hepatitis. The patient usually has general malaise, myalgia, arthralgia, easy fatigability, upper respiratory symptoms such as nasal discharge, pharyngitis, and severe anorexia out of proportion to the apparent degree of illness. An individual will frequently have nausea and vomiting, diarrhea or constipation, and a fever that is rarely higher than 39.5°C (103.1°F). As jaundice develops, fever often subsides. Abdominal pain tends to be mild but constant in RUQ or in midline and worsens with sudden movements. Not all of the above symptoms will be present; they vary with the individual.
   - Phase 2, or icteric phase: jaundice occurs approximately 5 to 10 days after onset of symptoms, although it may occur at the same time as the initial symptoms; a few patients never develop jaundice. If jaundice does occur, many may have an exacerbation of the prodromal symptoms and then gradual clinical improvement. Pruritus often accompanies jaundice.
   - Phase 3, or convalescent phase: the patient develops a very gradual increased sense of well-being; appetite returns and jaundice, fatigability, and abdominal pain gradually disappear. Caution the patient about "overdoing it" in this phase, he doesn't want to relapse.

The acute illness runs a 2- to 3-week course with full clinical and laboratory recovery in 9 weeks for hepatitis A, and about 16 weeks for hepatitis B and hepatitis C. The course of recovery may be longer in 10% of patients and some may even become chronic; fulminating hepatitis may develop, causing death in 1% to 3% of patients.

10. P.M. is living at home with his parents and 8 younger siblings. The youngest is a 4-year-old. His parents ask how to prevent the rest of the family from getting hepatitis. What specific instructions will you give? How will you know that these instructions are understood? **[I,E/an/PI,HP/ct,ni,tc]**
    - Thorough handwashing by all after defecating and urinating, and before eating; also thorough handwashing when helping P.M. or when doing his laundry.
    - Wear gloves if handling any feces/urine.
    - Clean toilet daily and flush twice after bowel movements.
    - Have a separate toilet for P.M. if at all possible.
    - Separately wash any contaminated laundry, such as bed linens.
    - Discuss "safe sex" with P.M., because hepatitis can be spread through sexual contact.
    - You will know they understand the instructions when they can paraphrase all that you told them in a clear, logical fashion.

    Instructor Note: P.M. and his parents will need to discuss with the infection control or general practice physician the advisability of postexposure prophylaxis for all members of P.M.'s family including his steady girlfriend and any other close personal contacts.

11. Given P.M.'s lifestyle, what specific patient teaching points must you emphasize? **[P,I/ap/S,PI,HP/ct,ni,tc]**
    - Must not drink ETOH during course of recovery; ETOH is a predictable hepatotoxin.
    - Must learn to rest; recovery is slow and may take 6 months to 1 year for full remission of symptoms and for liver function tests to return to normal. Overdoing physical activity may trigger relapse; expect easy fatigability for awhile.
    - Patient will be followed with periodic blood tests for 1 year after labs have returned to normal in order to monitor for relapse.
    - It would be preferable for P.M. not to return to work as a painter; many solvents are hepatotoxins. If he does return to painting, painting and stripping should be done only outdoors.
    - Follow his diet for optimal recovery.
    - P.M. must adhere to infection control procedures during his recovery; hepatitis is a very contagious disease that could endanger his family and community if it resurfaces during a relapse.

12. List 4 critical nursing diagnoses relevant to P.M.'s nursing care. **[PD/an/S,PI,PSI/ct]**
    - Altered nutrition: less than body requirements r/t anorexia, N&V, malaise, and fatigue.
    - Activity intolerance r/t fatigue, malaise, weakness, and arthralgia.
    - Pain and pruritus r/t bile salt accumulation.
    - Knowledge deficit: hepatitis A transmission r/t no previous education about hepatitis and inability/unwillingness to comprehend relevance and significance of risk.

Case Study 9: Alcoholic Hepatic Encephalopathy

Difficulty: **	*Setting:* Hospital
Index Words: Alcoholic hepatic encephalopathy, delirium tremens	

John Doe #6, an approximately 50-year-old man, is admitted to your floor from the ED. He is lethargic, has a cachectic appearance, does not follow commands consistently, and is mildly combative when aroused. He smells strongly of alcohol and has a notably swollen abdomen and lower extremities. This man was sent to the ED by local police who found him lying unresponsive along a rural road. He was aroused somewhat in the ED. Examination and x-rays are negative for any injury, and he is admitted to your unit for observation. He has no ID and is not awake enough to give any history or to coherently answer questions. Admitting orders are: admit to E3 with R/O hepatic encephalopathy; IV $D_5½$ NS with 20 mEq KCl at 75 ml/h; add 1 amp MVI (multivitamins) to each L IVF (IV fluid); Foley catheter to DD (down drain); HOB at 30 to 45 degrees at all times; tap water enemas until clear; abdominal ultrasound in AM; CBC with diff, Chem 20, NH_3 now and in AM; soft restraints prn; vitamin K 10 mg IM qd x 3 doses; thiamine 1 g IM qd; folic acid 5 mg IM qd; pyridoxine 100 mg PO qd; low-protein diet, eat with assistance only; call HO for any sign GI bleed, DTs, or 140<SBP<100, DBP< 50, P>120.

1. Which of the above orders must be done by the RN? By the aide? By the clerk? **[A/k/S/ct]**
   - RN: administer medications; start, monitor, add meds to IV; call physician with any changes in patient condition; check to be sure all orders are transcribed appropriately.
   - RN/LPN/aide: certain activities, such as inserting urinary catheters, giving enemas, and applying restraints may be done by the RN, LPN, or aide, depending on facility policies.
   - Aide: maintaining HOB, feeding appropriate diet, observing for anything unusual, such as elevated vital signs.
   - Clerk: transcribing orders, ordering labs, x-rays, and diet.

   Instructor Note: May vary according to state and location (e.g., VA hospitals)

2. The lab work drawn in the ED has come back, the blood alcohol level (BAL) is 320 mg/dl and the blood ammonia (NH_3) level is 85 μg/dl. What do these values indicate? **[A/c/Pl/ct]**
   - Any lab values must be interpreted in light of the patient's clinical condition. The BAL is far above the 100 mg/dl level considered to be intoxication in most areas, and it is still below the panic toxicity level of 400 mg/dl. The fact that this man can have this level of blood alcohol with *any* semblance of consciousness indicates that he has developed a high tolerance to alcohol.
   - The NH_3 level is considerably above normal (15-45 μg/dl) and is consistent with a significant degree of liver dysfunction. The danger of the high NH_3 level is that the ammonia will cross over the blood-brain barrier and cause hepatic encephalopathy.

While you are getting John Doe #6 settled, you continue your assessment. Neuro: PERRL, MAE sluggishly, pulling away during assessment, follows commands sporadically. CV: HR regular but tachy without adventitious sounds. All peripheral pulses palpable and 3+ bilat, 3+ pitting edema in lower extremities. IV of D_5½ NS with 20 mEq KCl/L at 75 ml/h in L forearm. Resp: breath sounds decreased to all lobes, no adventitious sounds audible, patient does not cooperate with cough and deep breathing, on RA (room air) with SaO_2 at 90%. GI: tongue and gums are beefy red and swollen, abdomen enlarged and protuberant, girth is 141 cm (64 in), abdominal skin is taut and slightly tender to palpation. BS x 4 quads. GU: Foley to DD with 75 ml dark amber urine since admission (2 hr). Skin: color pale to torso and LEs (lower extremities), heavily sunburned to UEs (upper extremities) and head. Skin appears thin and dry. Numerous spider angiomas on upper abdomen with several dilated veins across abdomen. VS are 120/60, 104, 32, 37.3°C. Toxicology screen and electrolytes have been drawn.

3. What is the significance of the spider angiomas, dilated abdominal veins, peripheral edema, and distended abdomen? **[PD/c/PI/ct]**
   - Taken together, these phenomena indicate significant portal hypertension, generally due to some form of liver disease.

4. How would you further assess the distended abdomen, and what is the clinical name for your findings? **[A/an/PI/ct,ni]**
   - Observe for any superficial abnormalities as has been done.
   - Measure the abdomen at its widest girth, marking the place measured bilaterally with ink. Record the girth. Leave the tape measure at the bedside or on the wall where other nurses can readily find it.
   - Percuss the abdomen for shifting dullness or for a fluid wave.
   - If these findings are present, the patient is collecting fluid within the peritoneal cavity; this condition is known as *ascites.*

5. Which of the following nursing diagnoses are appropriate for John Doe #6 based on the assessment given? **[PD/an/PI/ct]**

   ___ Altered nutrition, less than body requirements.
   ___ Impaired skin integrity.
   ___ Fluid volume excess.
   ___ Fluid volume deficit.
   ___ Altered thought processes.
   ___ Risk for injury.
   ___ Risk for impaired skin integrity.
   ___ Ineffective individual coping related to alcohol abuse.
   ___ Ineffective breathing pattern.
   - Diagnoses nos. 1,3, 5, 6, 7, and 9 are clearly present; there are not enough data to include the others yet.

6. What is your concern about John Doe's nutritional status? What are your objective reasons? **[E/an/PI/ct]**
   - Low protein (5.2 g/dl) and albumin (2.9 g/dl) lab values, poor muscle tone, cachectic appearance, beefy red tongue with fissures, atrophied or swollen and bleeding gums, and dry scaly skin, possibility of skin ulcers; less than appropriate weight for height will also hint toward malnutrition.
   - Midarm (halfway between the acromion and olecranon processes) muscle circumference of less than 20.5 cm (for men) also indicates malnutrition.
   - His lethargy will make oral feedings slow and difficult; he will be a candidate for additional nutrients by some other route, such as a nasointestinal tube with high calories and controlled protein intake.

7. Why is the low-protein diet ordered? How much protein is reasonable? **[PD/k/PI/ct]**
   - The dietary intake of protein is reduced to restrict the buildup of ammonia, a byproduct of protein digestion. Restrictions will vary from patient to patient; however, the usual amounts given range from 15 to 30 g/d.

8. How might you respond to fellow staff nurses' remarks, "Why are we wasting time with this 'wino.' He isn't worth the time or money. Why don't they let him die?" **[PD/ap/PSI/ct]**
   - This question requires a review of your principles. Then engage your coworkers in some values clarification (e.g., dignity, fairness, being judgmental, and confidentiality).
   - Be aware that many people drink to dull their pain or so they do not have to face unthinkable horrors of past physical, sexual, or psychologic abuse. Only the person who has been through it knows what it is like to live with that pain. As a professional, it is not for you to judge; a patient who is in pain or discomfort has the right to receive the best care that we can give. Remember that words, such as those above, can be deadly to the patient, his/her family, or to less experienced or less responsible personnel. Most of all, it affects our own integrity and humanity.
   - A brief review of facts might also be useful. Remember that a significant number of patients with cirrhosis are not alcoholics whether or not they were admitted smelling of alcohol! In this case, the BAL does point to alcoholism. Cirrhosis also arises from biliary problems, metabolic problems, and toxic effects of certain drugs, chemicals, and solvents. A certain number of cases have unknown etiology.

9. A nursing diagnoses that is appropriate for John Doe #6 is "Risk for Injury." Consider at least 3 areas of risk injury, and identify actions you will take to ensure his safety. **[P,I/ap/S,PI/ct,ni]**
   - Possibility of bleeding due to thrombocytopenia, decreased clotting factors, and esophageal varices. You should provide a safe environment and observe for evidence of bleeding (e.g., H&H trends, occult blood in stool, bruising, petechiae, tarry stools, hemoptysis, hematuria, bloody NG drainage, epistaxis).
   - Impaired skin integrity due to poor nutrition, edema, pruritus, pressure, friction, and shearing forces. You should monitor his skin for any signs of breakdown, control pruritus, turn q2h, but do not turn the patient too quickly or with insufficient personnel.
   - Delirium tremens (DTs), an episode of profound alcohol withdrawal that may occur anytime between 3 days and a week after the last drink. This can be avoided with the use of chlordiazepoxide (Librium); however, Librium may be contraindicated in a case of questionable level of consciousness (LOC).

10. What are the signs and symptoms of delirium tremens (DTs)? **[PD/k/PI/ct]**
    - The signs and symptoms of DTs herald a true medical emergency. Symptoms may begin with irritability, craving for alcohol, and a desire to simply leave the hospital. These progress to uncontrollable shaking, extreme restlessness, fear, and anxiety. Physiologically, brain metabolism has been interrupted, and this leads to confusion and hallucinations, often accompanied by dry heaves, anorexia, extreme wakefulness, excessive sweating, and seizures. The BP may rise dramatically and the pulse becomes rapid, between 120 and 140 bpm. Combinations of these symptoms can be life threatening; 5% of patients treated for DTs will die, and 15% of those not treated will die. Be alert and suspicious! Also, nurses and health care personnel can be injured.
    - It is important to recognize and prevent DTs.

11. Falls are particularly dangerous for a patient in John Doe #6's situation. Why? **[PD/c/S,PI/ct]**
    - Patients with liver disease are at high risk for subdural hematoma due to a lack of clotting factors or inadequate vitamin K. Even mild trauma can lead to intracranial bleeding that can have a rapid or a very delayed effect, resulting in an increase in intracranial pressure that can be lethal.

12. The aide asks you why the patient has tap water enemas ordered and how many to do "until clear." You reply with the following. **[PD/c/S,PI/ct,tc]**
    - "The enemas are given to decrease his ammonia level. He is lethargic because the extra high ammonia levels in his blood deactivates part of his brain. The enemas will wash out the colon bacteria that produce ammonia and also any sources of ammonia such as blood or stool. 'Until clear' means until no pieces of stool return with the enema drainage. Do not give more than 3 enemas without consulting the physician because enemas may wash out too many electrolytes. If he still has stool after 3 enemas, the physician may order a set of electrolytes before continuing."

John Doe #6 survives a rocky course of hepatic encephalopathy and near-renal failure. After 27 days, including a week in the Intensive Care Unit, he is discharged to a drug and alcohol rehabilitation facility. He is employed as a longshoreman; fortunately, his insurance covers his month of in-house intense rehabilitation.

Case Study 10: Reflux Esophagitis/Hiatal Hernia

Difficulty: ** *Setting:* Outpatient clinic

Index Words: Reflux esophagitis, hiatal hernia, hiatal hernia repair

J.S., a 57-year-old salesman, has come to his practitioner's office with a moderate amount of chest pain. He says this pain comes and goes and is worst at night, when it wakes him up. He looks haggard, with dark circles under his eyes, "I've got to get more sleep than this."

1. What are some common causes of "chest pain?" **[PD/k/PI/ct]**
   - Nonischemic cardiac causes (pericarditis, mitral valve prolapse, hypertrophic cardiomyopathy, aneurysm).
   - Pulmonary causes (pneumonia, asthma, pleurisy, pulmonary embolus, pneumothorax).
   - GI causes (esophagitis, esophageal reflux, peptic ulcer disease, gastric carcinoma, gallbladder disease, irritable bowel syndrome).
   - Musculoskeletal causes (costochondritis, thoracic osteoarthritis, muscle strain, fibromyalgia).
   - Psychologic causes (panic disorders, hyperventilation syndrome).
   - Herpes zoster.

2. What will you ask J.S. to better evaluate his pain? **[P,I/ap/PI/ct]**
   - COLDERRA: Characteristics, Onset, Location, Duration, Exacerbation, Radiation, Relief, and Associated signs/symptoms.
   - Past medical history.
   - Dietary habits and medications.
   - History of substance abuse.
   - Previous evaluation for chest pain.
   - Psychosocial issues (including depression, anxiety, physical or sexual abuse, current life stressors).

3. J.S. says the pain has been waking him up for 3 months. What would you want to know about J.S.'s lifestyle? **[A/c/PI/ct]**
   - What does he usually eat for supper and before going to bed?
   - How does he sleep? Is his bed flat?
   - Has he tried any medication or treatment on his own?
   - Does he do anything regularly before bedtime?
   - Does he drink alcohol?
   - Does he have any allergies to food or to anything?

J.S. indicates that he has tried taking antacids and some other medicine he bought at the drug store just in case these were ulcers but he gets no relief. He tried some sleeping pills but he just woke up groggy with a headache in addition to the chest pain.

4. What tests will be done to help determine the source of the problem? **[PD/c/PI/ct]**
   - Detailed physical examination and interview; pay attention to his affect to R/O anxiety and depression
   - R/O cardiac involvement: ECG, cardiac isoenzymes, echocardiogram.
   - R/O pulmonary causes: CXR, ABGs, nocturnal pulse oximeter study, if necessary a ventilation/perfusion scan.
   - R/O GI problems: barium swallow.

5. A barium swallow confirms a large sliding esophageal hiatal hernia. J.S. asks, "What is a hiatal hernia, and what do you mean its sliding?" How would you explain this to him? **[PD/k/PI/ct,tc]**
   - A hiatal hernia occurs when a portion of the bottom part of the esophagus and sometimes part of the stomach moves up into the chest through the opening in the diaphragm, the big muscle that separates your lungs and heart from your bowels. This is most likely due to weakness of muscles in the area of the hiatus, or opening in the diaphragm. This mass of herniated material slides back and forth relatively freely with changes in position.

6. J.S. asks, "Is 'heartburn' always caused by a hiatal hernia?" How would you respond? **[PD/k/PI/ct,tc]**
   - No, heartburn can also mean that you have cardiac disease. We have to R/O coronary artery disease first.
   - Many people have hiatal hernias and are never bothered by them.

7. J.S. would rather try more conservative medical treatment before having surgery. What measures can he try to minimize his pain? List at least 5. **[P/ap/PI,PSI/ct,ni]**
   - Have J.S. avoid eating for 4 hours before bedtime
   - Have J.S. elevate the head of his bed approximately 8" to 12" on blocks.
   - Do not lie down after eating.
   - Stop cigarette smoking and drink only a small amount alcohol, if at all.
   - Take medications as prescribed.
   - Take cholinergic drugs such as metoclopramide to increase gastric emptying.
   - Avoid fats, chocolate, orange juice, and tomatoes, which lower the cardiac sphincter pressure and allow reflux.
   - Avoid obesity; lose weight if overweight.
   - Avoid constipation, chronic coughing, and tight belts.
   - Try to avoid lying on his stomach or on his sides to sleep.

J.S. writes down all your instructions and is determined to conquer his problem without surgery.

8. What meds are most likely to be prescribed for J.S.? What will he need to know about them? **[P/c/S,PI/ct,tc]**
   - Several types of drugs may be prescribed: antacids, histamine (H_2) antagonists, cholinergics, and possibly proton pump inhibitors. An important point in counseling patients on hearburn to emphasize is to take their daily dose. If patients have heartburn at night, they should take their medication at night. They should experiment with administration times to achieve optimal results.

Two months later he reappears at your office, looking even worse than before. "I just can't keep the pain controlled, especially when I'm on the road."

9. After discussion, J.S. agrees on a date to have his hiatal hernia repaired. As he does this, he looks doubtful but desperate. What do you want to ask him right now? **[A/ap/PI,PSI/ct,ni]**
   - What is particularly bothering him about having the surgery? Has he known anyone who has had this surgery? Is there any past history that he is thinking about? Will knowing as much or as little as possible help him adjust to the idea of the surgery?

10. J.S. wants to know how the minilaparotomy (minilap) surgery is different from the larger laparotomy surgery. Using a picture you explain the following. **[PD/k/PI/ct,tc]**
    - "The Nissen-Fundoplication (NFP), or minilap, is the most common surgery done. The surgery is done through a slender tube containing fiberoptics. There are several quarter-inch incisions where the fiberoptic tube and a couple drains are introduced. These smaller incisions speed healing and will enable him to go home earlier than the patient receiving a traditional incision. After the surgery, he may experience some gas pain in his shoulders due to inert gas that was injected into the abdomen to help visualize the organs. Basically, the part of the stomach called the 'collar of the fundus' is drawn up and around the lower esophagus and sutured in place where the esophagus and stomach are held below the diaphragm."

11. J.S. is to have a mini-lap. What preop teaching will he need? **[P/c/PI,PSI/ct]**
    - J.S. needs to be aware that there will be postop pain and he will receive pain medications after surgery. He will need to keep his lungs clear by coughing and deep breathing at least q2h. If he is to have an incentive spirometer, he would benefit from using it before surgery. He will have an IV, an NGT, and possibly a Foley catheter. Explain these as needed. He will get out of bed to walk the day of surgery! If something unexpected occurs in surgery, he could possibly end up with a large incision. Ask if his surgeon discussed this with him.

J.S. went to surgery for an NFP by means of a minilap. The surgery was successful and J.S. went home on the second day postop. Two months later he stops back in when he comes in for an appointment with his surgeon. He has had complete relief of his gastric reflux and can sleep flat at night without waking up.

Case Study 11: Esophageal Varices

Difficulty: ***	*Setting:* Hospital
Index Words: Esophageal varices, portal hypertension, alcoholic cirrhosis	

J.D., with 2 years of sobriety behind him, has been promoted from longshoreman to nightshift foreman in a warehouse. He has new hope and new friends in his AA groups. Unfortunately, his cirrhotic liver has not recovered from 20 years of heavy drinking, and he still has residual effects. During the past 2 days he has had a "bad cough." This morning he coughed up bright red blood (BRB) and came into the ED. His coughing and bleeding have subsided for now. An IV of D_5 NS with 20 KCl/L at 100 ml/h is started and baseline labs are drawn. He is sent to the floor for observation. Shortly after you admit J.D., you hear coughing while passing his room. You enter and see BRB all over his gown and bed. He looks very frightened.

1. What needs to be done at once? **[I/an/S,PI,PSI/ct,ni,tc]**
   - Assess VS: speak calmly to J.D., and quickly take his VS to monitor cardiac status; check at least q 15 min.
   - Treat shock state: if he is showing signs of shock (low BP, rapid pulse and respiration, pale, diaphoretic), place J.D. with HOB flat and elevate foot of bed. *DO NOT* place J.D. in Trendelenburg because it will increase his portal hypertension.
   - Call MD: if J.D. is shocky, STAT page the physician; if he is stable, contact the physician. Several treatments are possible
   - Explain what you are doing while you are doing it. As the RN, you'll need to explain procedures quickly and simply help J.D. get through the procedure.

   Instructor Note: The bleeding is most likely coming from ruptured esophageal varices.

2. What specific tasks must be done? **[P,I/ap/S,PI/ct,ni]**
   - Several things need to be done simultaneously: check patency of IV (should be at least a 20 gauge), start O_2 at 4 L/nc or increase existing O_2 L flow, prepare suction set up with Yankauer tip to clear airway prn, start a second IV and hang LR, prepare an NGT to insert.

   Instructor Note: RNs should not insert NGT in patients with esophageal varices because of the likelihood of perforating a varix.

3. What do you think J.D.'s emotional state is? How would his body respond to this emotion? **[PD/ap/PSI/ct]**
   - Fear or terror; most people would be terrified. J.D.'s body would respond to the stress by releasing catecholamines, which would increase his blood pressure and may increase the esophageal bleeding. This may be counterproductive.

4. Recognizing his emotional state, what can you do to intervene? **[I/an/PSI/ni,tc]**
   - Tell J.D. that he is probably bleeding from his esophagus (the tube that runs from his throat to his stomach).
   - Tell him that the doctor is on his way to look in his esophagus and stomach, find the site of bleeding, and try to stop it.
   - Reassure him that you are going to stay with him and will help him through it. Be calm and encouraging but be realistic

5. What treatment options exist for esophageal varices? List in the order in which they are most likely to be tried. **[PD/c/PI/ct]**
   - Injection sclerotherapy via a fiberoptic endoscope.
   - Cauterization or freezing via fiberoptic endoscope.
   - Vasopressin therapy intravenously.
   - Balloon tamponade with a Sengstaken-Blakemore or Minnesota tube; this is done only to prevent a patient from bleeding to death until he can be taken to the OR.
   - Surgical ligation of varices and portacaval shunt to relieve portal hypertension (shunting the blood from the portal vein to the vena cava to decrease the pressure of the blood within the portal vein).

6. The gastroenterologist comes to the unit to perform an endoscopic exam. How will you prepare J.D. for this? **[P,I/ap/PI,PSI/ct,ni,tc]**
   - Tell J.D. that he will need to lie still on his side during the procedure.
   - The doctor will numb his throat. Then he will receive medication (Versed) that will help him relax and make it difficult to remember the procedure. Encourage him to try to relax and let the medication help.
   - Describe some of the likely sensations that will occur during the attempt to stop the bleeding; he may feel pressure or a burning sensation.
   - Send blood for labs and for T&C for possible blood transfusion.

7. The gastroenterologist performs the fiberoptic endoscopic examination. Neither cauterization nor sclerotherapy is successful for more than a few minutes and J.D.'s bleeding intensifies. The physician elects to use balloon tamponade to hold pressure on the varices until J.D. can more safely undergo surgery. What key rule will you observe with this tube? **[P,I/c/S,PI/ct,ni,tc]**
   - Monitor the pressure in the gastric and esophageal balloons to make sure they remain inflated at the proper level.
   - Regularly visualize the pharynx to make sure the esophageal balloon does not slip upward to obstruct the airway.
   - Make sure J.D. has the call light and instruct him to call if he begins to experience any difficulty.

   <u>*Instructor Note:*</u> Generally, a football helmet or traction device is used to maintain tension on the proximal end of the tube to maintain precise placement.

8. What is the major complication of balloon tamponade, and how can you help prevent this? **[PD,I/k,ap/S,PI/ct,ni]**
   - Aspiration is a major complication because the patient cannot swallow with the balloon inflated. You need to insert a catheter (NGT) through the opposite nostril and hook it to low suction or connect the esophageal suction port of the 4 lumen tube to suction.

9. J.D. looks at you and asks, "Am I going to die?" You know that the operative mortality is 5% to 15% in elective cases and 50% in emergency cases. Even the survivors have a curtailed lifespan because of an increased rate of hepatic encephalopathy and liver failure. How would you respond? **[PD/an/PSI/tc]**
   - Be honest but judicious in your response.
   - There is a possibility that he could die but his odds of surviving the surgery improve as he becomes more stable. Everyone is working to give him the best possible chance in surgery. You will keep him informed about his progress.
   - Talk to him a minute. Ask him if he believes in God. Tell him you would understand if he wanted to take a few minutes to make peace with his Maker. Ask if he would like to talk to anyone about dying or what he is going through.
   - Ask him about advanced directives. Ask him if he would like you to contact any family members.

   Instructor Note: Nurses must be honest with the patient at all times, even if the news is negative. The patient has the right to know his condition; he has the right to hear the truth. Being "midwives to the dying" is one of the greatest privileges nurses have.

10. What is shunt surgery and why is it done? **[PD/c/PI/ct]**
   - Esophageal varices arise as a result of increasing portal hypertension caused by compression or obstruction within the liver. These varices are actually collateral circulation between the portal vein and the vena cava. Varices rupture, and hemorrhage generally occurs when portal hypertension is significantly higher than inferior vena cava pressures.
   - Basically, the surgery consists of tying-off the varices and redirecting blood from the portal vein into the vena cava to lessen pressure within the portal vein.

11. J.D.'s current H/H = 8.6/26. He is to receive 2 units of fresh whole blood and 2 units of albumin (SPA). How will you know if J.D. is having any negative reactions to the transfusion, and what would you do to intervene? **[P,I/ap/S,PI/ct,ni]**
   - Determine baseline VS and assessment (location and intensity of pain, periorbital edema, ability to speak, respiratory difficulty, presence of rashes or discoloration of the skin). Ask J.D. to immediately turn his call light on if he experiences any changes.
   - Administer the blood very slowly, take VS in 15 minutes, and ask J.D. if he feels any differently than he did before the blood started.
   - Observe for changes, especially the presence of rash, hives, pruritus, periorbital edema, difficulty forming words, moderate to severe back pain, headache, or difficulty breathing.
   - If you note a reaction, immediately stop the blood, change the IV blood tubing and continue a slow NS infusion, administer O_2. Prepare for incipient anaphylaxis.
   - Notify the physician and obtain a prescription for diphenhydramine (Benadryl).
   - Send the unused portion of the blood to blood bank for follow-up analysis.

12. How much will you expect the hematocrit to rise after the transfusion of 2 units of whole blood? **[PD/k/PI/ct]**
    - Possibly as much as 6%; the average is 3% per unit.

13. Whole blood is rarely given today but might in a case of hepatic compromise. Why? **[PD/c/PI/ct]**
    - Administration of whole blood avoids the danger of ammonia breakdown products that may accumulate in packed red blood cells (PRBCs).

The blood has infused without evidence of reaction, his VS are stable, J.D. talked to the hospital chaplain at length, and then was sent to OR for a portocaval shunt. He will be transferred to ICU afterward for recovery.

Case Study 12: Inflammatory Bowel Disease with Small Bowel Obstruction

Difficulty: ***	*Setting:* Hospital
Index Words: Inflammatory bowel disease, small bowel obstruction, malabsorption problems, ileostomy	

C.W., a 36-year-old woman, was admitted several days ago with a diagnosis of recurrent inflammatory bowel disease (IBD) and possible small bowel obstruction (SBO). C.W. is married, and her husband and 11-year-old son are very supportive, but she has no extended family in-state. She had IBD x 15 years and has been on prednisone 40 mg qd for the last 5 years. She is very thin; at 5′2" she weighs 86 lb and has lost 40 lb over the last 10 years. She has an average of 5 to 10 loose stools per day. C.W.'s life has gradually become dominated by her disease (anorexia; lactase deficiency; profound fatigue; frequent nausea and diarrhea; frequent hospitalizations for dehydration; and recurring, crippling abdominal pain that often strikes unexpectedly). The pain is incapacitating and relieved only by a small dose of diazepam (Valium), Pedialyte, and total bed rest. She confides in you that sexual activity is difficult, "It always causes diarrhea, nausea, and lots of pain. It's difficult for both of us." She is so weak she cannot stand without help. You write CBR (complete bed rest) with side rails up on the Kardex.

1. Identify 6 priority problems for C.W. **[PD/ap/PI/ct]**
   - Chronic pain.
   - Diarrhea.
   - Malnutrition.
   - Risk for skin breakdown (perianal and pressure areas).
   - Fatigue.
   - Possible ineffective coping (individual or family).
   - Lactase deficiency.

2. You enter C.W.'s room and note that she has been crying. You ask what's wrong, and she explains that the nurse who admitted her to the hospital the last time said, "Welcome to death row!" C.W. says that she is knowledgeable about her condition, but she still can't seem to shake that "death row" feeling. She was afraid to come to the hospital this time. What can you do to help this woman? **[I/an,PSI/ni,tc]**
   - Let C.W. ventilate.
   - Ask her what meaning "death row" has for her.
   - Ask her what the nurses could do to be more helpful.
   - Mention to her that nurses on your unit often care for patients with her problem (if that is true). Ask her if she has anyone close to her who is supportive, and if she feels that the person needs to contacted. Offer to contact clergy if that would be helpful.
   - Continuity of care is an essential for this patient. She needs a primary nurse or a case manager to stay in close touch with her and with her care. Communication between staff nurses needs to be very clear in her case.

C.W. replies, "Treat me with respect, and as a person, not a disease. Act like I have the right and intelligence to understand my condition. Recognize that I probably know what I'm talking about when I try to refuse a delicious milkshake. When I'm either NPO or nauseated, please don't pop popcorn where I can smell it! It's pure torture!"

3. Considering C.W.'s weakness, chronic diarrhea, and lower-than-desired body weight, what interventions should minimize skin breakdown? **[I/an/PI/ct,ni]**
   - Use a fracture bedpan, and remove it as soon as she is finished.
   - Keep the perianal area clean and dry. Use a skin barrier (e.g., Desitin) as needed.
   - Use medicated wipes, such as Tucks or zinc oxide, on the anal area as needed.
   - Monitor pressure areas, especially those in contact with the bedpan.
   - Regular sitz baths may help.
   - Discuss instituting TPN with the physician with the eventual goal of high-protein, high-calorie, low-fat, low-residue diet. Also discuss a physical therapy (PT) consult for ROM and strength maintenance

C.W.'s condition deteriorates on the third day postadmission; she experiences intractable abdominal pain and unrelenting nausea and vomiting. C.W. is taken to the OR for probable SBO and is readmitted to your unit from the postanesthesia care Unit (PACU). Thirty-eight inches of her small bowel were found to be severely stenosed with 2 areas of visible perforation. Much of the remaining bowel is severely inflamed and friable. A total of 5 feet of distal ileum and 2 feet of colon have been removed and a temporary ileostomy established. She has a Jackson-Pratt drain to bulb suction in her RLQ and her wound was packed and left open. She has 2 peripheral IVs, an NGT, and a Foley. Her VS are 112/72, 86, 24, 38.2°C (ear).

4. You review the postop orders before the physician leaves the unit. One order reads vitamin A at 25,000 IU/d x 10 days. Why is C.W. to receive vitamin A? **[PD/c/PI/ct]**
   - The use of vitamin A for wound healing is controversial. Some people believe that vitamin A is needed for epithelial cell formation and maintenance. This fat-soluble vitamin is often deficient in patients with malabsorption problems such as C.W. has. Vitamin A is also given to patients who are on steroid therapy to help counteract the negative effects steroids have on wound healing. Vitamin A restores the local inflammatory response and the stimulus for epithelial migration that steroids destroy. Conversely, too much vitamin A can stimulate excess inflammatory response that can damage the wound.

5. You begin a thorough postop assessment of C.W.'s abdomen. What does your assessment include? List in the order that the assessment should be completed. **[I/ap/PI/ct,ni]**
   - Observe the dressing for drainage; abdominal distention or signs of inflammation; is the dressing intact, and does it contain drainage; color of the stoma, color and amount of drainage in the pouch, whether the seal is intact around the stoma, and if there is any skin exposed around the stoma and the drainage bag; and whether the JP fastened to it will not pull on the insertion site, is JP sutured in place, is the JP bulb connected to the JP drain, and, if suction is applied, the appearance and amount of drainage from JP drain?
   - Auscultate for BS around the periphery of the wound dressing.
   - Lightly palpate abdomen for any unusual tenderness or firmness.
   - Look around and under C.W. for drainage and bleeding.

6. A nursing student enters C.W.'s room and auscultates her abdomen. She looks at you and excitedly announces that she hears good bowel sounds. You take the opportunity to teach her the proper method of auscultating bowel sounds on a patient who has NGT to continuous LWS. How would you correct her error? **[E/an/PI/ct,ni,tc]**
   - Tell the nursing student that it is easy to forget that when the NGT is connected to suction, the suction will be misinterpreted as bowel sounds.
   - Show her how to pinch the NGT below the side port (blue side port) and listen for bowel sounds again. Explain that many people disconnect the NGT from suction before listening but this can still cause false positive sounds. Remind her that, generally, the more the bowel is manipulated, the longer it takes the peristalsis to resume. Bowel sounds should return between the third and the fifth day postop.

The nursing student follows your advice and listens again. She says "You're right, I didn't hear a thing." You tell her that she can impress her classmates while educating them in the correct technique.

7. C.W. is 4 days postop. During the routine dressing change you note a small pool of yellow green drainage in the deepest part of the wound. You realize the physician will want a wound culture. How will you culture C.W.'s wound? **[I/c/PI/ct,ni]**
   - As with any procedure, first explain to the patient what you are doing and why. Answer her questions. Irrigate the wound thoroughly with NS (never use an antiseptic solution), and use a sterile gauze to absorb any excess irrigant. The microbes that cause the infection rarely are found in the purulent drainage but instead cling to healthy, viable tissue for their sustenance. Therefore, swab only this healthy looking tissue for the specimen to culture. Avoid necrotic areas, eschar, and yellow fibrous slough. Use a prepackaged sterile culture tube with an appropriate transport medium. If microbes dry out, they die.
   - If medicated ointments or creams have been used on the wound, these must be thoroughly cleaned off before a reliable culture can be done.

8. You obtain a wound culture, complete the dressing change, obtain a full set of VS and note a temp of 38.1 °C, and assess increased tenderness in C.W.'s abdomen. You call to notify the physician and ask for additional orders. What prescriptions do you anticipate? **[P/an/S,PI/ct]**
    - Obtain full cultures, including blood, urine, sputum, and wound.
    - Flat plate x-Ray of abdomen now.
    - Change antibiotics or add a new one after obtaining cultures.

9. What information do you need to send to the lab with the wound culture specimen? **[PD/k/PI/ct]**
    - Patient's name, room number, date and time specimen was collected need to be attached to container. The exact origin of specimen (anatomical site) is needed, including type of specimen, such as swab from granulation tissue, or abscess fluid. The patient's diagnosis and any topical or systemic antibiotic therapy should also accompany the specimen.

10. The physician calls back and asks you to describe C.W.'s wound. What key aspects of the wound should be included? **[PD/c/PI/ct]**
    - Condition of skin around the wound.
    - Amount, color, odor of drainage on the dressing.
    - Tissue within wound: color, texture, odor, drainage, evidence of granulation or necrosis.
    - Size and depth of wound.
    - Any undermining or tunneling under edges or deep in wounds.
    - Remind the physician what antibiotics C.W. is taking.

11. The physician asks you how C.W.'s stoma and drainage look. What should a healthy stoma and usual drainage look like? **[PD/k/PI/ct]**
    - The stoma should appear to be a relatively uniform medium cherry red donut shape that rises above the level of the skin. There should be no blemishes or darker spots on the stoma, and the skin around the stoma, if visible, should also be intact. Drainage will be watery greenish brown and should be totally contained in the appliance pouch.

12. Will any aspect of C.W.'s history significantly affect the wound healing process? How? **[PD/ap/PI/ct]**
    - Her history of steroid use over 5 years and her chronic diarrhea both suggest that wound healing will be delayed. Steroids tend to delay healing by interrupting all phases of wound healing.
    - C.W. is clearly malnourished. Anorexia and weight loss are synonymous with malnutrition, which features a lack of cofactors and building blocks for wound healing.

13. With a fairly significant wound infection developing, why is C.W.'s temperature relatively low? **[PD/ap/PI/ct]**
    - C.W.'s inflammatory response is still below normal because of a long history of steroid intake. Infections may be masked until they are quite severe.

14. The physician tells you that she will be over to examine C.W. As you tell C.W. that her doctor is coming to talk to her, C.W. says that she feels something wet running down her side. You find the some leakage of intestinal drainage onto the skin, what should you do? **[I/an/PI/ct,ni]**
    - The appliance needs to be changed as soon as leakage is discovered. C.W. may be returning to the OR, but it is highly unlikely that the stoma will be revised. Gather materials and change appliance immediately.
    - At times it will be necessary or desirable to have the enterostomal nurse (ET) nurse do the change; at other times it will require some cooperation between shifts to get a timely change done. Few people plan their day to begin with an ostomy appliance change.

You change the ileostomy appliance before the physician arrives. C.W. is evaluated, and it is determined that she should return to surgery for exploratory laparotomy.

Case Study 13: Inflammatory Bowel Disease with Peritonitis

Difficulty: ***	*Setting:* Hospital
Index Words: Inflammatory bowel disease, malabsorption, ileostomy	

C.W., a 36-year-old woman admitted 7 days ago for inflammatory bowel disease (IBD) with small bowel obstruction (SBO). She underwent surgery 3 days postadmission for a colectomy and ileostomy. She developed peritonitis and 4 days later returned to the OR for an exploratory laparotomy. The lap revealed another area of perforated bowel, generalized peritonitis, and a fistula tract to the abdominal surface. Another 12 inches of ileum were resected (total of 7 feet of ileum and 2 feet of colon). The peritoneal cavity was irrigated with NS, and 3 tubes were placed: a Jackson-Pratt drain to bulb suction, a rubber catheter to irrigate the wound bed with NS, and a sump drain to remove the irrigation. The initial JP drain remains in place. A R subclavian triple lumen catheter was inserted.

1. C.W. returns from PACU on your shift. What do you do when her bed is rolled into her room? **[I/an/S/PI/ct,ni,tc]**
   - Tell C.W. that she is back in her room.
   - Take VS.
   - Check IVs for patency and amount of fluid remaining in the bag.
   - Connect the sump to wall suction.
   - Connect the irrigation solution to an infusion pump.
   - Empty the Foley drain of urine so you know how much urine she had out in OR/PACU and what has drained since her return.
   - Observe dressing/abdomen.
   - Obtain report from the PACU nurse.

2. You pull the covers back to inspect the abdominal dressing and find that the original surgical dressing is saturated with fresh bloody drainage. What should you do? **[I/an/S,PI/ct,ni]**
   - Reinforce the dressing with a heavy drainage dressing (trauma dressing), check C.W.'s VS, initiate treatment for shock if appropriate, and call the doctor.

3. C.W. has a total of 4 tubes in her abdomen as well as an NGT. What information do you want to know about each tube? **[PD/ap/PI/ct]**
   - Where does each tube go, are the tubes securely attached (sutured in place), are they patent and draining appropriately?

<u>Instructor Note</u>: For safety, all tubes should be clearly labeled.

4. The sump irrigation fluid bag is nearly empty. You close the roller clamp, thread the IV tubing through the infusion pump, check the irrigation catheter connection site to make sure it is snug, and then discover that the nearly empty liter bag infusing into C.W.'s abdomen is D_5W, *not NS*. Does this require any action? If so, give rationale for actions, and explain the overall situation. **[I/an/PI/ct,ni,tc]**
   - D_5W is not an appropriate solution to infuse into this patient's peritoneum. The solution is isotonic when administered intravenously but when instilled in the peritoneum, it acts hyperosmolar and pulls fluid into the abdomen from the vascular system. This could cause hypovolemia.
   - Glucose is a wonderful source of food for any bacteria left in the peritoneum.
   - The IV glucose may elevate the blood glucose on a transient basis, inhibiting wound healing.
   - Immediately change the IV tubing and solution, monitor VS, get a fingerstick blood glucose, notify the physician about what happened.
   - If C.W. appears anxious or asks what is going on, explain that the wrong solution was hung but you have corrected the error.
   - Notify the charge nurse, and complete an incident report.

The physician arrives on the unit and removes C.W.'s surgical dressing. There is a small "bleeder" at the edge of the incision so the physician calls for a suture and ties off the bleeder. You take the opportunity to ask her about a Demerol PCA pump for C.W., and the physician says she will go write the orders right away.

5. Postop pain will be a problem for C.W. after the anesthesia wears off. How do you plan to address this? **[P/ap/PI,PSI/ct,ni,tc]**
   - When C.W. is awake enough, get her to rate her pain on a 1 to 10 scale and rate the amount of relief she receives from the Demerol by way of the PCA pump. Teach C.W. that she needs to use the PCA pump to prevent the pain from becoming too intense. She should dose herself when the pain is starting to increase. If the prescribed medication does not work well, you will need to be a patient advocate to help C.W. get relief.

6. Pharmacy delivers C.W.'s first bag of TPN. The physician has written for you to start the TPN at a rate of 60 ml/h and decrease the maintenance IV rate by the same amount. What is the purpose of this order? **[PD/c/PI/ct]**
   - The physician does not want to fluid overload C.W.

7. The physician did not specifically order glucose monitoring but you know that it should be initiated. You plan to conduct a finger stick q2h for the first several hours. What is your rationale? **[PD/ap/PI/ct]**
   - You know that glucose intolerance can occur at the onset of treatment if the pancreas does not respond to the increased glucose load of the TPN solution. C.W. may require supplemental insulin injection or insulin added to her TPN solution to maintain a glucose level WNL.

8. C.W.'s blood glucose increased temporarily but by the next day it dropped to an average of 70 to 80 mg/dl and has remained there for 2 days. Her VS are stable but her abdominal wound shows no signs of healing. She has lost 1 kg over the 3 days. What do these data mean? **[E/an/PI/ct]**
   - Given her critical illness, C.W. is not receiving adequate nutrition. If C.W. were receiving adequate nutrition, she should gain 0.25 to 0.5 lb/d. C.W. has lost 1 kg (2.2 lb), and her wound is not showing signs of healing.

You discuss your concerns with C.W.'s physician, and she agrees to request a consult from a registered dietitian. After gathering data and making several calculations, the dietitian made recommendations to the attending physician. The TPN orders were adjusted, C.W. began to slowly gain weight and her wound showed signs of healing. Nutritional problems in clinical populations can be complex and often require special attention.

9. You and a coworker read the following in C.W.'s progress notes: "Wound healing by secondary closure. Formation of granular tissue with epithelialization noted around edges. Have requested dietitian to consult on ongoing basis. Will continue to follow." Your coworker turns to you and asks if you know what that means. How would you explain? **[PD/an/Pl/ct,tc]**
   - The physician is describing the first phase of healing, called the proliferative phase. "Granular tissue" is the beefy red tissue that fills in the surgical wound because it contains newly formed collagen and blood vessels. The "epithelialization noted around edges" means that the epithelial cells migrate and proliferate around the edges of the granulation tissue. The epithelial tissue looks silvery. Adequate nutrition is essential to the healing process.

10. Both of you start to discuss what specific digestive difficulties C.W. is likely to face in the future. What problems might C.W. be prone to develop after having so much of her bowel removed? **[PD/ap/Pl/ct]**
    - The ileum is responsible for absorbing bile salts, vitamins C and B_{12}, and chloride. The large colon is responsible for absorbing water and electrolytes. Therefore, if C.W. lost 7 feet of ileum and 2 feet of colon, she would be at-risk for dehydration, an electrolyte imbalance, and may be at risk for developing pernicious anemia.
    - People who lose more than 50% of the small intestine develop "dumping syndrome." Fortunately C.W. has only lost about 30% but with her IBD she will undoubtedly lose more in the future and may develop dumping syndrome at that time.

11. The dietitian consults with C.W. about dietary needs. You attend the session so that you will be able to reinforce the information. What basic information is the dietitian likely to discuss with C.W.? **[P/ap/Pl/ct]**
    - Avoid dehydration, drink at least 2500 to 3000 ml (or 10 to 11 8-oz glasses) per day.
    - Eat slowly and chew thoroughly to slow down passage of food.
    - Take a multivitamin tablet daily.
    - Avoid high-residue or high-fiber foods for 4 to 6 weeks, and gradually add new foods carefully.

12. After 3 days of dressing changes, C.W.'s skin is quite irritated, and a small skin tear has appeared where tape was removed. How can you minimize this type of skin breakdown and help this area heal? **[P,I/ap/Pl/ct,ni]**
    - Use Montgomery straps to hold dressing on, and replace changing tape each shift.
    - Use Benzoin/skin prep to keep Montgomery straps on *OR* use a mesh tube to hold the dressings on.
    - Use a skin barrier to prevent damage to skin from ileostomy drainage; ileostomy drainage is very caustic, and skin must be monitored frequently for damage.
    - Prevent skin damage with a properly fitted pouch/appliance.

13. What specifics of ostomy teaching do you plan to do. **[P/ap/PI,PSI/ct,ni,tc]**
    - Have C.W. and her husband look at the stoma.
    - Instruct C.W. and her husband in the use of ileostomy equipment.
    - Help C.W. and her husband provide ostomy care.
    - Provide support and assistance while C.W. and her husband develop skills in caring for stoma.
    - Have both of them demonstrate the use of the equipment.
    - Encourage C.W. to express her feelings and concerns about changes in body image.
    - Encourage visitation by someone from the ileostomy club.
    - Instruct C.W. where she can obtain ileostomy supplies.
    - Instruct C.W. on methods of reducing odor.
    - Instruct that drainage from the stoma will vary slightly with changes in diet.

    - Never irrigate the stoma, and do not use laxatives.
    - Empty the pouch when it is one-third to one-half full.
    - Change the pouch every 5 to 7 days at a time when the stoma is inactive.
    - Change the pouch at the first sign of a leak in the seal.
    - Refer C.W. to the community nursing service or to an enterostomal therapist for follow up.
    - Encourage C.W. to contact local ostomy support groups (*Iowa Intervention Project,* 1992).

C.W. successfully battled peritonitis. Gradually tubes were removed as she grew stronger with TPN and time. C.W. learned how to change her ostomy appliance and was discharged to home.

Case Study 14: Acute Pancreatitis

Difficulty: ***	*Setting:* Hospital
Index Words: Acute pancreatitis, pleural effusion	

B.B., a 72-year-old woman, is admitted from the ED with complaint of constant, severe abdominal and lower back pain x 2 days and SOB over the last 24 hours. "I've had to rest 4 or 5 times gettin' back to the house from the shed—it's gotten real hard to manage all by myself." A niece stopped by and insisted B.B. come into the county hospital ED. B.B. has never received any medical care of any kind. She lives by herself "up the mountain" off of a dirt road in rural Pennsylvania. She is restless, nauseated, and in pain. Everything around her is new and frightening to her. VS are 108/72, 128, 30, 37.9°C (ear), SaO_2 84% on 2 L O_2/nc. B.B. is admitted to your unit at 1900.

1. What possible diagnoses would you suspect with a presentation of severe abdominal pain? **[PD/ap/PI/ct]**
   - Peptic ulcer disease (gastric or duodenal ulcer, gastritis, duodenitis).
   - Gastroesophageal reflux.
   - Gastric cancer.
   - Biliary tract disease (cholecystitis, common bile duct obstruction).
   - Pancreatitis.
   - Irritable bowel syndrome.

2. The ED nurse giving you report says that B.B.'s admitting diagnosis is R/O pancreatitis. You know that pain control is difficult in patients with pancreatitis. What information will you want to ask the ED nurse before hanging up? **[A/c/PI/ct]**
   - Has B.B. received any pain medication in the ED? If so, how much and how long ago? Did it seem to help? Would he suggest a larger dose, or not?

3. B.B. arrives on your unit. As she is getting into bed you notice that her eyes are very wide and she is looking all around. She seems totally overwhelmed in response to the ED nurse's instructions about how to operate the bed. What of the above information may be used to guide the manner in which you approach B.B.? **[A/an/PSI/ct]**
   - She is 72 years old and has never before seen the inside of a hospital.
   - She lives by herself in the mountains.
   - She is used to doing things in her time.
   - It is likely that this woman is used to an outhouse and pumps her water from a well. It is unlikely that she has ever seen the standard pieces of equipment in her hospital room, let alone know what they are for or how to use them.

4. What approach would you use to obtain a psychosocial history and complete your assessment? **[P,I/ap/PSI/ct]**
   - B.B. is in pain, but you need to ask a few very basic questions to get a sense of how this woman lives and her level of understanding.
   - It is unlikely that you will be able to use your routine hospital talk with this woman.
   - Start by asking her, "What do you want me to call you?" Write it down, and have everyone use the same method of address.
   - Ask her if she has an outhouse at home (she'll tell you if she has indoor plumbing).
   - Ask her if she has her own well. If she does, ask her "Where is your pump? Inside or outside?"
   - Tell her that this is her room, that she will be staying here while she is in the hospital. Show her the indoor bathroom and your indoor running water. Tell her when she passes water or when her bowels move, she needs to call you to come see it.
   - Show her the call light and have her practice turning it on. Explain that you will see the light and come to her. Explain that it might take a few minutes because you have other folks to attend to. Tell her to stay put because you will come.
   - Ask her if she has any questions and answer them very simply. Remember, the woman is not stupid, just unfamiliar with your world; you would be equally lost in her world.
   - Complete your assessment. Tell her "I want to check you over like the doctor did. We're going to try to find out what's wrong with you and fix it so you can go home. First, I want to listen to your heart and lungs, feel your skin, see if you have any trouble with swelling. Then I'm going to check your belly last. That's the part that hurts you the worst so we'll check that out carefully."

You complete an assessment and note the following abnormalities: restless, prefers to sit on side of bed, leaning forward and tightly clutching her handbag. States pain has decreased "some after that lady jabbed me with that needle downstairs." Skin cool, diaphoretic, and pale. Heart rate irregular and tachy. Peripheral pulses weakly palpable x 4 extremities. Resp rapid but unlabored on 2 L O_2/nc, SaO_2 85%, breath sounds absent at the base of the LLL (left lower lobe) posteriorly. Reports marked nausea without emesis. BS hypoactive x 4 quads. Abdomen distended and exquisitely tender throughout to light palpation, guarding noted. Has not voided but states that she has "made less water than usual." Poor skin turgor, dry mucous membranes, mild scleral jaundice.

5. How are you going to assess B.B.'s pain? **[P,I/ap/PI/ct,ni,tc]**
   - Diplomatically determine if B.B. can read. Do not assume literacy among any population.
   - B.B. is unlikely to be familiar with the abstract concept of rating pain on a scale of 1 to 10.
   - If B.B. can read, you might try a word scale.
   - If she cannot read, you might try drawing a line and explain that one end is no pain and the other end is the worst pain she could ever have. Ask her to make a mark on the pain line. She will think you are crazy but that's OK.
   - You may have to settle for a description of the pain. Remember, do not suggest words to her. Let her tell you and you try to put them together in a meaningful way.
   - If you find something that works, be sure to "pass it on" so that other nurses can use the same approach.

B.B.'s admission labs return: Na 148 mEq/L; WBC 17.2 mm^3; amylase 200 U/L; K 4.2 mEq/L; Hgb 12.5 g/dl; Hct 38%; lipase 375 U/L; Cl 114 mEq/L; LDH 160 U/L; HCO_3 98 mEq/L; platelets 306 mm^3; AST 54 U/L; BUN 26 mg/dl; ALT 46 U/L; creatinine 1.0 mg/dl; ALP 96 U/L; glucose 185 mg/dl.

6. Indicate which lab values are important in the diagnosis of pancreatitis. **[PD/k/PI/ct]**
   - Amylase and lipase.

7. Reviewing the CBC and Chem 7 results, what results are consistent with your observations on her physical exam? **[PD/an/PI/ct]**
   - Mild dehydration is consistent with electrolyte concentration, slightly low BP, tachycardia, weak pulses, reported decreased urine output (UOP), poor skin turgor, and dry mucous membranes.
   - Infection is consistent with elevated WBC, desaturation, abdominal distention, tenderness to light palpation, and guarding.
   - Anemia is consistent with desaturation and low-normal H&H; once B.B. is rehydrated, her H&H will drop below normal levels.

8. B.B. voids 150 ml dark brown urine 2 hours after admission to your unit. What will you do? **[P,I/ap/PI/ct,ni]**
   - Check urine for specific gravity and guaiac. Call results to MD.

9. The physician orders a 500-ml bolus of NS and Foley to down drain. What do these orders mean, and why are they appropriate at this time? What priority assessment must be done when a fluid bolus is given? **[P,I/ap/PI/ct,ni]**
   - A bolus of fluid is given to challenge the kidneys to see if they are functioning and to see if patient's output will increase with the bolus. The Foley is a catheter into the bladder to drain urine so you can more accurately assess B.B.'s hydration status. Carefully assess breath sounds before administering the bolus; reassess q1h for several hours to monitor for fluid overload.

You deliver the NS bolus over an hour and insert a Foley catheter. You are surprised that the color of B.B.'s urine is dark amber, instead of the dark brown urine that you saw in the commode. You send a specimen to the lab.

10. The next time you answer B.B.'s call light, she states that her pain is, "Getting bad again." You are puzzled because she is not used to taking narcotics and it has been only 2 hours since her last injection of meperidine (Demerol) 100 mg. What can be done to improve her pain management? **[P/c/PI/ct]**
    - Increase the dose or frequency of the narcotic.
    - Change to another narcotic.
    - Add an NSAID such as ketorolac (Toradol) IM q6h.

NSAIDs are added to the pain regimen. You administer the first dose and notice that her bedpan is under the covers and it contains the same dark brown fluid that you noted in the commode. You ask B.B. about it and she states, "Aw honey, that's just my chewing tobacco." She spit, the dark fluid lands in the pan.

11. Is there any connection between heavy tobacco use and the effectiveness of medications used for pain control? **[PD/c/PI/ct]**
    - Tobacco increases the metabolism of drugs cleared through the liver, increasing the rate of metabolism of Demerol.

12. Based on your discovery, what action would you take? **[P,I/ap/PI/ct,ni,tc]**
    - Consult the pain management team to determine your next approach. You can either have her stop chewing or increase the medication dose or frequency.

13. B.B.'s oximeter alarms at 83% saturated, her respiratory rate is 34, and the IV bolus has infused. You auscultate no breath sounds from the scapula down on the L. You percuss B.B.'s lung posteriorly and hear a dull thud up to the scapula on the L and percuss resonant on the R. What is the significance of your findings? **[PD/an/PI/ct]**
    - Absence of breath sounds plus a dull thud on percussion indicates either the accumulation of fluid (blood or serous) in the pleural space or consolidation (e.g., pneumonia, pulmonary edema, lung abscess).

14. What 2 actions would you take next and why? **[I/ap/PI/ct]**
    - Increase B.B.'s oxygen liter flow to increase the availability of oxygen for diffusion.
    - Elevate the head of the bed to allow expansion of the thorax during inspiration.
    - Call the physician and inform him what has transpired.

The physician orders a STAT CXR, which shows a significant pleural effusion developing over the LLL.

15. Based on the diagnosis of pleural effusion, what treatment will the physician likely perform next and what is your responsibility throughout the treatment? **[P,I/c,ap/PI/ct,ni,tc]**
    - A thoracentesis will be performed to remove the pleural fluid.
    - You responsibilities include the following: helping B.B. sit on the side of the bed and remain still while the trochar is being inserted. Coach B.B. to sit still until the fluid has drained. Then make sure the specimen is properly labeled and sent to the laboratory for analysis.

Patients with subdiaphragmatic inflammatory processes frequently present with pneumonia or pleural effusion. Cloudy, yellow fluid (250 ml) was removed. B.B. was placed on broad-spectrum antibiotics until the cultures returned. She was found to have acute pancreatitis and was eventually released to home. As she is wheeled out of the hospital B.B. tells you, "I'll die up on my mountain before I'll come back here." She probably did.

CHAPTER 5. GENITOURINARY DISORDERS

Case Study 1: Urinary Tract Infection

Difficulty: *	*Setting:* Hospital
Index Words: Urinary tract infection	

You are working on a medical unit in an acute care hospital and have been assigned to care for M.Z., an 89-year-old widow. She was admitted after experiencing a sudden onset of R-sided weakness, followed by mental confusion and expressive aphasia. This combination of factors leads to problems with urinary continence. A Foley catheter is placed to facilitate urinary drainage.

1. Insertion of the catheter places M.Z. at risk for a urinary tract infection (UTI). What are the signs and symptoms of UTI? **[A/k/PI/ct]**
   - Urine color, odor, hematuria, back pain, increased WBC in urine, bacteria in urine, fever, chills, nausea.

2. If M.Z. did not have a Foley catheter, how would your list of signs and symptoms be different? **[A/k/PI/ct]**
   - Urgency, frequency, and dysuria, in addition to the responses to question #1.

3. M.Z. developed diarrhea. What special instructions are you going to give the nursing assistant assigned to give basic care to M.Z.? **[P,I/c/PI/ni,tc]**
   - Careful attention to perineal care. Carefully wash around the catheter with soap and water and dry thoroughly. This should be provided at least twice a day and after each bowel movement.
   - Encourage fluid intake.
   - Monitor intake and output carefully.
   - Observe for and report signs of UTI.

4. The nursing assistant reports that M.Z.'s 8-hour intake is 520 ml, the output is 140 ml. Is this significant? Generate at least 3 possible factors that could account for the difference. Next to each identify which item would be assessed and how. **[PD/c/PI/ct]**
   - Tubing kinked or obstructed: check tubing for kinks, blockage (follow agency policy regarding irrigation of catheter if needed); assess for bladder distention.
   - Dehydration: assess skin turgor and mucous membranes, monitor lab values, check total intake and output record for the last several days.
   - Inaccurate recording of intake and output: double-check with those caring for M.Z. about any discrepancies.

5. What factors will you teach M.Z. and her daughters about her Foley catheter. **[P,I/c/PI/tc]**
   - Its purpose and reasons for use in this situation.
   - Positioning of tubing/bag.
   - Projected length of placement.

6. You are the nurse assigned to M.Z.'s care. You notice that the nursing assistant emptying the gravity drain is not wearing personal protection devices. You also observe that the spout is contaminated during the process. What issues need to be considered in protecting M.Z.'s safety? Describe your actions in working with the nursing assistant. **[P,I/ap/S,PI/ct,ni,tc]**
   - M.Z.'s safety must be maintained. The Foley catheter is a direct route for contamination and a potential source of infection. Fortunately, the contamination of the spout should not represent a problem because most gravity drain bags have an antireflux value that prevents bacteria from moving through the tubing in a retrograde direction into the bladder. Urinary drainage bags have varying features. It is necessary to become familiar with the equipment and the special precautions for use.
   - Approaching the nursing assistant is a delicate matter. First, establish her/his knowledge of the specific procedures, such as the use of personal protection devices and the correct procedure for emptying a gravity drain. Teach and review rationale and principles inherent in both matters. Discuss possible consequences of poor procedure including spread of infection to either party and to other residents and staff.

7. M.Z. is scheduled for a CXR. You help the transportation technician transfer M.Z. onto a stretcher and notice that he raises the gravity drain to chest level to make sure the tubing is not caught on anything, then lays the bag on its side on top of M.Z.'s legs. The air vent becomes wet with urine. What breach of technique have you witnessed and what is your next responsibility? **[PD,P,I/c/S,PI/ni,tc]**
   - Immediately change the gravity drain bag. Once the air vent (usually located in the upper corner of the bag) becomes wet, it no longer serves as a barrier against bacteria/viruses.
   - Educate the transportation technician about the risk of infection that a contaminated gravity drain poses to the patient. Stress that he is in an excellent position to educate his coworkers and protect patients.

8. As you are changing M.Z.'s Foley gravity drain, she says to you, "Honey, I'm just a lot of trouble. I'm not much use to anyone anymore. Why don't you just let me go?" How are you going to respond? **[P/an/PI,PSI/ct,ni,tc]**
   - Ask her to tell you a little about her life. What she's done, what she likes to do.
   - Her condition will improve to some degree with rehabilitation. You do not know how much. Suggest that she wait and see how much function she regains. Tell her that in rehabilitation they will help her understand what she will be able to do.
   - Talk to her about advanced directives and tell her to make her wishes know to the physician.
   - Ask her if she feels ready to die. Patients often know more than we do and recognize when it's "their time."

   Instructor's note: It is essential to differentiate a developmental readiness to die from depression. Depression should be evaluated and treated appropriately.

Case Study 2: Chronic Renal Failure

Difficulty: *	*Setting:* Hospital
Index Words: Chronic renal failure	

K.B. is a 32-year-old woman who is being admitted to the medical floor for complaints of fatigue and dehydration. While taking your nursing history you discover that she has diabetes and has been insulin-dependent since the age of 8. She has been in chronic renal failure (CRF) and undergoing hemodialysis for the past 3 years. Your initial assessment of K.B. reveals a pale, thin, lethargic woman in no acute distress. Her admitting chemistries are Na 145 mEq/L, K 5.5 mEq/L, Cl 93 mEq/L, HCO_3 27 mEq/L, BUN 40 mg/dl, creatinine 3.0 mg/dl, glucose 238 mg/dl. Her skin is warm and dry to touch with poor skin turgor, and her mucous membranes are dry. Her VS are 140/88, 116, 18, 99.9°F. She tells you she has been nauseated for 2 days so she has not been eating or drinking. She denies vomiting.

1. What aspects of your assessment support her admitting diagnosis of dehydration? **[PD/c/Pl/ct]**
   - The patient's history supports an admitting diagnosis of dehydration because she told you she has not been drinking for 2 days. Her skin is warm and dry with poor skin turgor and dry mucous membranes, all of which can be physical assessment findings of a patient with dehydration. Most of her laboratory findings are elevated, which can result either from concentration when intravascular hematocrit volume is decreased or elevated secondary to CRF.

2. Identify 2 possibilities for K.B.'s low-grade fever. **[PD/an/Pl/ct]**
   - The first possibility is from her dehydration because dehydration frequently causes low-grade fevers. A second possibility could be that she has a viral illness, which could also explain her complaints of nausea.

The rest of K.B.'s physical assessment is within normal limits. She tells you she has an AV fistula in her left arm.

3. What is a fistula? Why does K.B. have one? **[PD/c/Pl/ct]**
   - *Fistula* is a term used to describe when two separate body parts are connected. In K.B.'s case, her fistula is an arteriovenous (AV) fistula. This fistula is surgically created by connecting an artery with a vein and allows access for her hemodialysis.

4. In assessment of an AV fistula, what physical findings would you expect during auscultation and palpation? Why? **[PD/c/Pl/ct]**
   - A functioning AV fistula has a "thrill" evident with palpation and a bruit present with auscultation. Both of these assessment findings are present because of the turbulence caused by the mixing of blood between the artery and vein.

Over the next 24 hours, K.B.'s nausea subsides, and she is able to eat normally. Her physician believes she experienced a viral illness because there was no other etiology found for her nausea. While you are in helping her with her AM care she confides in you that she never really understood what "diet I'm supposed to be on anyway."

5. What information would you seek from K.B. now? **[A/c/PI/ct]**
   - Before beginning any patient teaching, you should assess what knowledge the patient already has. This concept is especially important with your patients who have chronic illnesses because they will have had a lot of information that has been given to them throughout the years. Information that was accurate 10 years ago may have been replaced with updated or new information. By understanding "where the patient is" you can better individualize your teaching plan.

6. Because K.B. is on chronic hemodialysis what are her special nutritional needs? **[PD/c/PI/ct]**
   - Patients on chronic hemodialysis need to limit their K and protein. They should limit their total daily K intake to $\leq$ 2 g, and they should avoid high-potassium foods, such as citrus fruits, prunes, nuts, chocolate, and green leafy vegetables. Protein intake should be limited to 0.6-1.0 g/kg of body weight a day. Protein is broken down into nitrogen wastes in the blood that are not adequately filtered out in patients with CRF.
   - If K.B. has a tendency toward retaining fluid, her physician may limit her Na intake as well. It is important to teach your patients not to use salt substitutes because these are usually KCl instead of NaCl.
   - Adequate caloric intake (35-50 kcal/kg/day) is also important to avoid endogenous protein catabolism. Complex carbohydrates, including pasta and rice, provide good sources of protein for patients in CRF.
   - Magnesium is excreted by the kidney and also accumulates in CRF. K.B. should be cautioned about taking additional magnesium. Magnesium is most commonly found in vitamins, some antacids, and cathartics.
   - Enlist the help of other health care team members, such as the registered dietician, to help augment your patient instruction.

K.B.'s complete blood count yields the following results: WBC 7.6 mm^3, RBC 3.4 mm^3, Hgb 8.1 g/dl, Hct 24.3%, and platelets 333 mm^3.

7. Are these values normal? If not what are the abnormalities? **[A/c/S,PI/ct]**
   - K.B.'s WBC and platelets are normal. Her RBC, Hgb, and Hct are all low.

8. K.B.'s physician notes that she is anemic and this is most likely the cause of her increasing fatigue. Why is K.B. anemic? **[PD/k/PI/ct]**
   - Anemia is common in CRF and occurs because the diseased kidney is unable to manufacture an adequate amount of erythropoietin. Erythropoietin stimulates the bone marrow to produce red blood cells.

The following day K.B. is discharged feeling much better and with a good understanding of her dietary restrictions. Her iron stores have been evaluated and found to be adequate. Her physician has instructed her to continue her same medications before her admission except for the addition of recombinant human erythropoietin 50 units/kg 3 times a week with dialysis.

9. What information would you tell K.B. about her new medication? **[P,I/c/S,PI/ni,tc]**
   - Recombinant human erythropoietin is being prescribed for K.B. for her anemia. She will receive the medication after her dialysis and over time it should help with her complaints of fatigue. Other symptoms that respond to erythropoietin therapy include poor appetite, coldness, disordered sleep patterns, depression, and sexual disinterest. Patients usually require chronic therapy. The most common side effects include hypertension and iron deficiency anemia due to the mobilization of large amounts of iron.

Case Study 3: Oral Contraceptives and Domestic Violence

Difficulty: *	*Setting:* Women's homeless shelter clinic
Index Words: Oral contraceptives, domestic violence	

M.J., a 36-year-old caucasian woman, comes into the homeless shelter clinic where you work as an RN. She says she needs a prescription for birth control pills to help with her "cramps." She says she is from out of state, "between jobs," and tells you her boyfriend threw her out last night. She says she has 2 children who live with her mother "back home" and tells you she's had 3 "miscarriages." Her LMP was "3 to 4 months ago and irregular, but I don't think I'm pregnant." She denies any chronic conditions or current health problems. Her knowledge of family health history is sketchy. You smell cigarette smoke on her clothing and she admits to smoking 2 packs of cigarettes a day. She vehemently denies ETOH and drug use, and says she does not take any prescription or over-the-counter medication. Her hair is dull, her skin is dry and sallow. She appears to be hyperalert and oriented x3, her eyes dart around the room nervously. You watch her eyes as she looks around the room: the pupil sizes appear to respond appropriately to the ambient light and are equal bilaterally. She is 5'6" but she weighs only 106 lb. Although it is a hot and humid day, she is wearing blue jeans and a man's long-sleeved flannel shirt. When she responds to your request to roll up her sleeve so you can take her VS, you notice she's watching your face for any sign of a reaction. Her arm is covered with bruises that range in color from yellow and yellow-green to brown and blue. As you insert the thermometer into her mouth, you make a mental note of several scars and bruises on her face and a recent cut on her lip. Her teeth do not appear to have been cared for in a long time.

1. How would you summarize the above information for the chart? **[A/k/S,PI,PSI/ct]**
   - "Client is 36 y.o., WF P5, G2 presented at the clinic with a request for BCP. She is transient, unemployed, homeless, and states she was 'thrown out by her boyfriend last night.' VS are 108/64, 92, 22, 98.0°F (oral). Client denies ETOH, drug intake, OTC or Rx drugs. Smokes 2 ppd. Wt 106 lbs, 66". Appears nervous, hypervigilant, AAOx3. Speech is appropriate and without hesitation. Pupils appear normal and bilaterally responsive to light. Dressed too warm for conditions, with long-sleeved, flannel shirt. Bruises appear to show gradations in color indicating 1-14d old."

2. List 3 reasons she may be requesting the oral contraceptives. **[A/c/S,PI,PSI/ct]**
   - She has cramps that are alleviated by OCs.
   - She is having to prostitute herself to get money to live or for drugs and doesn't want to get pregnant.
   - She is aware of her risk and vulnerability for rape.
   - She may be getting them for someone else.

3. From the above description, state 3 pieces of information that indicate she is malnourished. **[A,D/c/PI/ct]**
   - Height for weight is lower than normal.
   - Hair and skin are dry and lifeless (possible protein deficiency).
   - Current living situation and absence of menses for 3 to 4 months (menses ceases when the body fat content goes below a critical level).

In all clinical settings you encounter individuals who are fearful and suspicious of health care workers as part of "the system." Because of their past experiences, they are hypervigilant to the possibility or perception of harm, insult, or betrayal. This includes victims with a background of domestic or political abuse, prisoners, homeless, illegal aliens, or non-US citizens (particularly if police and health care workers worked together to torture or interrogate), and minority groups. Often there are questions you would like to ask clients, but it is necessary to wait until you have been able to build an atmosphere of trust.

4. List 4 questions you would like to ask someone like M.J., if you knew it wouldn't threaten her. **[A/c/S,PI,PSI/ct,ni,tc]**
   - Have you been having sex with multiple partners or with someone who may have had multiple partners?
   - Have you used condoms every time you have had sex (oral, anal, or vaginal) and has anyone ever showed you how to use them correctly?
   - How are you earning money for living?
   - Have you been involved in prostitution?
   - Are you taking any kind of drugs or ETOH?
   - Where did you get those bruises and scars?
   - Have you been in any other shelters or in detention in the past few years?

5. You are very concerned about the possibility of abuse, but want to approach the question gently so you don't frighten her. Instead of asking her directly about her bruises and scars, what other questions could you use that might be less threatening and could lead you to what you need to know? **[A/c/S,PI,PSI/ct,ni,tc]**
   - Has anyone ever touched you in a way that made you feel uncomfortable or that you didn't like?
   - Has anyone threatened you or hit you?
   - Have you been involved in using ETOH or drugs to help you "cope" with your pain?
   - Is there any place you can go where you know you will be safe?
   - Have you ever gone to the police for help before? If so, what happened?

The family nurse practitioner (FNP) comes in and introduces herself to M.J. She sits eye-to-eye and asks M.J. a few questions about how she has been feeling. She asks M.J. if she ever had a vaginal exam performed in the past and how it made her feel. She explains to M.J. she would like to do a physical and vaginal exam as part of the evaluation. The FNP and you leave the room to give M.J. privacy for changing into the examination gown.

6. Explain why the FNP talked with M.J. first, before having her change into the examination gown. **[P/c/PSI/ct,ni,tc]**
   - By setting a less authoritarian atmosphere, the FNP wants to signal M.J. that both she and what she says are important. By meeting "face-to-face" while still wearing her street clothes, M.J. is less likely to feel vulnerable and victimized. The FNP knows that physical touch of any sort may be frightening and threatening for someone with a background of abuse. The goal is to create a milieu of client-centered support.

7. As you present your assessment to her, the FNP tells you that M.J. is not an appropriate candidate for OCs because of her age and her smoking. Explain the rationale behind this statement. **[A,PD/c/S,Pl/ct]**
   - OCs are not advised for older women, especially if they are sedentary because of the increased risk of thromboembolism that they present.
   - The risk of thromboembolism is greatly increased by smoking.
   - The combination of risks is especially lethal.

8. The FNP tells you that her goal is to see if M.J. will allow her to test for HIV status, TB, STDs, take an H&H, and let her do a Pap smear. Explain the rationale for each of these tests in the current setting. **[A/c/Pl/ct]**
   - HIV: M.J. probably has directly or indirectly been exposed to multiple sex partners at risk (substance abusers, those who have been in prison, possibly IV drug transmission in the past).
   - TB: individuals in homeless shelters are frequently exposed to TB through transients and illegal aliens.
   - STDs: M.J. probably has been exposed to several STDs through her ex-boyfriend or through prostitution.
   - H&H: M.J. has several characteristics that may indicate anemia, such as (1) poor nutritional status, (2) somewhat higher pulse and respirations, (3) sallow facial coloration, and (4) absence of period for past several months.
   - Pap smear: A prior history of early and frequent sexual partners, such as the FNP suspects in M.J., also places her at higher risk for cervical cancer.

As the FNP conducts a general physical examination on M.J., she explains what she is going to do and how it should feel. She also explains the tests she would like to do and why they would be important to M.J. She makes it clear that there is no charge for the tests. During the course of the examination, M.J. admits that she has not eaten a good meal "for longer than she can remember." She also admits that her ex-boyfriend really was her pimp and he beat her when she didn't bring in enough money. She is afraid he is going to come after her and kill her as he threatened. She doesn't know anyone she can trust; her mother "got custody of the kids several years ago while I was on crack and got sent-up for possession" and she won't talk to her. M.J. also alludes to the probability that she will be engaging in prostitution to "pick up a little cash" by saying, "I gotta earn a living the only way I know how." About your offer to teach her about condoms, she says, "It's OK, honey. I've heard it all."

M.J. allows the tests to be taken. To your surprise, the FNP gives her a 1-month paid prescription for OCs and encourages her to come back for the test results, check-up, and prescription renewal. The FNP also gives her a pass for a good meal and directions to the domestic violence shelter for the night. As M.J. goes out the door, she turns to you both and says, "Hey thanks...you've been real nice to me."

9. Why do you think the FNP gave M.J. the OC prescription despite the clear contraindications? **[P/c/S,Pl/ct,ni]**
   - The chance of a pregnancy for M.J. right now would be far more disastrous for mother and baby than the possibility of a cerebrovascular accident (CVA) or stroke. Sometimes the best choice we can make is to select the lesser of two evils.

Unfortunately, M.J.s body was found along the interstate 10 days later. She had been sexually molested and bludgeoned to death. No one ever claimed the body, and no one was ever arrested or charged in her death.

Case Study 4: Acute Renal Failure

Difficulty: *	*Setting:* Hospital
Index Words: Acute renal failure	

You are working on a medical-surgical floor when you assume the care of K.S., a 52-year-old man who is 3 days postoperative from an appendectomy. K.S. was admitted to the hospital with acute R lower quadrant pain, and R/O appendicitis. During surgery it was noted K.S.'s appendix had ruptured and he experienced a brief episode of hypotension. Hemostasis was immediately restored and he has been stable since that time. K.S.'s VS are 106/70, 88, 12, 100.8°F. His most recent laboratory data are Na 144 mEq/L, K 4.8 mEq/L, Cl 100 mEq/L, CO_2 25 mEq/L, BUN 84 mg/dl, creatinine 8.4 mg/dl, glucose 106 mg/dl. Yesterday K.S.'s physician had noted in his progress note that K.S. had acute tubular necrosis.

1. What is acute tubular necrosis (ATN)? **[PD/k/Pl/ct]**
   - Acute tubular necrosis (ATN) is the most common cause of acute renal failure (ARF). Although these terms are used interchangeably, they are not the same because ARF can occur without ATN. ATN is usually caused by ischemia or, to a lesser degree, nephrotoxic agents. ATN occurs most frequently after surgery (40% to 50% of cases) but is also associated with sepsis, severe burns, and obstetric complications.

K.S.'s medications include gentamicin (Garamycin) 80 mg IVPB q8h. MSO_4 1-10 mg IV q4h prn for pain, and acetaminophen (Tylenol) 650 mg q4h prn for fever.

2. K.S. has 3 potential causes for ATN. What are they? **[PD/c/Pl/ct]**
   - The most likely cause of K.S.'s ATN would be his documented hypotension during surgery. ATN could also occur if he is septic from his ruptured appendix. Lastly, aminoglycoside administration can cause ATN, and since K.S. is receiving gentamicin routinely, this could cause or exacerbate ATN. As K.S.'s nurse, it would be your responsibility to question the physician about his rational for ordering gentamicin for him.

   Instructor Note: Gentamicin dosing and ARF is somewhat tricky. Typically, patients are given a 3 mg/kg loading dose, then a peak level is drawn and a 12 hour random level is drawn to determine the appropriate dose and dosing interval. A dose of 80 mg IV q8h would lead to a high trough level and would contribute to ototoxicity and nephrotoxicity.

3. K.S. informs you he is having incisional pain. What information should you assess before administering his MSO_4 that is ordered? **[A/c/S,Pl/ct]**
   - Before administering his MSO_4 you should first verify the order on his medication administration record as well as the last time he received a dose. If sufficient time has elapsed since his previous dose (in this case 4 hours) then you can prepare an additional dose. Whenever there is a dosage range (1-10 mg), you should verify what the previous dose was and then ask your patient if the last pain medication adequately controlled his pain. With this information you can adjust the medication dose up or down depending on your patient's response.

4. What correlation do rising creatinine (Cr) levels have with the number of functioning nephrons? **[PD/k/PI/ct]**
   - The normal kidney can lose 25% to 50% of its functioning nephrons before there is any elevation in the serum creatinine because the functioning 50% to 75% will increase their workload. Once 50% of the nephrons are affected, the serum creatinine level will usually double. If a patient loses 75% of his nephrons, the creatinine will elevate to about 8 times normal. If a patient has lost 90% of the functioning nephrons, creatinine will elevate to about 10 mg/ml. These elevations represent end-stage disease where kidney transplant or dialysis is required.

5. K.S.'s BUN and Cr are markedly elevated. Do these elevations correlate with his risk of developing chronic renal failure? **[PD/k/PI/ct]**
   - No. In ATN you can't correlate the creatinine levels with the degree of nephron loss because all of the nephrons are damaged at one time so there are no nephrons to compensate.

6. S.M. calls you into his room and states, "My arm hurts where the IV is." What should you do? **[A/k/S,PI/ct,ni]**
   - Anytime a patient has an indwelling IV catheter, there is a potential for infiltration or infection. Your first response should be to evaluate the site for signs and symptoms of infiltration or infection, which include erythema, tenderness, swelling, or drainage at the site. Usually the IV will not be infusing or it will be infusing more slowly than expected.

7. You inspect S.M.s's IV site and note the site has no erythema, drainage, or swelling. The IV infuses freely when the dial a flow is wide open. S.M. continues to complain of tenderness at the site. What is another potential cause for his pain, and what are appropriate nursing interventions? **[PD/c/S,PI/ct]**
   - Another potential cause could be related to his IV Gentamicin. All IV medications can cause vein irritation and tenderness at the site without the IV being infiltrated. Appropriate nursing interventions include asking the physician if the IV rate could be decreased, and continue to monitor his IV site frequently to ensure it has not infiltrated or have another IV inserted. As always, document his complaint, your assessment, your intervention (including patient teaching), and the plan and evaluation in the patient's medical record.

8. What are general nursing priorities for patients in ATN? **[P,I/c/S,PI/ct,ni]**
   - Monitor I&O and daily weights. Monitor for any hypertension or other symptoms of fluid overload including tachypnea, decreased SaO_2, or congestive heart failure in those patients predisposed to cardiac complications. Monitor laboratory data, especially BUN, Cr, and serum K levels, all of which elevate with ATN.

Case Study 5: Transurethral Resection of the Prostate

Difficulty: *	*Setting:* Emergency department
Index Words: Transurethral resection of the prostate	

You are working in the ED when M.B., a 72-year-old man, enters with a chief complaint of inability to void. His initial VS are 168/92, 70, 20.

1. Are M.B.'s vital signs appropriate for a man his age? If not, what are the abnormalities and offer possibilities for the abnormality. **[A/c/PI/ct]**
   - M.B.'s blood pressure is elevated, and his respirations are borderline increased. Both of these elevations are probably caused by the pain response or anxiety about having to go to the hospital.

While taking your nursing history, you discover he is in general good health and leads an active life. His current medications include finasteride (Proscar) 5 mg daily and vitamin supplements. He reports that he hasn't been able to void in 12 hours and is very uncomfortable. He asks if there is anything you can do to help him.

2. During your initial assessment what finding would you expect in regard to his chief complaint? **[A/c/PI/ct]**
   - If M.B.'s symptoms are caused by complete outflow obstruction, you would expect to find a distended bladder on palpation of his lower abdomen.
   - Anxiety r/t hospitalization and inability to void.

3. What are your nursing priorities for this patient? **[PD/ap/S,PI/ct,ni]**
   - M.B.'s symptoms are due to distention of the bladder so obtaining an order to insert an indwelling catheter should alleviate his symptoms. Although rare, bladder rupture can occur, so placement of the catheter must be completed as soon as possible.
   - Another priority includes pain control with the use of prescribed analgesics.
   - Help reduce M.B.'s anxiety by keeping him informed about what is happening and updating him on his treatment plan.

4. After examining M.B., the ED physician asks you to insert a indwelling urinary catheter. What should you include in M.B.'s teaching regarding the placement of a indwelling urinary catheter? **[P,I/k/PI/ct,ni,tc]**
   - M.B. should be instructed that placement of the catheter will allow his urine to flow through the catheter into a collection bag. This procedure will require you to cleanse the head of his penis so that the risk of causing an infection will be decreased
   - Obtain lidocaine jelly for placement of the Foley; liberally lubricate the catheter before inserting.

Insertion of the catheter is usually not painful although, he will feel pressure while the catheter is advanced up the urethra. Once the catheter is in place, he should have a rapid relief of his symptoms, and the catheter will be secured into place.

5. After 2 attempts at placing the catheter you are frustrated because you are unable to advance the catheter without forcing it. What is your next intervention? Why? **[P/c/S,PI/ct,ni]**
   - The ED physician should be notified that you are unable to pass the catheter. When there is total urethral obstruction, catheterization frequently can be difficult and often you are unable to pass the obstruction. It is imperative that the catheter never be forced, or internal trauma with resultant inflammation and bleeding can occur, making additional attempts at catheterization more difficult.

After successful placement of the urinary catheter, M.B. reports he is much more comfortable. M.B. informs you he is scheduled for surgery in the coming week because "the doctor told me the pills were not working." M.B.'s urologist calls with the following orders: admit to urology, condition stable; diet as tolerated; NPO after midnight; consent for transurethral resection of the prostate (TURP).

6. What general preoperative teaching would you provide for M.B.? **[P,I/k/PI/ct,ni,tc]**
   - First you must identify what type of anesthesia M.B. will have. Many TURP procedures are performed under spinal anesthesia, which requires different teaching than general anesthesia. Independent of the anesthesia type, education should be provided regarding pain control, prevention of pulmonary complications, intravenous therapy, oxygen therapy, general information about tentative length of surgery, and where significant others can wait during the surgery. Be sure to ask M.B. if all his questions have been answered before ending the preoperative teaching session.

7. What specific preoperative teaching would you provide regarding a TURP? **[P,I/c/PI/ct,ni,tc]**
   - M.B. will have a catheter postoperatively. Inform him you will be checking his urinary drainage frequently after surgery, and depending on the amount of bleeding and his surgeon's preference, irrigations may be performed.

8. What psychosocial issues should be addressed with M.B.? **[P,I/ap/PSI/ni,tc]**
   - You would teach M.B. that a TURP should not affect his ability to have an erection or alter his sexual performance. Often patients are reluctant to ask these questions because they are embarrassed. By discussing the topic in a straightforward manner, you will help M.B. feel more comfortable and less reluctant to bring up his other concerns.

Case Study 6: Sexually Transmitted Disease

Difficulty: **	*Setting:* Outpatient clinic
Index Words: Sexually transmitted disease, pelvic inflammatory disease, human immunovirus	

You are the nurse in a walk-in clinic. A.P. is being seen this morning for a 2-day history of diffuse but severe abdominal pain. She complains of nausea without vomiting but denies vaginal bleeding or discharge. A.P. claims to have had unprotected sex with several partners, some of whom complain of penile discharge. Her last menstrual period ended 3 days ago. She has no known medication allergies and denies previous medical or psychiatric problems. VS are 108/60, 110, 20, 100.6°F (tympanic).

Physical exam finds her abdomen is very tender. The slightest touch of her abdomen causes her to "jump off the exam table." Bowel sounds are normal in all quadrants. Pelvic exam found purulent material pooled in the vaginal vault, it appeared to be coming from the cervix. A sample of the vaginal drainage was obtained and sent for culture.

1. What medical interventions can you anticipate? **[P/ap/PI/ct]**
   - Administer pain medications. A.P. will likely receive IV meperidine (Demerol) for rapid pain control.
   - Treatment of probable infection. Starting dose will be given in the clinic with take-home prescription.
   - A.P. will be rehydrated with PO fluids to offset fluid loss from her elevated temperature.

2. Based on A.P.'s stated history and the results of the vaginal exam, the physician suspects a *Chlamydia* infection. Formulate a nursing plan for A.P. that can be shared with the community agency for follow-up. **[P,I/ap/S,PI/ni,tc]**
   - Patient teaching. A.P. must understand that *Chlamydia* is a sexually transmitted disease and that her partners must be treated. She needs to understand that the disease may be present even if no symptoms are present.
   - Consequences. *Chlamydia* is a pelvic inflammatory disease that, if left untreated, may result in sterility. The liver capsule may be involved, causing perihepatitis. Systemically it may result in arthritis and dermatologic problems.
   - Unfortunately, compliance with any medical regimen requires that the patient believe in the treatment and that the treatment will be effective, and the patient must be willing to pay for the prescription(s).

3. Based on the previous question, identify the potential issues for noncompliance and what other action might encourage successful compliance. **[P/c/PI/ct]**
   - A.P. may not be willing to discuss the problem with her partners or help them understand the importance of seeking treatment. She may also be unwilling to practice safe sex for present or future partners.
   - There is potential that when the symptoms diminish, she may also not be willing to continue the medication.
   - Follow-up by community nursing or a home health nurse may help monitor for further problems and compliance.

The physician has the option of treating A.P. by one of two different methods. First, the physician could prescribe treatment over a period of 1 week; A.P. would be given the first dose of doxycycline (Monodox) 100 mg PO then would be given a prescription for the same to be taken PO bid x 7 days. Second, the physician could prescribe a one-time dose of azithromycin (Zithromax) 1 g PO which could be administered in the clinic.

4. A one-time dose of azithromycin 1 g PO is ordered for A.P.. Why is this a good choice for her? **[PD/c/S,Pl/ct]**
   - This medication is now being prescribed for treatment of *Chlamydia* infections. The one-time dose is the full course of treatment. For that reason it eliminates the concern with her compliance with the medication regimen part of treatment.

5. *Chlamydia* is considered a sexually transmitted disease that has not been mandated to be reported to the Public Health Department (PHD). Why would the PHD wish to see this become a reportable disease? **[PD/c/S,Pl/ct]**
   - *Chlamydia* is responsible for dramatic clinical manifestations in men and in women.
   - Transmission from mother to fetus can result in newborn morbidity; most frequently conjunctivitis and pneumonia.
   - It is often not microbiologically confirmed and may be asymptomatic; therefore, it is difficult to assess the incidence of infection in men or women.
   - 1990 statistics indicate that over 800,000 cases of symptomatic *Chlamydia* occur in men annually. The incidence in women is estimated to be about the same. With these estimates in mind, it is suggested that *Chlamydia* is the most prevalent STD in the United States.

   Instructor Note: This issue may be used as a classroom activity, with small groups representing each side of the issues.

6. You ask if someone has talked with her about "safe sex." She laughs and tells you there is nothing safe about sex. Undaunted, you ask if she would be willing for you to discuss the use of condoms with her sexual partners. She tells you that she's already careful; if she doesn't know the guy, she uses condoms every time. How are you going to respond? **[A,P,I/c/S,Pl/ct,ni,tc]**
   - Tell her you understand she tries to be careful but you are very concerned about her. Pregnancy is not the only problem.
   - You cannot tell by looking at someone if he/she has a STD or HIV.

7. You ask her if she has been tested for HIV. She says, no, she doesn't know anyone with AIDS, and she doesn't do sex with gay men. Now what are you going to say? **[A,P,I/c/S,Pl/ct,ni,tc]**
   - Tell her HIV is not limited to gay men. It may have started in that group, but one of the fastest growing groups getting HIV is women with multiple sex partners.
   - PID is one of the primary presenting manifestations of HIV in women.

8. You ask her if she would like to be HIV tested; it won't cost her anything and no one has to know—it's completely confidential. She agrees to the test and it comes back positive. What is her prognosis? **[PD/c/PI,PSI/ct]**
   - HIV-infected women seek medical care later than do men. All women who have PID should be HIV-tested. The course of the disease varies, depending on the degree of immunocompetence reflected by the CD4 count. However, A.P.'s long-term outlook is dismal.

Case Study 7: Benign Prostatic Hyperplasia

Difficulty: **	*Setting:* Clinic
Index Words: Benign prostatic hyperplasia	

S.M. is a 68-year-old man who is being seen at your clinic for routine health maintenance and health promotion. He reports that he has been feeling very well and has no specific complaints except for some trouble "emptying his bladder." He had a CBC and chemistry survey completed 1 week before his visit, and the results are as follows: Na 140 mEq/L, K 4.2 mEq/L, Cl 100 mEq/L, HCO_3 26 mEq/L, BUN 22 mg/dl, creatinine 0.8 mg/dl, glucose 94 mg/dl, RBC 5.2 mm^3, WBC 7.4 mm^3, Hgb 15.2 g/dl, Hct 46%, platelets 348 mm^3. His VS at this visit are 148/88, 82, 16.

1. What can you tell S.M. about his lab work? **[PD/k/PI/ct]**
   - All of S.M.'s lab results are within normal ranges.

While obtaining your nursing history, you discover that there is no family history of cancer or other genitourinary problems. During further questioning you discover that S.M. has had progressive symptoms over the past 6 months, which include the urge to urinate frequently, decreased ability in starting the stream of urine, and decrease in the force of the urinary steam. The health care provider examines S.M. and reports that his prostate is enlarged and gives a tentative diagnosis of benign prostatic hypertrophy (BPH). The health care provider also orders a clean-catch urine and PSA test.

2. S.M. is curious why this condition would affect his urination. What would you teach him? **[P,I/c/PI/ct,ni,tc]**
   - BPH is caused by nodular hyperplasia (increase in the number of cells), as well as hypertrophy (increase in size of the existing cells) of the prostate gland. As the gland increases in size, the tissues that surround the prostatic urethra compress it, causing the symptoms of urethral obstruction.

3. Why were the additional tests of the UA and PSA ordered? **[PD/c/PI/ct]**
   - The UA was ordered to rule out a urinary tract infection as the cause of his symptoms. The PSA is a blood test used in combination with examination to detect prostate cancer.

4. What concepts would you include in teaching S.M. to obtain a clean-catch urine specimen for UA? **[P,I/k/PI/ct]**
   - S.M. should not touch inside the collection container to prevent contamination. He should wipe from the meatus outward using the towelette provided (usually packaged with the clean-catch collection container). S.M. should initiate his stream of urine and then collect the sample midstream. After the sample has been collected, the lid should carefully be replaced, taking care not to touch the inside of the lid or container.

S.M.'s UA returns with results that are within normal limits (wnl). His PSA is 2.0 ng/mL. The health care provider informs S.M. his blood work was normal. S.M. tells you he still has several questions. What information would you include in answering his following questions?

5. S.M. asks you, "Do I have cancer?" **[PD/c/PI,PSI/ct,ni,tc]**
   - Frequently patients' biggest fear is that they have cancer. Until this fear is alleviated, they will not be ready to learn additional information. You should tell S.M. that his test results indicate he does not have cancer and again reinforce the previous teaching about BPH.

6. "Will this condition affect my relationship with my wife?" What do you tell him? **[PD/c/PSI/ni,tc]**
   - Patients are often embarrassed to ask questions about their condition and how it may affect their sexuality. The nurse needs to be aware that phrases such as "relationship with my wife" frequently refer to the ability to have an erection or ejaculate. You need to clarify your patient's question and offer answers in a professional clear manner. BPH should not affect S.M.'s ability to have an erection or other normal sexual function.

7. Before being discharged, the health care provider gives S.M. a prescription for doxazosin (Cardura) with instructions to take 1 mg/d x 7 days, then 2 mg/d x 7 days, and then 4 mg/d thereafter. What type of drug is Cardura, and what are other indications for the use of this drug? **[PD/k/PI/ct]**
   - Cardura belongs to the drug class of alpha-1-adrenergic blockers. This class of drugs has long been used for hypertension, but over the past few years has been found effective for the treatment of BPH.

8. What are the most common side effects for this drug class? **[PD/k/S,PI/ct]**
   - Hypotension, especially orthostatic hypotension. Other side effects include dizziness, drowsiness, somnolence, syncope, and palpitations.

9. From a safety standpoint, what information does S.M. need to know about his treatment with Cardura? **[PD/c/S,PI/ct]**
   - The most common side effect is orthostatic hypotension. It is imperative for the nurse to teach patients to go from a lying to sitting to standing position slowly. In an effort to decrease this side effect, Cardura is usually begun at a low dose and tapered upward over a few weeks. The most profound blood pressure effect occurs 2 to 6 hours after dosing, so taking the medication at bedtime can help alleviate some of the symptoms. Patients should be cautioned about the potential for falling, especially when they get up at night to urinate.

Case Study 8: Renal Calculi

Difficulty: **	*Setting:* Emergency Department
Index Words: Renal calculi	

It is a hot summer day and you are an afternoon nurse in an ED. S.R., an 18-year-old woman, presents at the ED with severe L flank and abdominal pain, nausea, and vomiting. S.R. looks very tired, her skin is warm to touch, and she is perspiring. She paces about the room doubled-over and is clutching her abdomen. S.R. tells you that the pain started early this morning and has been pretty steady for 6 hours. Her abdomen is soft and without tenderness but her L flank is extremely tender to touch/palpation. She is obviously in a great deal of pain. You place S.R. in one of the exam rooms and take the following VS: 138/88, 90, 20, 99°F. Urinalysis shows hematuria. A flat plate x-ray of the abdomen and an intravenous pyelogram (IVP) confirm the diagnosis of a kidney stone low in the L ureter.

Her mother is in the waiting area and seems to be intoxicated. She is quite noisy, belligerent, and has a strong smell of alcohol. She is obviously upsetting her daughter and is disturbing other patients and their families. The mother is berating you and the other staff members in her loudest voice, "You need to do something, NOW. Don't you know how to do anything?"

1. What is your first priority and why? **[P/c/Pl/ct,ni]**
   - Your first priority is to intervene to control S.R.'s pain. Complete an assessment of her pain, obtain appropriate orders, and administer pain medication as soon as possible. S.R. will need clear and explicit instructions about the medication and its expected effects.
   - Working with the mother will be more of a challenge. Talk to S.R. and ask if there is a family member or friend who could come to stay with and calm her mother. S.R.'s mother will need reassurance that you are actively working to make her daughter comfortable. Information should be offered in small understandable pieces and repeated. Hospital personnel (staff or security) may be helpful in keeping her mother settled.

S.R. is seen by a urologist. His plan is to control her pain, prevent infection, and encourage fluids to flush out the stone. She received a dose of intravenous meperidine (Demerol), which eases her pain for the time being. His orders are as follows: discharge to home, encourage fluids, and strain all urine. Prescriptions include oxycodone (Percocet) 1 or 2 tabs PO q3-4h for pain and ciprofloxasin (Cipro) 250 mg PO q12h.

2. What specific instructions will you give S.R. about her urine, fluid intake, medications, and activity? **[P,I/ap/S,PI/ni,tc]**
   - Strain all urine (provide with strainer), and instruct S.R. to keep all stones. Inform her that the urologist can examine the stones to determine the type of stone and that this information is helpful to determine the plan for preventing stones in the future.
   - Fluids: S.R. should increase her intake to 3000 to 4000 ml per day with urine output of at least 2000 ml/day. She should understand that this is the primary method of flushing the stone from the urinary tract. A written record may help her keep track of her actual intake; constant sipping of water is usually more tolerable than drinking large amounts less frequently. Compliance with such instructions can be increased when you help the client set simple achievable goals, such as drink 1 ½ quarts (approximately 1500 ml) by 1200, 1 ½ quarts by 1600, and another quart by 2000.
   - Activity: ambulation may facilitate movement of the stone through the urinary tract.
   - Medications: she should take the pain medication regularly. She should also understand not to operate machinery while taking the medication. Narcotics may slow bowel activity and result in constipation. Fortunately, her increase in fluid intake and ambulation may offset the effects of narcotics on bowel activity. You may counsel her to increase fiber intake to prevent constipation. The antibiotic should be taken until gone. Avoid antacids with ciproflux.

3. What factors may impede S.R.'s comprehension of your instructions, and how can you increase her retention of important information? **[P/ap/S,PI/ct,ni]**
   - S.R. is under the influence of IV narcotics and she is under a great deal of stress. Both of these factors will influence S.R.'s retention of information.
   - When teaching patients, remember that retention can be increased by engaging several senses in the instruction. Use of written instructions (handouts) will serve as a reminder and help with retention. Ordinarily, including family members when explaining instructions can be helpful. This allows them to discuss specific information and formulate plans for compliance with instruction. In S.R.'s case, however, the mother is not likely to enhance learning.

4. S.R. is quite young to develop a renal calculi. She may need to understand how she can prevent the development of stones in the future. What factors lead to development of the stones. **[PD/k/PI/ct]**
   - Climate: high atmospheric temperature leads to increased fluid loss, thus increasing the urine concentration and the concentration of the solutes that result in stone formation. There is a higher incidence of calculi formation in the summer months.
   - Diet: generally, limited fluid intake may precipitate the formation of stones. Most patients are encouraged to increase fluid intake. Before offering specific dietary instructions, you need to know what type of stone the patient has developed. Ninety percent of all stones formed contain calcium. Until recently, most patients were advised to reduce calcium-rich diets. It was previously thought that by simply reducing the concentration of calcium, stone formation could be prevented; just the opposite may be true. About 40% of all stones are calcium oxalate; thus, high calcium intake may decrease the absorption of oxalate in the intestine, thereby decreasing stone formation.

5. The urologist schedules S.R. for a follow-up visit in 2 days. He informs her that if the stone has not passed by then he will schedule her for extracorporeal shock-wave lithotripsy (ESWL). The physicians' explanation to S.R. is quite technical and confusing to her. In appropriate terminology explain to S.R. the concepts and principles of ESWL. **[I/c/PI/ni,tc]**
   - ESWL is noninvasive and it does not require any incisions or tubes. A machine called a lithotriptor generates high-energy sound waves to shatter the stone without hurting the surrounding tissue. She will be able to pass the smaller pieces in her urine.
   - Other techniques may use a more direct route. The percutaneous ultrasonic lithotriptor is introduced into the renal pelvis and positioned against the stone. Ultrasonic waves break up the stone, and saline is used to flush the stone fragments out.

6. S.R.s' pain has been controlled by the use of IV narcotics. Her mother is still obviously intoxicated. What ramifications might this have on discharging S.R.? Discuss the issues, and generate several possible actions. **[P/c/S,PI/ct,ni]**
   - The judgement of both individuals is impaired, and neither should drive an automobile. Legally you should do what you can to ensure the safe return home for S.R.
   - Students should generate lists of alternatives that might ensure her safe return home. The following list is only the ideas of the author and are not exhaustive. Call a friend or family member to transport. Check if social services has a "slush fund" for taxi or bus fare. Retain S.R. and her mother for several hours until the mother is able to drive.

7. In view of her mother's condition, you are concerned with sending S.R. home with narcotics. How would you discuss this issues with S.R.? **[P,I/c/S,PI,PSI/ct,ni,tc]**
   - Caution her that ETOH and narcotics may be a lethal combination. Her mother must not have access to her pain medication, although she may put a lot of pressure on S.R. She must do this for her mother's protection.

8. You notice S.R. appears to be embarrassed to discuss her mother with you. How will you respond? **[P,I/c/S,PSI,HP/ct,ni,tc]**
   - Situations like this are common in American families and especially in ED's. You know many people who are trying to live with this kind of confusion.
   - Ask her if she has ever attended "Alateen" meetings (call Alcoholics Anonymous for information)? If so, did she find them useful? Encourage her to go back. If not, suggest she needs support and encouragement in dealing with her mother's problems. She needs to do this for herself.

Case Study 9: Renal Calculi

Difficulty: ***	*Setting:* Emergency department
Index Words: Renal calculi, noninsulin-dependent diabetes mellitus	

F.F., a 58-year-old with noninsulin-dependent diabetic mellitus (NIDDM), presents at the ED with severe R flank and abdominal pain, nausea, and vomiting. The abdomen is soft and without tenderness. The right flank is extremely tender to touch and palpation. VS are 142/80, 88, 20, 99.0°F; urinalysis shows hematuria; an IV of .9 NS is started and is to infuse at 125 ml/h. An intravenous pyelogram confirms the diagnosis of a staghorn-type stone in the R renal pelvis. The right kidney looks enlarged. He states that he did not sleep well last night and has not eaten much today. He is obviously very fatigued. His laboratory results are as follows: Na 144 mEq/L; K 4.0 mEq/L; Cl 101 mEq/L; CO_2 26 mEq/L; BUN 30 mg/dl; creatinine 3.6 mg/dl; glucose 260 mg/dl; Uric acid 5.0 mg/dl; Ca 9.0 mg/dl; Phos 2.6 mg/dl; total protein 7.8 g/dl; Albumin 4.0 g/dl; total-bili 0.3 mg/dl, direct-bili 0.1 mg/dl; Chol 200 mg/dl; Alk phos 61 U/L; LDH total 100 U/L; AST (SGOT) 13 U/L; ALT (SGPT) 13 U/L; GGTP 40 U/L; Amylase 98 U/L.

1. F.F. is treated with IV morphine for pain. It is late afternoon before he is admitted to your unit and scheduled for lithotripsy in the morning. What specific priorities do you identify for F.F.? **[P/ap/Pl/ct,ni]**
   - Pain control: F.F. C/O R flank pain, tenderness, and nausea.
   - Control his glucose: the stress of his illness will alter his metabolism of glucose. Although he has not eaten much, his glucose is elevated 260 and he needs sliding-scale insulin coverage to control his glucose.
   - Sleep/rest: F.F. looks exhausted and stated that he did not sleep well last night.
   - Monitor his hematocrit and hemoglobin: he is losing blood in his urine.
   - Monitor fluid status: F.F.'s BUN and creatinine are elevated, which indicates underlying renal damage.

2. The physician has prescribed gentamicin 80 mg IVPB q8h. You question the physician about giving this large a dose of gentamicin to F.F. You are met with angry and belittling statements. Articulate why you *should* question this specific order for F.F. **[PD/c/Pl/ct]**
   - The ordered dose of gentamicin has the capacity to be nephrotoxic. F.F.'s renal function is already impaired as reflected by the elevated BUN and creatinine.
   - Also, the enlarged R kidney could already represent the development of hydronephrosis.

3. How should you handle the situation with the physician in order to protect the patient and promote a collegial relationship? **[P,I/an/S,Pl/ct,ni,tc]**
   - The communication should be direct, private, and respectful.
   - Tell the physician that you are trying to understand the rationale for his decision, you are interested in sharing new information, and you are both interested in meeting the needs of F.F.
   - Share with him the factors you have identified as placing F.F. at risk for further renal impairment: impaired renal function, presence of the staghorn calculi, and the already enlarged R kidney.

4. Hydronephrosis is a potential complication for F.F. What may be the impact of this problem on his long-term kidney function. **[PD/ap/PI/ct]**
   - Complete obstruction of urine flow results in increased pressure that affects the function of the proximal tubule and the glomerulus. Glomerular filtration is decreased. Complete unilateral obstruction may reduce the GFR to 30% of normal. F.F.'s creatinine clearance is already abnormal.

5. Analyze the relationship between creatinine and GFR and predicting kidney function. **[PD/c/PI/ct]**
   - Creatinine is constantly released by muscle cells. The glomerulus in the intact nephron will clear creatinine from the body as it is produced, keeping the level constant. If the GFR decreases, the serum creatinine level will increase. Therefore, creatinine concentration or creatinine clearance can be used to indicate change in glomerular function. It is important to monitor the BUN:creatinine ratio for F.F. (normal is 10 or 15:1).

6. Later, as you walk past his bed, you notice F.F. crawling off the end of the bed. What are you going to do? **[P,I/ap/S/ct,ni,tc]**
   - As you help him back into bed, you tell him he could hurt himself if he tries to get out that way.
   - Ask him why he was trying to get up. Ask him if he has to go to the bathroom.
   - Lower the siderail, help him to stand up at the side of the bed, hold onto him, and give him a urinal (you'll probably have to hold it in place for him—*be sure to wear gloves*).
   - Return him to bed, raise his side rails, and give him a call light. Tell him, if he needs anything, he needs to call.
   - If he has family in the waiting room, ask him who he would like to have come back to stay with him.

F.F. is going to be admitted. You call the unit nurse to give report. You tell her he's been up all night with pain that has just been relieved by IV morphine. You don't know whether he's going to have lithotripsy or surgery; surgery is unlikely because the stone is so large.

7. You tell F.F. he is going to be admitted and will probably need surgery for his kidney stone. He looks at you, panicked, and says, "I can't do that. I don't have any insurance. This is costing me a wad already." How are you going to respond? **[P,I/an/S,PI/ct,ni,tc]**
   - Tell him that if this is not treated appropriately, it can completely obstruct his kidney and he could end up in intensive care or die.
   - Evaluate your usual resources. Reassure him this is an increasingly common problem. If he is indigent and there is a city/county hospital, he could be transferred there for treatment. Your ED also has a social worker who is experienced in facilitating reasonable payment options.
   - Inform him that this cannot be ignored. The longer he waits, the more it is going to cost.
   - If he insists on leaving, explain the consequences of his signing out AMA (against medical advice).
   - Document this discussion on the chart.

Case Study 10: Acute Renal Failure

Difficulty: ***	*Setting:* Hospital, ICU
Index Words: Acute renal failure, percutaneous transluminal coronary angioplasty	

You are working in the ICU of an acute care hospital and assume the care of E.B., a 78-year-old woman who is 3 days postinferior wall MI. E.B. had been healthy before admission except for a long-standing history of osteoarthritis treated with piroxicam (Feldene) 20 mg daily, and severe long-standing hypertension treated with atenolol (Tenormin) 50 mg daily. She also takes ranitidine (Zantac) to prevent NSAID-induced duodenal ulcers. On presentation to the ED, E.B. had severe hypertension (210/122 mm Hg); therefore, thrombolytics were contraindicated and she was taken directly to the cardiac catheterization lab for acute percutaneous transluminal coronary angioplasty (PTCA). Her angioplasty was successful and she has been pain-free since the PTCA. You are reviewing E.B.'s lab work and note the following values: Na 142 mEq/L, K 4.9 mEq/L, Cl 100 mEq/L, CO_2 26 mEq/L, BUN 28 mg/dl, creatinine 2.2 mg/dl, glucose 158 mg/dl.

1. What abnormalities are there in E.B.'s lab work? **[A/k/PI/ct]**
   - E.B.'s BUN, Cr, and glucose are all elevated.

2. What are possible causes for these abnormalities? **[A/c/PI/ct]**
   - Glucose levels rise during stress and then slowly return to normal. E.B.'s glucose was probably elevated because of the stress of her impending MI. E.B.'s elevated BUN and Cr could be from several causes. First, hypertension can result in stenosis of the renal arteries, which reduces blood flow to the nephrons causing less effective filtration. Second, long-term treatment with nonsteroidal antiinflammatory drugs, such as Feldene, can cause a chronic renal insufficiency. Finally, if E.B. experienced a hypotensive episode from her MI before her admission to the ED, she could have had decreased blood flow to the kidney with resultant decrease in filtration.

3. Describe prerenal, intrarenal, and postrenal causes of acute renal failure (ARF). Given the potential causes of E.B.'s elevated BUN and creatinine, how would they be categorized? **[PD/ap/PI/ct]**
   - Prerenal causes of ARF include those conditions that originate outside the kidney causing a net effect of decreased blood flow to the glomeruli. Because blood flow is inadequate, filtration is less effective. Intrarenal conditions include damage to the nephrons from ischemic or toxic insult (e.g., aminoglycoside antibiotics or radiocontrast dye). Postrenal conditions block the flow of urine creating greater pressures in the kidney's collecting tubules, which ultimately results in decreased filtration.
   - Hypotension is an example of a prerenal condition. Hypertension can be classified as prerenal if it has caused renal artery stenosis or intrarenal by direct effect on the nephron. NSAID use is classified as an intrarenal cause of ARF.

You are given the results of E.B.'s lab work from today. The results are: Na 140 mEq/L, K 5.3 mEq/L, Cl 104 mEq/L, CO_2 24 mEq/L, BUN 68 mg/dl, creatinine 3.0 mg/dl, glucose 104 mg/dl. You have also noted her urine output for the past 8 hours is 160 ml.

4. Based on these values, what is your next action going to be? **[PD/an/S,PI/ct,ni]**
   - Because E.B.'s lab work is significantly changed from yesterday and her urine output is inadequate (less than 30 ml/h) you should immediately notify her physician.

5. Define oliguria and anuria. Which term best describes E.B.'s renal function? **[PD/c/PI/ct]**
   - Oliguria is urine output less than 30 ml/h or 400 ml/24 hours. Anuria is defined as urine output less than 50 ml/24 hours. E.B. is currently oliguric.

6. In reviewing E.B.'s vital signs you cannot identify any episodes of hypotension since her admission. What might be a possible explanation for her increase in BUN and creatinine? **[PD/an/PI/ct]**
   - Radiocontrast media (x-ray media) can be an intrarenal cause of ARF. Patients who have preexisting renal insufficiency will frequently lapse into ARF from the nephrotoxic effects of the radiocontrast. E.B. would have received radiocontrast during her acute angioplasty.
   - Her MI may have resulted in decreased cardiac output and decreased perfusion of the kidneys.

7. What are your nursing interventions and priorities for a patient in ARF? **[P,I/ap/S,PI/ct,ni]**
   - Careful monitoring of VS, I&O, and daily weights. If a patient begins to retain too much fluid, you will see an increase in weight, blood pressure, and a potential for respiratory difficulty. Monitor all of your patient's lab work but specifically BUN, creatinine, and K. K levels can rise in ARF to critical levels, leaving your patient at-risk for life-threatening cardiac dysrhythmias.

8. E.B. has been very quiet. Suddenly she asks you, "Am I going to die?" How will you respond? **[P/an/PSI/ct,ni,tc]**
   - First recognize how frightening these events must have been for her.
   - Yes, people can die from the things that are happening to her. That is why she is in the hospital, and she is being watched carefully. Nobody knows for sure, but you are doing everything possible to prevent that.
   - Talk about advanced directives.
   - Ask her how she feels about dying.

9. You talk to her about the possibility of dialysis, which may be a treatment for her. She responds, "You know, I'm 78 years old. I've had a pretty good life and I don't want to be hooked to a machine." What will you say? **[P/an/PI,PSI/ct,ni,tc]**
   - Explain that if dialysis is initiated early in the treatment of ARF, she may regain kidney function.
   - Explain the difference between hemodialysis and peritoneal dialysis. You don't know which one she would be eligible for because she hasn't been evaluated. With peritoneal dialysis, she would receive her treatments at home and would be able to walk around.
   - Tell her that is certainly her choice and she should discuss *all* her options with her physician.
   - Encourage her to be assertive about her feelings and opinions when she talks to her physician. See if she would like a family member, a clergyperson, or you to be there when she talks with him.

Case Study 11: Urinary Tract Infection

Difficulty: ***	*Setting:* Extended care facility
Index Words: Urinary tract infection	

M.Z., an 89-year-old widow, recently experienced a left cerebrovascular accident (CVA). She has R-sided weakness and expressive aphasia with swallowing difficulty. M.Z. has a PMH of L CVA 2.5 year previous, chronic atrial flutter, hypertension, and noninsulin-dependent diabetes (NIDDM). M.Z. has a negative psychiatric history and has lived with her daughter's family in a rural town since her previous stroke. Since admission to an acute care facility 5 days ago, M.Z. has gained some strength, has become oriented to person and place, and is anxious to begin her rehabilitation program. M.Z. is transferred for rehabilitation to your skilled nursing facility with the following orders: hydrochlorothiazide (HydroDiuril) 25 mg PO qd, digoxin (Lanoxin) 0.125 mg PO qd, aspirin (Halfprin) 81 mg PO qd, warfarin (Coumadin) 5 mg PO qd, Tylenol 325 mg q6h prn for pain, zolpidem (Ambien) 5 mg PO hs prn for sleep. Diet: mechanical soft 1800 ADA low Na with ground meat; maintain Foley catheter to down drain; and speech, occupational, and physical therapy to evaluate.

1. What lab orders would you anticipate as a result of this specific list of orders? With each response describe your rationale. **[PD/ap/PI/ct]**
   - Chemistry studies to monitor the Na, K, Cl, and CO_2. Hydrochlorothiazide can dramatically effect K, Na, Cl, glucose, BUN, and creatinine.
   - Prothrombin time to monitor the anticoagulant effects of the Coumadin.
   - Digoxin level should be kept within therapeutic range (0.5-2.0 ng/ml) to prevent significant cardiovascular side effects such as dysrhythmias and bradycardia.

2. Based on the information given, what are the 3 priority nursing diagnoses for M.Z.? **[PD/an/S,PI,PSI/ct]**
   - Impaired verbal communication related to CVA as evidenced by inability to express thoughts verbally.
   - Toileting self-care deficit related to impaired mobility and transfer ability, decreased strength, and neuromuscular impairment.
   - Impaired physical mobility related to neuromuscular impairment as evidenced by right sided weakness, decreased strength and endurance.

3. At the interdisciplinary care conferences you report that bladder training is progressing and recommend removing the catheter if M.Z.s mobility and communication abilities have progressed sufficiently. The group and M.Z. agree that she is ready. The Foley is removed. Identify 3 problems that M.Z. is at risk of developing following catheter removal. Describe specific nursing interventions for each problem. **[PD,P/ap/S,PI,PSI/ct]**
   - Incontinence: place the call light in reach, and respond rapidly to her request. Establish a q2h (regular) voiding schedule with use of verbal cuing; offer the bedpan or transfer to the commode q2h and clean genital area after each voiding. Provide fluids according to schedule and limit fluid intake 2 to 3 hours before bedtime. Monitor intake and output carefully. Encourage M.Z. to conduct Kegel exercises for 5 to 10 minutes qid. Place incontinent pads as appropriate. Provide M.Z. with positive feedback when episodes of incontinence decrease.
   - Safe ambulation: schedule ambulation after voiding to reduce the need to hurry. Dress M.Z. in nonrestrictive clothing. Help M.Z. use footwear that facilitates walking and prevents injuries. Help M.Z. sit on the side of the bed to facilitate postural adjustments. Consult physical therapist regarding ambulation plan as needed. Use a gait belt to help with ambulation as needed. Provide assistive devices (cane, walker, wheelchair) for ambulation until M.Z. is steady on her feet. Monitor M.Z.'s use of the assistive devices. Help M.Z. stand and ambulate a specified distance and with a specified number of staff. Help M.Z. establish realistic increments in distance for ambulation. Encourage M.Z. to sit up in the chair as much as tolerated (Iowa Intervention Project, 1992).
   - Bladder retention. Monitor intake and output carefully. Monitor for bladder distention and discomfort. Help to bedside commode at regular intervals. Flush toilet, run water, or place M.Z.'s hands in warm water while she is on the BSC.

4. Two days after the Foley is removed you observe that M.Z.'s urine is cloudy and concentrated and has a strong odor. What are your immediate actions? **[P,I/an/PI/ct,ni]**
   - Assess for other signs and symptoms of urinary tract infection.
   - Obtain order for a clean-catch specimen for culture and sensitivity.
   - Encourage fluids.
   - Obtain order for antibiotics.

5. M.Z. is started on sulfamethoxazole 400 mg/trimethoprim 160 mg (Bactrim DS) 1 tab PO bid x 3 days. However, 2 days later you find M.Z. in the bathroom on the toilet, and she is very upset. There is blood on the floor next to the toilet, and the water is bright red with clots. You help her clean herself, help her into bed, and provide emotional support. Describe your assessment steps. What complications do you anticipate? **[P,I/an/PI/ct,ni]**
   - Examine the perineal area to determine if the blood is originating from the urethra, vagina, or rectum.
   - Take full set of vital signs.
   - Assess the abdomen for pain, tenderness, or rigidity.
   - Obtain recent urinary elimination history from M.Z. (intake/output, frequency of urination, presence of dysuria, nausea/vomiting, chills).

6. You complete your assessment and report your findings to the physician. You obtain an order for a straight catheterized specimen for culture and sensitivities. Identify at least 2 causes for M.Z.'s hematuria. **[PD/ap/PI/ct]**
   - The urinary tract infection that is not responding to the antibiotic presently prescribed.
   - Prolonged anticoagulation time from the Coumadin and Halfprin; both interfere with normal clotting mechanisms. Coumadin depresses the hepatic synthesis of vitamin K-dependent coagulation factors (II, VII, IX, X).
   - Bactrim DS interacts with warfarin and may cause hypothrombinemia.

7. M.Z.'s UTI is responding to antibiotics and you want to prepare M.Z. and her daughter for eventual discharge. What specific issues must be considered in the teaching/discharge planning to prevent a recurrence of infection? **[P,I/ap/PI/ni,tc]**
   - Proper perineal cleaning after toileting (clean from front to back).
   - Proper intake of fluids.
   - Void every 2 to 3 hours and completely empty bladder, and try not to delay voiding.
   - Wear cotton panties; they decrease perineal moisture.
   - Watch for signs and symptoms of UTI, and seek medical attention if they are present.

8. You talk with M.Z.'s daughter about her understanding of caregiving responsibilities for her mother. What kind of questions are you going to ask to assess whether she is capable of taking on this additional burden? **[A/an/S,PI,PSI/ct,ni,tc]**
   - Does she work outside the home? If yes, is she dependent on this job for financial support and benefits? If yes, is management accepting of employees taking family leave time when needed?
   - Does she have room in her house? What is the structural layout or floor plan of the house? Will her mother be able to get in and out of the house, are there steps, is there a bathroom close by and is it accessible.
   - Will anyone be available to help her or relieve her in caring for her mother. Remind her that this is a 24-hour-a-day, 7-day-a-week job. If yes, how committed is that help?
   - Tell her about respite care. There are adult day care facilities.
   - What kind of financial resources does her mother have? Have they consulted an attorney about long-term financial needs and resources? They also need to talk to the social worker to see about the availability of assistive devices.
   - Does she have personal resources of support who are willing to let her express her needs and frustrations?

Case Study 12: Abdominal Surgery

Difficulty: ***	*Setting:* Hospital
Index Words: Hysterectomy	

T.C. is a 30-year-old woman who, 3 weeks ago, underwent a vaginal hysterectomy, right salpingo-oophorectomy for abdominal pain, and endometriosis. Postoperatively she experienced an intraabdominal hemorrhage and her Hct dropped from 40.5% to 21%. She was transfused with 3 units of PRCs. Following discharge she continued to have abdominal pain, chills, and fever and was subsequently readmitted twice: once for treatment of postop infection and the second time for evacuation of pelvic hematoma. Despite treatment, T.C. continued to have abdominal pain, chills, fever, and N/V.

T.C. has now been admitted to your unit following an exploratory laparotomy. V.S. 130/70, 94, 16, 37.6°F (tympanic). She is easily aroused and oriented to place and person. She dozes between verbal requests. She has a low-midline abdominal dressing that is dry and intact and a Jackson-Pratt (JP) drain that is fully compressed and contains a scant amount of bright red blood. Her Foley to down drain has clear yellow urine. She has an IV of 1000 ml D_5.2 NS infusing at 100 ml/h in her L forearm, with no swelling or redness. T.C. is receiving IV morphine sulfate for pain control through a patient-controlled analgesia pump (PCA). The settings are: dose 2 mg, lock-out interval 15 min, 4 hour maximum of 30 mg. When aroused, she states that her pain is an 8 on a 1 to 10 scale. She also has 2 L O_2/nc, and her SaO_2 by pulse oximeter is 93%.

1. During your assessment you note that T.C.s' respiratory rate is 16 and shallow. Articulate your plan for a more complete assessment of T.C.s' condition. Include factors to be considered, the supporting rationale, and your nursing actions. **[P/an/Pl/ct,ni]**
   - T.C. has several factors that may influence her respiratory status. First, she is immediately postop. Anesthetic agents and other medications given intraoperatively affect both rate and depth of respiration. The most commonly utilized general anesthetics are administered, absorbed, and excreted through the respiratory tract. In addition, muscle relaxants are administered during abdominal surgery to aid surgical access. Second, postoperative medication used for pain control affect the respiratory system, especially immediately postop. Intravenous narcotics can dramatically effect the character, depth, rhythm, and rate of respiration. When caring for a patient receiving this type of pain control, respiratory rate, rhythm, and depth should be monitored frequently. Third, lying in the same position for extended periods of time can lead to stagnation of pulmonary fluids during surgery. These factors tend to induce ateletectasis.
   - Interventions include encouraging T.C. to breathe deeply to expand all lung fields and facilitate the pulmonary excretion of anesthetic agents. Also, T.C. needs to cough and turn side to side to facilitate the mobilization of pulmonary fluids. A pulse oximeter should be used to continuously monitor oxygen saturation levels.

The unit is very busy when T.C. is returned from the postanesthesia care unit (PACU). Staffing is minimal. You are concerned about monitoring T.C. carefully enough. Your present patient load is 6, 2 patients are newly postop, and 1 is getting ready for discharge. You have a nursing assistant that you share with another R.N. You are most concerned with T.C.s' respiratory status and the possibility that she may, in her drowsy state, self-administer a dose of narcotic that would further reduce her respiratory status.

2. Formulate a plan, given the resources mentioned above. **[P/an/S,Pl/ct,ni]**
   - First, make sure the control to the PCA pump is not accessible to T.C. until she is completely awake. Second, following a complete assessment, work out a schedule with the nursing assistant so that one of you will monitor VS, LOC, and SaO_2 q15min until T.C. is more awake.

3. Pain control using the PCA can be very tricky. Throughout the first post-op day it has been difficult to juggle T.C.'s need for pain medication and depression of her respiratory status. Discuss the concepts of controlling pain with IV narcotics and factors that may be adjusted to better control her pain. **[PD/c/S,Pl/ct]**
   - PCA attempts to administer low doses of analgesic at frequent intervals to deliver a more continuous level of pain control. A loading dose is delivered initially to raise the blood level to an effective range. The patient then self-administers to maintain the blood level within an effective range, based on his/her perception of the pain. The type of medication, amount of medication delivered with each dose, and time interval between doses may need to be adjusted to achieve the greatest effectiveness. Sometimes the additional administration of nonsteroidal antiinflammatory medications or PO analgesics may prove effective when used in conjunction with PCA. Remember, no single drug is effective for everyone.

   Instructor Note: PCAs can also be set to deliver a specified amount of drug at regular intervals.

4. T.C. is beginning to withdraw from conversations with you and the other staff, she sleeps most of the day, and is not eating. At times she is tearful and is irritable with her husband. You believe that she is showing signs of depression. What actions should you take to help her? **[P,I/an/S,PSI/ni,tc]**
   - Document the specific behaviors, and report them to the physician.
   - Allow her to verbalize her feelings, and make the situation emotionally safe for her.
   - Consistency in staff assignments will help develop relationships in which she can verbalize her feelings.
   - Use other members of the health care teams (pastoral care, social workers) to provide opportunities for her to work through her issues.

5. T.C. and her husband are talking one evening and you overhear that they are very dissatisfied with the care provided by the physician. They believe that he has mismanaged T.C.'s care. They are discussing getting an attorney. They ask you what you think. What do you do? **[PD/an/PSI/ni,tc]**
   - Many legal conflicts are preventable and stem from two parties not communicating or understanding each other, or from a difference between expectations and actual outcomes. Many agencies have risk managers who are skilled at helping both parties work through potential problems. Your role is to provide the best opportunity for the patient and the physician to work through their differences. You may encourage T.C. and her husband to write down their issues to help them clarify them and schedule a time when the physician can sit down and discuss them. You should not take sides. Promoting communication is the key.

You realize threats of legal action are based on many issues. Anger and disappointment are among the most common. You sit down to communicate to them that you are willing to listen.

6. You state, "Legal action won't fix how you're feeling or what you need *now*. Tell me what's going on with you. Maybe I can help." What would be the benefit of taking this approach? **[PD/c/PSI/ct,ni,tc]**
   - In situations like this, people usually are emotionally "loaded." They have not felt listened to or acknowledged.
   - Situations like this frequently arise from misunderstandings or lack of communication.
   - They may just need a chance to ventilate their confusion and frustrations.
   - You are acknowledging they are human beings and have legitimate needs.

7. Mr. C. says, "No one is telling us anything. My wife came in here for a simple hysterectomy, she ends up with 4 surgeries, she still has pain, and she's worse off than when she started. *Somebody* has screwed up big time. Then they have the nerve to send me a bill. This morning they demanded $185,000. I'm not paying a dime until she gets better." How are you going to respond? **[PD/c/PSI/ct,ni,tc]**
   - Tell them they have legitimate concerns and, if it were you, you would have the same questions.
   - Endometriosis can be very complicated. When endometriosis is involved, there is no such thing as a simple hysterectomy. You understand their concerns and they have a right to know what's going on.
   - You tell them you are going to call the physician, Dr. "X" (use the attending physician's name) immediately and tell him that the family is very upset. From their perspective, she came in for a hysterectomy, has had 4 surgeries, and is worse than when she started. To top it off, they just got a bill for $185,000 from the hospital. There is an urgent need for him to talk to them and explain what's been happening to T.C.
   - Ask them if they would like a social worker to discuss their hospital bill and payment with them. Hospital billing personnel often are not trained in crisis management and interpersonal relationship skills and often escalate the situation. Try using an experienced intermediary, and then give the social worker the background.
   - Ask them if there is anything you can do for them right now to make them more comfortable. (Addressing physical needs also facilitates "deescalation" of crises.)
   - Chart this discussion and action taken.
   - Risk management people need to be notified of this situation.

CHAPTER 6. NEUROLOGIC DISORDERS

Case Study 1: Alzheimer's Disease

Difficulty: *	*Setting:* Extended care facility
Index Words: Alzheimer's disease	

M.E. is a 62-year-old woman who has a 5-year history of progressive forgetfulness. She is no longer able to care for herself, has becomes increasingly depressed and paranoid, and recently started a fire in the kitchen. After extensive neurologic evaluation, M.E. was diagnosed as having Alzheimer's disease. Her husband and children have come to your extended fare facility's (ECF) Alzheimers Unit for information about this disease and to discuss the possibility of placement for M.E. You reassure the family that you have experience dealing with questions and concerns that most people in their situation have.

1. How would you explain Alzheimer's disease to the family? **[A/k/Pl/tc]**
   - Alzheimer's disease is a progressive, degenerative disorder of the brain. It causes irreversible loss of memory and loss of mental functions. The brain atrophies, or shrinks, and brain cells and nerve endings (cerebral cortex neurons) are destroyed. Currently, there is no known cure.

2. The husband asks, "How did she get Alzheimer's? We don't know anyone else who has it." How would you respond? **[A/k/Pl/tc]**
   - We don't known what causes Alzheimer's disease. Scientists have linked Alzheimer's to many different possibilities (aluminum toxicity; viruses; autoimmune disease; genetics; and neurotransmitter deficiencies, such as acetylcholine, somatostatin, substance P, and norepinephrine), but no one knows for sure. People usually show symptoms between the ages of 40 to 60, and it usually takes 3 to 15 years for a person to become mentally and physically disabled or incapacitated. People with Alzheimer's disease often die from infection or aspiration pneumonia.

3. After asking the family to describe M.E.'s behavior, you determine that she is in stage 2 of Alzheimers' three stages. Describe common signs and symptoms for each stage of the disease. **[A/k/Pl/ct]**
   - The appearance and severity of signs and symptoms vary for each individual. The following describes each of the 3 stages of Alzheimer's.
     - Stage 1, early stage (2 to 4 years): forgetfulness, declining interest in the environment and people, hesitancy in starting activities, poor work performance, and may lose job.
     - Stage 2, middle stage (2 to 12 years): progressive memory loss, mild aphasia, difficulty with following directions and simple calculations, irritable, evasive, may have increased physical activity, particularly active at night with wandering behavior, loses way around home or when in familiar environment and hallucinations may occur due to misperceptions of the environment, loses important papers and forgets to pay bills, unable to keep up with housework or manage familiar activities, loses possessions and claims they were stolen, neglects personal hygiene, and loses social graces.
     - Stage 3, final stage (up to 1 year): marked weight loss from not eating; loss of written and verbal communication; doesn't recognize family or common objects; bowel and bladder incontinence; chance for major seizure activity; grasping, sucking, and snorting reflexes easily elicited; loss of ability to stand and walk and becomes bedridden; no conscious awareness of surroundings; and death from complications of immobility.

4. The daughter expresses frustration at the number of tests M.E. had to undergo and the length of time it took for someone to diagnosis M.E.'s problem. What tests are likely to be performed and how is Alzheimer's disease diagnosed? **[PD/k/Pl/ct]**
   - Diagnosis is made by neurologic and mental status examination.
   - CT scan of the brain shows atrophy or shrinking of the brain.
   - Magnetic resonance imaging (MRI) can show anatomic and biochemical changes.
   - Positron emission tomography (PET) can measure regional blood flow, oxygen uptake, and the uptake and metabolism of glucose.
   - Electroencephalogram (EEG) may show abnormally slow waves.
   - These tests also rule out other disorders such as brain tumors, hydrocephalus, metabolic problems, and drug toxicities.
   - There is also a series of psychologic diagnostic tests administered by a Licensed Clinical Psychologist.

The husband states, "How are you going to take care of her? She wanders around all night long. She can't find her way to the bathroom in a house she's lived in for 43 years. She can't be trusted to be alone any more; she almost burnt the house down. We're all exhausted; there are 3 of us and we can't keep up with her." You acknowledge how exhausted they must be from trying to keep her safe. You tell the family that there is no known treatment and that Alzheimer's units have been created to provide a structured, safe environment for each person.

5. Describe the Alzheimer's-related nursing interventions related to each of the following nursing diagnoses: self-care deficits, sleep pattern disturbance, impaired verbal communication, impaired cognitive function, risk for injury. **[P,I/c/S,PI,PSI,HP/ct,ni,tc]**
   - Self-care deficits: continuously assess M.E.'s self-care needs and her ability to participate in her care; provide direct care as needed.
   - Sleep pattern disturbance: control her activities so she is awake during the day; provide measures to facilitate sleep at night; maintain an environment conducive to sleep at night; administer appropriate medications.
   - Impaired verbal communications: develop alternative patterns for communication; watch for subtle communication clues; anticipate her needs; make sure you get M.E.'s attention when speaking to her.
   - Impaired cognitive function: don't ask M.E. to perform cognitive skills above her level of ability; control environmental stressors and reduce environmental stimuli; develop and maintain daily routine; provide continuity of care.
   - Risk for injury: provide constant supervision; maintain a safe environment; administer prescribed antiseizure, antipsychotic, antidepressive, or sedative medications (ordered to control symptoms or behaviors).

6. M.E.'s son asks why different medications might be prescribed for M.E. How would you describe the purpose of antiseizure, antipsychotic, antidepressive, or sedative medications for a patient like M.E.? **[PD/c/S,PI,PSI/ct,tc]**
   - Antiseizure medication: as the disease progresses and more brain cells and nerve endings are destroyed, there is a chance the M.E. will develop seizures.
   - Antipsychotic medication: M.E. has exhibited paranoid behavior; this medication would minimize her distress and minimize her antisocial behavior.
   - Antidepressive medication: this medication should relieve M.E.'s depression.
   - Sedative medication: this medication should allow M.E. to sleep at night and decrease her continuous daytime wandering.

You try to comfort the family by telling them that the problems they are experiencing are very common. You explain that family support is a major focus of your program.

7. List 4 ways that M.E.'s family might receive the support they need. **[P,I/c/PSI/ct,ni,tc]**
   - Provide ongoing, up-to-date information about Alzheimer's disease and specifics related to M.E.
   - Encourage the family to attend a family support group at your facility or a local chapter of the Alzheimer's Disease and Related Disorders Association.
   - Encourage the family to seek legal advice on financial and legal measures to protect the family and M.E.
   - Provide information on community resources and social services available.
   - Encourage professional counseling as appropriate.
   - Encourage the family to spend as much time as they want or can with M.E. Acknowledge how difficult it must be to be in their situation. Do not be judgmental if they are unable to spend much time.

Note: Alzheimer's disease support groups:

Alzheimer's Disease and Related Disorders Association
919 North Michigan Ave., Suite 1000
Chicago, IL 60611
1-800-272-3900

American Association of Retired Persons
Fulfillment Services
601 E. St., N.W.
Washington DC 20049
1-202-434-2534

Case Study 2: Myasthenia Gravis

Difficulty: *	*Setting:* Hospital
Index Words: Myasthenia gravis	

D.S. is a 74-year-old retired social worker who has been on your floor for several days receiving qod plasmapheresis for myasthenia gravis (MG). She has a PMH of NIDDM for 3 years and low back pain secondary to spinal stenosis. She received 2 steroid injections into her spine for pain 2 to 3 weeks before her admission, which was followed by progressive, symmetric, weakness in her lower extremities proximal > distal, R foot numbness, poor eye-hand coordination, and significant hand weakness. On admission, D.S. was unable to bear any weight or take fluids through a straw. There have been periods of exacerbation and remission since admission.

1. You are visiting with D.S.'s grandson who tells you he is just starting medical school and he would like to know more about MG so he can discuss it with his grandmother. What do you tell him? **[A/k/PI,PSI/ct,tc]**
   - M.G. is an autoimmune disorder that affects the neuromuscular junction at the skeletal muscle motor endplates. It is postulated that humoral antibodies bind to acetylcholine receptors so there are fewer receptors available for the acetylcholine. This is manifested by weakness in the skeletal muscles usually affecting eye movement, chewing, swallowing, speech, breathing, and head control. The weakness in the muscles increase as they are used and recover fairly rapidly with rest.

2. He asks you to explain how plasmapheresis works. How would you explain this treatment? **[A/k/PI/ct,tc]**
   - This is a method where the circulating antibodies are removed from the blood. There is a special piece of equipment and a specially trained nurse who performs the treatment. It takes 2 to 5 hours to complete; an antecubital vein or shunt may be used for access.

3. He asks what drugs are used to treat MG. You explain that although neostigmine (Prostigmin) and pyridostigmine (Mestinon) are often used in combination, drug regimens and doses are highly individualized. Identify the appropriate drug classification for and explain the action of these two drugs to D.S.'s grandson. **[A/k/S,PI/ct,tc]**
   - These are anticholinesterase drugs. The neostigmine enhances the cholinergic action by facilitating transmission of impulses across the neuromuscular junction and inhibits the destruction of acetylcholine by cholinesterase. Pyridostigmine also inhibits the destruction of cholinesterase.

4. D.S. told her grandson that after taking her morning medications she often experienced nausea, heartburn, slight shortness of breath, sweating, and felt her heart beating rapidly. What can you tell him about this? **[PD/c/PI/ct,ni,tc]**
   - These are muscarinic-type side effects and are fairly common. Remind him that doses often have to be adjusted to maximize the therapeutic effect while minimizing side effects. Inform him that she is monitored closely after receiving medications, and everything will be done to minimize the number of side effects and the discomfort associated with the side effects.

5. Describe a myasthenic crisis. **[A/k/S,PI/ct]**
   - This refers to an exacerbation of the myasthenic motor weakness characterized by acute respiratory difficulty and acute motor weakness of the voluntary muscles. In addition to the respiratory symptoms, the patient often experiences difficulty swallowing, speaking, and moving other body parts. During a myasthenic crisis, the patient is at-risk for aspiration and respiratory arrest.

6. List 6 nursing diagnoses that would be appropriate for D.S. **[PD/an/S,PI,PSI,HP/ct,ni]**
   - Risk for ineffective airway clearance and aspiration r/t weak respiratory muscles.
   - Ineffective breathing pattern r/t weak respiratory muscles.
   - Risk for alteration in nutrition r/t difficulty swallowing and GI hypermotility associated with drug therapy.
   - Risk for altered bladder and bowel elimination.
   - Impaired verbal communication.
   - Activity intolerance.
   - Impaired physical mobility r/t voluntary muscle weakness.
   - Risk for injury.
   - Knowledge deficit: medications.
   - Knowledge deficit: plasmapheresis and other treatment modalities.
   - Knowledge deficit: proper care during a crisis.
   - Knowledge deficit: self- and home-care measures.

7. List 5 factors that could predispose D.S. to an exacerbation of her illness. **[A/c/PI/ct]**
   - Infection, surgery, stress, increased or hard physical activity/exercise, sedative medications, enemas, strong cathartics.

8. D.S. asks you what the doctors meant when they were talking about some kind of a challenge test. You realize they must have been discussing the possibility of performing an edrophonium (Tensilon) challenge. What is a Tensilon challenge and what information will it yield? **[PD/k/S,PI/ct]**
   - Often, the first step is a normal saline challenge, used to determine if a patient reports a change in symptoms. The patient is injected with normal saline and asked to report any changes/sensations he/she experiences. If the patient reports no change, a larger dose of normal saline is administered, and the patient is asked to report the same. The NaCl test is used by many physicians to determine if the symptoms may be psychologic/emotionally related. This is one of the few cases in which administration of a placebo can be justified.
   - A Tensilon challenge is used to determine the presence of and differentiation between myasthenic and cholinergic crisis. Tensilon is administered in the same way; initially a 2-mg dose is injected, and if the patient reports no change, then an 8-mg dose is administered. Tensilon prevents the breakdown of acetylcholine and increases skeletal muscle tone; the myasthenic patient's experiences improved muscle strength that lasts for several minutes. If the patient gets worse (experiences increased weakness, diaphoresis, oral or pulmonary secretions, dyspnea, N/V, diarrhea, or bradycardia) he/she is having a cholinergic reaction and may require atropine as an emergency intervention. Emergency supplies and respiratory support should be in the immediate area.

9. D.S.'s grandson wants to know when she'll be able to go home. How do you respond? **[P,I/ap/PI,PSI/ct,ni,tc]**
   - Most patients with MG are managed at home once the crisis is resolved, treatments are complete, and medication regimen is optimized. Explain that D.S. will continue to need assistance once she is home. Discharge planning will involve working with and teaching D.S. and the family members who will be involved in her care at home. Social services are involved in identifying needs and arranging for use of community resources.

10. What supportive measures can you suggest to D.S.'s grandson that he can undertake or arrange on behalf of his grandmother? **[P/ap/PSI/ct,ni,tc]**
   - This is obviously an intelligent woman. He might take her to an MG support group.
   - Discuss with her what she would like to do for intellectual stimulation if she cannot get out as much.
   - Suggest he spend a day each with a neurologic nurse, a social worker, a physical therapist, and an occupational therapist to understand what parts they play in caring for patients like D.S. This may help him better understand how to address her needs. Not incidentally, it may help him be a more sensitive and effective physician.

Before D.S.'s grandson leaves, you give him the following address:

Myasthenia Gravis Foundation
222 S. Riverside Plaza Suite 1540
Chicago, IL 60606
1-800-541-5454

Case Study 3: Seizure Disorder

Difficulty: *	*Setting:* Rehabilitation facility, home care, case management
Index Words: Seizure disorder	

J.G. is a 34-year-old PI GI woman who underwent an emergency cesarean delivery after a prolonged labor, during which she exhibited a sudden change in neurologic functioning and started seizing. Since that time, she has experienced 3 tonic-clonic (grand mal) seizures, diagnosed as having a basal ganglion hematoma with infarct, and was started on phenytoin. Postdelivery, J.G. demonstrated dyskinesia, resulting in frequent falls with ambulation. When the seizure disorder appeared to be under control, she was transferred to a rehabilitation facility for evaluation, and 2 weeks of intensive physical therapy. She is now home, where she is doing quite well but still has occasional falls and is receiving physical therapy 3 times a week in her home. She remains on phenytoin and has had no seizures since her release from the rehabilitation facility. As case manager for J.G.'s HMO, you visit her and her family at home for evaluation of long-term, follow-up care.

1. A seizure is not a disease in itself but a symptom of a disease. What is the term for chronically recurring seizures? **[PD/k/PI/ct]**
   - Epilepsy.

2. Does J.G. have epilepsy? **[PD/k/PI/ct]**
   - No. She has a seizure disorder related to the basal ganglion hematoma with infarct.

3. The 3 main phases of a seizure are the preictal, ictal, and postictal. Differentiate between the 3 phases, and list clinical symptoms you may observe when a patient is having a seizure. **[A/k/PI/ct]**
   - The preictal period occurs immediately before a seizure, ictal occurs during, and postictal occurs following the seizure.
   - Clinical symptoms can include altered mental function, decreased LOC, altered sensations, decreased coordination, and convulsive movements. Any or all of these symptoms can occur in different combinations.

4. What is the pathophysiology of a seizure? **[A/k/PI/ct]**
   - A seizure is abnormal and excessive electrical discharge of the neurons in the brain. This electrical activity can be limited to one specific area or spread diffusely across brain tissue.

5. J.G. had grand mal, or tonic-clonic, seizures. Describe this type of seizure. List 5 other types of seizures. **[A/k/PI/ct]**
   - Tonic-clonic seizures are characterized by LOC due to rapid spread of electrical activity. In the tonic phase, the total body stiffens, respirations are temporarily interrupted, hands and jaw are clenched (may bite tongue), pupils are dilated and nonreactive, and the person may be incontinent. This is followed by the clonic phase which has violent rhythmic contractions of all muscle groups. The respirations are uneven. The seizure usually lasts 2 to 4 minutes followed by total relaxation and a period of unresponsiveness.
   - Other types of seizures are absence or petit mal, myoclonic, clonic, tonic, infantile, febrile, atonic, partial or Jacksonian, focal, and psychomotor.

6. Some patients know they are about to have a seizure. What is this preseizure warning called, and what form does it take? **[A/k/PI/ct]**
   - It is called an aura. It is usually a brief sensory change and may be a smell, a feeling of weakness, dizziness, numbness of a part of the body, or GI pain.

7. Besides the brain injury, what are some other possible conditions that could be contributing to J.G's lowered seizure threshold? **[A/k/PI/ct]**
   - Infection, recent pregnancy, metabolic and/or nutritional disturbances, and stress.

8. List 5 classifications of antiseizure medications. **[A/k/PI/ct]**
   - Barbiturates, benzodiazepines, hydantoins, succinamides, and valproates.

9. J.G.'s husband comes to visit and asks you what he should do if she has a seizure at home. What would do you tell him? **[P/ap/S,PI/ct,ni,tc]**
   - Stay with her, ease her to the floor, loosen her clothing, protect her head from injury, try to keep the airway open with head position (do not force anything into her mouth and *do not* put your fingers in her mouth), do not restrain her but protect her arms and legs from injury, try to place her on her side in case she vomits or has excessive oral secretions. If the seizure does not stop in 1 minute call 911. These instructions should be given to the family in writing.

10. Her husband states that he is afraid for J.G. to take care of the baby. What would you say to him? **[PD/ap/S,PI,PSI/ct,ni,tc]**
    - Explain that finding the most effective medication regimen is an individualized process. It usually starts with small doses of one drug, and the dose is increased until there are no more seizures and blood levels remain below toxic levels. A second drug will then be added, and so on. J.G. is being regulated on medication so that the likelihood of having a seizure is decreased.
    - Tell him that it would be a good idea for someone to stay with her and the baby for several weeks.
    - Tell him that the likelihood of having a seizure decreases with time and medication if the cause is addressed.
    - Discuss the issue of bonding with her baby. Explain that she needs time with the infant to bond, because her hospitalization interrupted this process.
    - As a case manager, you would arrange for a maternal-child nurse practitioner to work with J.G.

11. J.G.'s husband tells you that his wife is not good at remembering to take medication. What are some strategies that you should review with J.G. and her husband to increase the likelihood of compliance? **[I/an/S,PI/ct,ni,tc]**
    - Inform her that the drug must be taken as prescribed to maintain constant drug levels in the blood. Suggest that she use a compartmentalized pill box and set an alarm clock to take her medications at the prescribed time, or place it in a location where she will see it and be reminded to take the medication.
    - Inform her that serum drug levels are necessary at regular intervals.
    - Inform her that her doctor is required to inform the state's Division of Motor Vehicles that she has a seizure disorder. Although requirements vary from state to state, there is a specified amount of time that she needs to be seizure free (often 1 to 3 years) before the license will be issued or reissued.

12. J.G. asks, "If I get my blood level under control will it stay at the same level as long as I take my medicine?" How would you answer her question? **[PD/ap/S,PI/ct,ni,tc]**
    - Not necessarily. Your drug levels may fluctuate, and the dosages may need to be altered if you are under emotional stress, become ill, need surgery, or suffer trauma.
    - It is important to keep your physician informed about major changes in your life.
    - It is very important for you to ask your pharmacist or physician before taking any other drugs or medications, whether they are prescriptions or over the counter (OTC). Phenytoin interacts with many other types of drugs.

13. J.G.'s husband asks if the drugs could harm his wife in any way. What general information would you give them about anticonvulsants? **[PD/c/S,PI/ct,ni,tc]**
    - Instruct them that some drugs may cause blood, liver, or kidney problems. Instruct J.G. to observe and report easy bruising, petechiae, jaundice, dark urine, burning on urination, and/or abdominal pain.
    - Stress that it is very important for J.G. to wear a Medic Alert bracelet and/or identification that identifies her seizure disorder.
    - Inform them that the drugs may affect J.G.'s level of fatigue.

14. J.G.'s husband says, "I was watching 'Emergency' last night and they showed this guy who just kept on having a seizure. That doctor had to give him lots of medicine before he came out of it. What is that called?" How would you explain status epilepticus, and why is it a medical emergency? **[PD/K/S,PI/ct,ni/tc]**
    - Status epilepticus refers to seizure activity that is constant and without periods of recovery or consciousness. This patient is at-risk for total airway collapse and hypoxia causing brain damage. Emergency management includes maintenance of a patent airway (may need to be intubated), supplemental oxygen, prevention of secondary injury, and administration of drugs to stop the seizure activity (lorazepam or diazepam). The health team will also try to determine and treat the underlying cause.

Case Study 4: Multiple Sclerosis

Difficulty: *	*Setting:* Outpatient Clinic
Index Words: Multiple sclerosis	

You have been asked to see D.V. in the Neurologic Clinic on referral from his internist, who thinks his patient is having symptoms of multiple sclerosis (MS). He is a 20-year-old man who has experienced increasing urinary frequency and urgency over the past 2 months. Because his female partner was treated for a sexually transmitted disease, D.V. also underwent treatment, but the symptoms did not resolve. D.V. has also recently had 2 brief episodes of eye "fuzziness" associated with diplopia and brightness. He has noticed ascending numbness and weakness of the R arm with inability to hold objects over the past few days. Now he reports rapid progression of weakness in his legs.

1. MS is an inflammatory disorder of the nervous system causing scattered, patchy demyelinization of the CNS. What does myelin do? What is demyelinization? **[A/k/PI/ct]**
   - Myelin allows nerve impulses to travel quickly through the CNS. Demyelinization occurs in response to an inflammation of the myelin nerve sheaths resulting in separation of the myelin from the axon cylinders and interruption of nerve transmission.

2. MS is characterized by remissions and exacerbations. What happens to the myelin during each of these phases? **[PD/c/PI/ct]**
   - During remission, the myelin can regenerate, and transmission of the nerve impulse is restored. Symptoms decrease or disappear during this phase. The inflammation can recur and cause exacerbations. If it is severe, it can cause irreversible destruction of the myelin with dense scar tissue forming sclerotic plaques. The plaque permanently damages the CNS.

3. Isn't D.V. too young to get MS? What is the etiology? **[A/k/PI/ct]**
   - The etiology is unknown but autoimmune processes and/or viral infections have been identified as possible causes. MS is more common in cold, temperate climates, is 12 to 15 times more common among first-degree relatives, and women are slightly more affected than men. The highest rate of incidence is between the ages of 20 and 40.

4. What assessment data from the case study caused the physician to suspect a possible diagnosis of MS? **[PD/c/PI,ct]**
   - Urinary symptoms (damage to motor and sensory control centers); ocular symptoms; and arm numbness, tingling, and weakness (damage to motor and sensory nerve tracts). There can also be symptoms associated with damage to the cerebellar region, cerebral cortex, or sacral cord lesions.

Diagnostic tests are often done to rule out other disorders with similar symptoms. A diagnosis will be made when other disorders have been ruled out, when the patient has 2 or more exacerbations, there is slow, steady progression, and/or the patient has 2 or more areas of demyelinization or plaque formation.

5. What are 4 common diagnostic tests you can begin to teach D.V. about?
   [P/c/PI/ni,tc]
   - MRI to reveal presence of plaques.
   - CT scan to demonstrate plaques and rule out other lesions.
   - Lumbar puncture and CSF analysis to look for elevated and specific proteins.
   - Positron emission axial tomography (PETT).
   - Evoked potential studies (EPS) to observe nerve transmission.

6. D.V. asks you, "If this turns out to be MS, what is the treatment?"
   [PD/k/PI,PSI/ct,ni,tc]
   - There is no standard therapy, and individual therapies vary widely. Drug therapy for exacerbations may include antiinflammatory agents (steroids), immunosuppressive agents, such as azathioprine (Imuran), and antineoplastic agents such as cyclophosphamide (Cytoxan). Antispasmodics and muscle relaxants may be given to help manage symptoms (baclofen, dantrolene sodium, diazepam). Bethanechol (Duvoid) or propantheline (Pro-Banthine) may be given to help manage urinary symptoms. Physical medicine and physiotherapy are a large part of the treatment plan with the goal of keeping the patient as independent as possible for as long as possible. Other experimental treatments include interferon drug therapy and plasmapheresis.

7. As part of your teaching plan you want D.V. to be aware of situations or factors that are known to cause an exacerbation of symptoms. List four.
   [PD/k/S,PI,HP/ni,tc]
   - Fatigue, stress, excessive exertion, overheating (fever, hot weather, hot baths/showers), excessive chilling, infections of any kind, and pregnancy.

8. The National Multiple Sclerosis Society, 733 3rd Ave., 6th Floor, New York, NY 10017-3288(1-800-344-4867),is a great resource for D.V. What are some resources available in the community that D.V. may need referrals to?
   [P,I/ap/PI,PSI/ct,ni]
   - Local MS chapter or support groups, public health nurse, social workers, physical therapists, psychologic therapists, vocational rehabilitation agencies, financial counselors, and many others.

D.V. confides in you that he tried to commit suicide at the age of 14 when his parents got a divorce. He tells you that he knows his girlfriend hasn't been faithful but he is afraid of living alone. He admits that she occasionally hits him, but he's afraid if he tells her about his M.S. diagnosis she'll leave him for good. You recall seeing yellowish bruises on his arms when you took his admission blood pressure.

9. What are you going to do with this information? **[P,I/ap/S,PSI/ni,tc]**
   - Thank D.V. for having the courage to share something so sensitive and personal. Tell him you feel that he deserves better and that you are confident that he will be able to develop relationships that are supportive and healthy. Inform him that the problem of women abusing men is not uncommon but most men are ashamed to admit it.
   - Suggest to him that his current relationship is abusive and destructive to him and that you would like to see him get help with feeling better about himself as well as developing positive relationships.
   - Tell D.V. you plan to ask his physician about obtaining a psychiatric nurse specialist (or social worker who specializes in abuse) referral to help him with some of his personal issues. You will also ask the physician about a psychiatric consult for medications (if necessary) to help him through this phase of adjustment.
   - Reassure D.V. that the fact that he was open with you about what is happening in his life tells you that he has the courage to make a better life for himself in spite of his MS diagnosis.

   Instructor Note: Legally, you are obligated to tell his physician what he shared with you. However, by explaining in this manner, it helps him see that the purpose is to protect and help him; it's not a punitive measure or a violation of confidence.

10. In view of his personal history and current diagnosis, what two critical psychosocial issues are you going to monitor for in his follow-up visits? **[E/an/S,PSI/ni]**
    - Beware of continued signs of abuse if he stays in his current relationship.
    - Watch for indications of suicidal intent.

D.V. took advantage of his time with the psychiatric nurse specialist, joined a local MS support group, and told his girlfriend to move out. He later married a woman from the support group.

Case Study 5: Subdural Hematoma

Difficulty: *	*Setting:* Hospital
Index Words: Subdural hematoma	

S.B. is a 28-year-old married woman with a PMH of seizure disorder controlled with phenobarbital (last seizure was 15 years ago), hypothyroidism controlled with Synthroid, and a recent URI. She was on a day outing with her family, slipped and fell, landing on the back of her head. She experienced a loss of consciousness at the scene. She was taken to a local hospital where a CT scan revealed a L subdural hematoma. She has been transferred to your regional medical center, which has a neurosurgeon on call.

1. The ED RN gives you the above information during a phoned report. What other information do you need to prepare for this patient? **[A/c/S,PI,PSI/ct,tc]**
   - Her current neurologic status and vital signs; presence of IV access; treatments she has received; lab tests or diagnostic tests other than the CT that are completed; medications she has received, including any pain medication or narcotics; the presence of any family; and if she has been evaluated by the neurosurgeon.

2. Because you always have trouble remembering the layers of the brain and different hematomas, you look up subdural hematoma before S.B. arrives. What do you find? **[A/k/PI/ct]**
   - A subdural hematoma is a collection of venous blood between the dura mater (outer meninges) and arachnoid membrane (middle meninges). This blood is not reabsorbed and, therefore, creates a space-occupying lesion that creates pressure on the underlying brain and causes increased intracranial pressure (IICP). Approximately 10% to 15% of head-injured patients develop subdural hematomas.

3. S.B.'s subdural is considered acute because symptoms appeared within 24 hours of injury. What are the other classifications of subdural hematomas? **[PD/k/PI/ct]**
   - Subacute: when symptoms appear 2 to 10 days later.
   - Chronic: when symptoms appear weeks or more later.

4. What are common signs and symptoms of an acute subdural hematoma? **[A/k/PI/ct]**
   - Headache, drowsiness, agitation, decreased LOC and confusion, and the ipsilateral pupil dilates and becomes fixed. All of these symptoms may gradually worsen. Late indicators can include hemiparesis and loss of consciousness.

5. Why are the elderly and alcoholics at-risk for chronic subdural hematomas? **[PD/c/PI/ct]**
   - Cerebral atrophy from aging or ETOH risk causes separation of the cortex from the dura, and fragile veins are more prone to tear. There is a larger space for bleeding to occur in, so it takes longer for symptoms to appear because of the atrophy.

6. How would you monitor for neurologic change? **[P,I/c/S,Pl/ct,ni]**
   - Trends of Glasgow Coma Scale (GCS).
   - Pupils (size, shape, symmetry, and reactivity).
   - Level of consciousness and orientation.
   - Recent memory, attention span, long-term memory, mood, affect, and behaviors.
   - VS.
   - Respiratory status: ABGs; SaO_2; depth, pattern, rate, and effort.
   - Reflexes: corneal, cough, gag.
   - Muscle tone, motor movement, gait, proprioception, bilateral symmetry.
   - Tremor.
   - Facial symmetry and tongue protrusion.
   - Extraocular movements (EOMs), gaze characteristics, and tracking response.
   - Visual disturbance.
   - Complaint of headache.
   - Speech characteristics.
   - Response to stimuli.
   - Sensory perception: sharp/dull.
   - Paresthesia.
   - Smell.
   - Pattern of diaphoresis (Iowa Intervention Project, 1992).

7. Why is it especially important to make sure S.B. is taking her phenobarbital and has a therapeutic serum level? **[A/c/S,Pl/ct,ni]**
   - IICP can predispose S.B. to a lower seizure threshold.

8. The decision was made in S.B.'s case not to do a craniotomy. When would a neurosurgeon decide to treat medically vs. perform surgery? **[A/k/Pl/ct]**
   - Small subdural hematomas can be treated medically because they often can be absorbed. Large subdural hematomas must be surgically evacuated so that IICP and tentorial herniation are avoided.

9. Burr holes work only for acute subdurals, and a craniotomy must be done for subacute and chronic subdurals. Why? **[A/k/Pl/ct]**
   - After the acute phase, the hematoma becomes gelatinous, and a membrane has developed that must be dissected away from the dural and arachnoid layers.

10. Why would hypotonic IV solutions such as D_5W be avoided? **[A/k/Pl/ct]**
    - They increase cerebral edema.

11. How would you position S.B. in bed? **[P,I/ap/S,Pl/ct,ni]**
    - With HOB elevated at least 25 degrees to promote venous drainage and help reduce cerebral edema.

12. If S.B.'s level of consciousness started to decrease, what information would you give the neurosurgeon when you call him? **[I/ap/S,Pl/tc]**
    - Identify yourself and give a brief patient history. Then give current VS, GCS, details of the neurologic exam, including things that are changing and over what time period.
    - Document who you talked to, when, what information you gave, orders received, and action taken.

13. How would you provide support to the family? **[P,I/ap/PSI/ni,tc]**
    - Keep them up-to-date on current findings, plan of care, and potential complications. Because they are from out of town, they may need the assistance of a social worker to find local resources and a place to stay. Allow them to stay with S.B. and become involved in her care as much as possible or desired. Begin early assessment and discharge planning as it may be more difficult if they are from out of town or live in a small community.

14. The neurosurgeon has ordered codeine IM as a pain medication. Why did he order codeine? **[PD/c/PI/ct]**
    - Codeine is less likely to have sedating effects, mask symptoms of IICP, or cause respiratory depression than other narcotics.

Case Study 6: Intracranial Hemorrhage

Difficulty: **	*Setting:* Rehabilitation facility
Index Words: Intracranial hemorrhage, cerebrovascular accident, rehabilitation	

R.B. is an 80-year-old English woman who is visiting a friend in the United States. One morning her friend noticed that upon awakening, R.B. had slurred speech, a R facial droop, and was disoriented. She was transported to the hospital where a CT scan confirmed the diagnosis of intracranial hemorrhage. Because of the location of the bleed, surgery was not possible and over the next couple days R.B.'s R facial droop progressed to a totally flaccid R side. R.B. was transferred to your rehabilitation facility for therapy. Ten days after the initial insult, R.B. still has some confusion, memory problems, difficulty swallowing, slurred speech, and profound R sided weakness. She is hoping to be able to return to England soon.

1. Define CVA. **[A/k/Pl/ct]**
   - A cerebrovascular accident, commonly called a stroke, is the sudden disruption of the oxygen supply to some brain cells. It is usually caused by an obstruction in or rupture of one or more blood vessels that supply the brain. CVA is the 3rd leading cause of death and the most common cause of neurologic disability.

2. List 3 main causes of a CVA and describe how they disrupt the O_2 supply. **[A/c/Pl/ct]**
   - Thrombus is caused by an atherosclerotic plaque or inflammation within the vessel wall causing a narrowing of the vessel and decreased blood flow to the brain tissue.
   - Embolus is a portion of a thrombus that has broken loose and become lodged in a smaller cerebral vessel. The embolism could originate in the L heart or a cerebral vessel.
   - Hemorrhage occurs when there is a rupture of a cerebral vessel. This may occur anywhere within the brain causing either an intracerebral bleed or bleeding into the subarachnoid space.
   - Systemic hypoperfusion resulting in decreased cerebral blood flow is due to circulatory failure from too little blood, too low a blood pressure, or failure of the heart to adequately pump.

3. List 10 factors that increase the risk of a CVA. **[A/k/Pl/ct]**
   - Hypertension (HTN); diabetes; increased serum cholesterol and/or triglycerides, cardiac disease, especially cardiac valve disease; gout; blood dyscrasias; anticoagulant therapy; neck vessel trauma; obesity; cigarette smoking; stress; oral contraceptives; transient ischemic attacks (TIAs); previous CVA.

4. What is the overall goal of rehabilitation? **[P/k/S,Pl,PSI,HP/ct,ni]**
   - To help the patient achieve the highest level of independence possible and maintain a satisfying and productive life with dignity and self-respect. Care is directed at prevention of complications and maximizing optimum function.

5. List 12 potential members of the rehabilitation health care team. **[P/k/S,PI,PSI,HP/ct]**
   - The individual affected, his/her family, nurse, physician, physical therapist, registered dietitian, social worker, speech therapist, occupational therapist, vocational counselor, recreation therapist, and clergy.

6. Why is positioning with proper body alignment so important for a patient like M.E.? **[P/c/S,PI/ct,ni]**
   - Positioning and alignment are important in the prevention of musculoskeletal deformities, such as contractures and ankylosis; prevention of skin breakdown; and prevention of problems associated with decreased vascular supply, such as thrombosis and edema.

7. An aggressive exercise program must be part of the rehabilitative process to maintain and improve muscle tone and function and to prevent further disability. Describe the following exercise classifications: passive, active, active assistive, active resistive, and isometric. **[A/k/PI/ct]**
   - Passive motion is provided by another person or outside force without voluntary participation by the patient.
   - Active or voluntary motion is independently performed by the patient.
   - Active assistive motion to a joint is performed by the patient with assistance from another person.
   - Active resistive is voluntary motion performed against resistance.
   - Isometric is the alternative tightening and relaxing of a muscle or muscle group without joint movement.

8. What are some nursing interventions for R.B. related to the patient problem of weight loss r/t continued swallowing problems and risk for aspiration r/t swallowing difficulty. **[P/ap/PI/ct]**
   - Obtain consultation for a registered dietitian (RD). Until the patient is no longer at risk for aspiration, tube feedings must be maintained to meet nutritional needs. The RD will calculate R.B.'s nutritional needs and select the appropriate tube feeding. Occupational and speech therapists should evaluate R.B's swallowing and provide ongoing swallow retraining. Until swallow has returned to normal, R.B. should not be allowed to take anything PO without supervision, and suction equipment should be available at all times.

9. Discharge planning begins upon admission to any facility. What special discharge needs does R.B. have and who needs to be involved? **[P,I/an/S,PI,PSI/ct,ni,tc]**
   - This case is complicated by the fact that R.B. lives in England. The social worker should be contacted when R.B. is first admitted and should be working on special arrangements for transfer back to England. The consulate from a particular country is usually contacted very early on, because they can help with details about immigration, customs, government interface needed, and any national health insurance plan. R.B. will need to be stable enough to withstand an international flight and complex arrangements need to be made for placement in a facility in England. Because her memory has not totally returned, the friend she was visiting will be instrumental in helping find and contact her family in England.

Once the family is located and contacted, the nurse and the physician should talk to them. Offer to have a physician from the receiving facility in England call and talk to the discharging physician from your institution. FAXes are a common way of communicating from the United Kingdom to the U.S.

10. R.B. seems to be homesick. What nursing interventions could you plan to help her homesickness? **[P/an/PSI/ct,ni]**
    - Most large cities have a British-American Club. See if R.B.'s friend could arrange for a few British expatriots to visit her and bring "old time" British songs on tape. Videotapes of British TV shows (such as Benny Hill, Fawlty Towers) may also help.
    - Ask R.B. what she would like and be patient for the answer.

Case Study 7: Neuropathy

Difficulty: ** *Setting:* Hospital

Index Words: Obesity, herniated disk, laminectomy

You are assigned to take care of M.X. this evening's shift. In report you are told that she is a 40-year-old obese (112 kg) woman who arose from a sitting position and experienced acute and severe low back pain 3 weeks ago. She was diagnosed with herniated disks L4-S1. Dr. W., who performed a lumbar laminectomy 3 days ago, is concerned because her WBC count has gone from 8.1 mm^3 to 19.6 mm^3.

1. What is meant by the term *herniated disk* (herniated nucleus pulposus)? **[A/k/Pl/ct]**
   - The intervertebral disk is a semifluid-filled fibrous capsule that acts as a shock absorber and facilitates spinal movement. Some pressure on the disk may cause elastic material from the center to break or herniate through the rim of the disk, causing pressure on and irritation of the spinal nerve roots or the spinal cord itself. This is usually the result of an injury or a series of insults to the vertebral column. It can also be caused by degenerative changes.

2. What tests may be performed to detect and diagnose the herniation? **[A,PD/k/Pl,ct]**
   - X-ray of the spine, myelogram, electromyelogram, magnetic resonance imaging (MRI), CT scan of the spine, and possibly a lumbar puncture (LP).

3. What is a laminectomy? **[A/k/Pl/ct]**
   - A surgical procedure performed by making an incision over the involved vertebral area through the fascia and muscles to the laminae to remove the disk or other tissue that is exerting pressure on the spinal cord.

4. Identify 2 general objectives of postoperative nursing care of M.X.? **[P/c/Pl/ct,ni]**
   - The postoperative nursing objectives are prevention of complications and initiation of rehabilitation.

5. What is meant by "log-rolling?" **[I/k/S,Pl/ct,ni]**
   - Log-rolling is a method of turning a patient so that spinal alignment is maintained. The body is rolled with the assistance of several nurses and a turn sheet that keeps the spine straight and the neck aligned. The arms are bent across the chest. The patient assists by contracting the long muscles of the back to keep the shoulders and pelvis in straight alignment. Pillows are placed for maximum support of all body parts in proper alignment including one between the legs.

6. You ask 4 coworkers to help you log-roll M.X. As one nurse enters the room she makes a statement about breaking her back trying to move M.X. You are a little overweight yourself and watch M.X.'s face when she hears the remark. How would you handle the situation? **[I/ap/PSI/ni,tc]**
   - First, log-roll M.X.
   - Second, take the nurse outside the room and ask her what is bothering her. Tell her that you were shocked at her inappropriate and unprofessional behavior. Also, tell her that if she has a disability, she should let it be known so that she could handle the patient's head or feet. Tell her that she owes M.X. an apology.
   - Third, go back into M.X.'s room after the other nurses have left. Sit down and acknowledge how she must feel and explain how you would feel if you were in her place. Give her the opportunity to ventilate her frustration at the stigma of being overweight.

7. Patients who have undergone a lumbar laminectomy frequently experience paralytic ileus and urinary retention. Why? **[PD/c/PI,ct]**
   - Stimulation of the sympathetic nervous system leads to decreased peristalsis in the GI tract and anesthetic agents and autonomic stimulation lead to bladder distention.

8. What are 4 possible sources of infection that may account for M.X.'s elevated WBC? **[PD/ap/PI/ct]**
   - Surgical wound infection, respiratory tract infection, urinary tract infection, bacteremia (infection in the blood), meningitis.

9. M.X. asks you how you would know if her wound were infected. Differentiate between signs and symptoms of wound infection for M.X. **[PD/c/PI/ct,tc]**
   - Tell M.X. that signs are things you can determine without asking her. The signs of wound infection are swelling, redness, drainage or discharge, warmth at the site, fever, and increased WBC.
   - Symptoms are determined by asking her for information. A symptom of wound infection would be local pain.
   - Inform M.X. that you are monitoring both signs and symptoms.

10. Discharge planning should begin the day M.X. is admitted to your unit. What factors should discharge planning include? **[P/ap/S,PI,PSI/ct,ni]**
    - A home assessment should be completed. What is the physical layout of the house; is she required to climb stairs; what are the distances between the bedroom, living room, bathroom, and kitchen; are there handrails along stairways; are there grab bars in the shower or near the toilet; are there throw rugs; is it feasible for M.X. to stay at her home or should other arrangements be made?
    - Does M.X. have help at home for the recovery period, or have arrangements been made for assistance at home?
    - Assess transportation needs for PT, grocery shopping, etc.
    - Assess immediate financial needs and get social services involved if needed.
    - Assess learning needs of M.X. and her family, and initiate discharge teaching.

11. List 7 written home care instructions that should be reviewed and given to M.X. before discharge. **[P,I/ap/S,PI,PSI/ct,ni,tc]**
    - Information about prescribed medications: rationale, dose, schedule, potential side effects, and specific information about not drinking with narcotics or other sedating medications (risk for injury to themselves and others, legal ramifications of driving under the influence, and that alcohol potentiates narcotics and sedatives).
    - Prescribed PT, OT follow-up for an exercise regimen.
    - Surgeon-directed activity restrictions considering prolonged sitting, sexual activity, stairs, driving or riding in a car, and bathing.
    - Lifting and carrying limitations (per individual surgeons) are usually not more than 10 to 15 pounds for several weeks.
    - Signs and symptoms of a wound infection that which require medical attention. Name and phone number of contact person and surgeon should problems or questions arise.
    - Diet instructions, including constipation prevention.
    - Pain management.
    - Signs and symptoms of neurologic deterioration and when to call the surgeon.
    - Information on follow-up appointment.

M.X. was treated with aggressive antibiotic therapy for a urinary tract infection (UTI). With the help and support of her family, M.X. was discharged to home where she made a complete recovery. After talking to you, M.X. started on a healthy low-fat diet and lost 52 pounds over the next 9 months. When you were arranging her discharge papers, you discovered that M.X. was a script writer for soap operas! Six months after her discharge, she calls to meet you for coffee. She asks if you would like to supplement your income by consulting with her on improving the image of nurses in soap operas. She said it was your professionalism that gave her this idea.

Case Study 8: Brain Tumor

Difficulty: **	*Setting:* Hospital
Index Words: Brain tumor	

F.N. is a 57-year-old housewife, happily married with grown children, and 2 new grandchildren. F.N. made an appointment with her optometrist to explore a progressive OS visual loss over a 9-month period. Her eye exam was essentially normal, and the optometrist referred her to a neurologist. After workup, a 2.5 cm brain mass was found, and surgery was scheduled. Her only past medical history (PMH) is hypertension, for which she takes nifedipine XL 60 mg qd and potassium chloride (K-dur) 10 mEq bid, and her past surgical history (PSH) includes T&A as a child, cholecystectomy, and a TAH at age 42. She also takes a conjugated estrogen (Premarin) 0.625 mg qd.

1. Name 4 tests that can be done to evaluate for brain tumor. **[A/k/PI/ct]**
   - Skull x-rays, CT scan of brain, MRI, EEG, brain scan, cerebral angiography, positron emission tomography (PET), echoencephalogram.

There is no standardized, universally accepted system of classifying brain tumors. They can be classified according to histologic basis, intraaxial vs. extraaxial, or malignant vs. benign.

2. Using the term *benign* when discussing brain tumors is somewhat misleading. Why? **[PD/c/PI/ct]**
   - A complete cure is not always possible with a benign tumor; it is still a space-occupying lesion that may not be surgically accessible. The benign tumor will continue to grow and cause increased intracranial pressure (IICP), neurologic deficits, herniation, and finally death. The last outcome is not "benign."

3. Onset of neurologic symptoms is usually insidious, and they exhibit symptoms in relation to the area of the brain where the tumor is located. List 6 general symptoms associated with many brain tumors. **[PD/k/PI/ct]**
   - Headache, nausea, vomiting (often projectile), papilledema and vision changes, lethargy, forgetfulness, personality changes, and seizure activity.

4. Dexamethasone (Decadron) is commonly prescribed when a tumor is diagnosed and the presence of increased intracranial pressure (IICP) is demonstrated. It is administered preoperatively and postoperatively, and in conjunction with radiation and chemotherapy. Why is Decadron prescribed, and why should it not be abruptly stopped? **[A/c/S,PI/ct]**
   - Decadron is a long-acting steroid that suppresses the immune response. It is given in IICP to decrease cerebral edema and reverse symptoms. Abrupt withdrawal from Decadron can precipitate an adrenal crisis. Patients must be cautioned not to stop taking Decadron; it must be slowly tapered. The patient should also be educated as to the other side effects of steroids.

5. Other common supportive medications include antiseizure, diuretics, antacids and H_2 blockers, analgesics, antiemetics, and antidepressants. Indicate why each is used. **[PD/ap/PI/ct]**
   - Antiseizure medications prevent seizures.
   - Diuretics decrease cerebral edema and ICP.
   - Antacids and H_2 blockers prevent/treat stress ulcers.
   - Analgesics control headaches and other pain.
   - Antiemetics control nausea, which is a common symptom.
   - Antidepressants are given to combat depression.

6. Once the diagnosis is made, the patient and family must be involved in the plan for treatment. Treatment depends on the type and location of the tumor and can include surgery, radiation, chemotherapy, or any combination of these. The patient also has the right to refuse treatment. Identify 4 other considerations the medical team, patient, and family will consider in devising a treatment plan. **[P/an/PI,PSI/ct,tc]**
   - Size of tumor, prognosis, symptoms, general condition of the patient, finances, social support system, religious beliefs.

7. Describe common responses to a diagnosis of a brain tumor. **[A/c/S,PI,PSI/ct]**
   - Diagnosis can cause extreme physical and emotional stress.
   - Diagnosis often means profound changes in life for the patient and the family.
   - The patient's self concept and body image become altered.
   - Responses can range from anger, denial, extreme sadness, and fear.
   - Thoughts of mutilation, incapacitation, and death are overwhelming for some patients.
   - Fear of abandonment or loss by the spouse.
   - Denial; everything is going to be fine.

8. List 2 role-relationship nursing diagnoses for F.N. **[PD/an/PI,PSI/ct,ni]**
   - Anticipatory grieving r/t loss of functioning, and possible death.
   - Risk for impaired verbal communication r/t brain injury.
   - Risk for impaired social interaction r/t brain injury.
   - Altered family processes r/t role changes.

9. F.N. drew up a living will and health care power of attorney after she heard the diagnosis. She also sat down with her family and made her wishes known. Why is this important for F.N. in particular and for everyone in general? **[P,I/an/S,PI,PSI/ct,tc]**
   - A brain tumor is a potentially devastating disease that may result in profound loss or may be terminal. It is possible that F.N. will be unable to make her own health care decisions, and it is important to have those responsible for her care and her family know what those wishes are.

10. You enter F.N.'s room to take VS and she says, "What if I come out of surgery and I'm different? Or what if I die? My grandbabies will never know me." You hear the concern in her voice. Suggest several ways that F.N. can communicate with her loved ones in the event that her surgery is unsuccessful.
[P,I/ap/PSI,HP/ct,ni,tc]
    - Write letters to her grandchildren. Indicate on the envelope the time or event that you want each letter to be opened and read (birthdays, first date, wedding, religious events, birth of their first child, etc.).
    - Videotape a special message to your husband, children, and grandchildren.
    - Arrange a family meeting when they can discuss their lives, finish unfinished business, reminisce, share stories, laugh, and cry. If something does happen to F.N., the family will have those memories to carry with them.
    - Arrange for the husband to have some intimate time with his wife before surgery.

11. F.N. had the surgery and was admitted to ICU postop. She did very well and remained neurologically intact (q1h neuro checks), her BP was slightly elevated (147/68), the rest of her VS were normal, she had 2 peripheral IVs, TED hose, O_2 at 4 L/nc, and a Foley. Postoperatively, F.N.'s K level dropped to 2.7 mEq/L and glucose was 202 mg/dl. Describe possible reasons why these 2 laboratory values are abnormal, and identify what treatment will be ordered to correct each.
[P,I/an/PI/ct,ni,tc]
    - The K could be decreased due to NG loss and/or diuresis, which is induced to decrease cerebral edema. K needs to be administered but the patient will be NPO. You need to call and notify the physician. The physician will order KCl 40 mEq to be added to each liter of IV fluid and a "K-Rider" or "K-flash" of 40 mEq in 100 ml D_5W to be infused over 4 hours.
    - The glucose could be elevated due to steroids and/or IV fluids. It will be necessary to monitor serum glucose levels and a sliding scale for regular insulin may be needed.

F.N. did suffer mild neurologic damage as a result of the surgery. She was discharged to a rehabilitation facility, and eventually was able to recover most of her lost function. She continues to enjoy an active life, and has become involved in helping others facing similar experiences.

For additional information contact:
Brain Injury Association Help Line
1776 Massachusetts Ave. N.W., Suite 100
Washington, DC 20036
1-800-444-6443

Case Study 9: Carotid Endarterectomy

Difficulty: **	*Setting:* Hospital
Index Words: Carotid endarterectomy, atrial fibrillation	

You walk in to T.E.'s room on initial rounds and find Mrs. E. in tears. She says, "He is having such a rough time, I wonder if I'll ever have the same man back." You heard in report that T.E. is a 63-year-old man who, while at breakfast with his wife several days ago, developed slurred speech, became severely confused, and collapsed to his R side. The acute episode began resolving in approximately 15 minutes while en route to the ED. Mrs. E. was almost hysterical because her husband had had 2 episodes of "being revived from sudden cardiac death" 5 years ago. A CT scan revealed an acute L middle cerebral aneurysm (frontal/parietal) stroke. Heparin therapy was started right away and the next day an angiogram revealed high grade L carotid artery stenosis with very stagnant flow. The heparin was discontinued, and he was taken to the OR for a carotid endarterectomy. After 2 days in the ICU, he is on your floor. T.E. has R-sided paralysis and expressive aphasia.

1. What is an angiogram and why was it important to perform an angiogram in T.E.'s case? **[PD/c/PI/ct]**
   - The radiologist places a sheath into blood vessels in a special angiogram room in the radiology department. A radiopaque dye is then injected into the blood vessels and images are taken to note how the dye flows through the vessels. In a known or suspected CVA, carotid and cerebral angiography can pinpoint the site of lesions, ruptures, occlusions, aneurysms, and arterial-venous malformation and it can identify collateral circulation. T.E.'s angiogram revealed a high grade L carotid artery stenosis, which gave the medical team and family specific information to develop a treatment plan.

2. Describe a carotid endarterectomy. **[PD/k/PI/ct]**
   - Once a temporary bypass shunt is created to provide blood supply to the brain, the atherosclerotic plaque from the innermost lining of the carotid artery is removed. After removal of the atherosclerotic plaque, circulation is reestablished. The goal of surgery is to prevent occlusion of the artery or emboli formation from the plaque.

3. Because T.E. already suffered a CVA, why is the carotid endarterectomy being performed? **[PD/c/PI/ct]**
   - Because the diagnostic tests revealed stagnant flow along with a high-grade lesion, T.E. was at very high risk for having another CVA or extending the present one.

4. Why is a baseline neurologic exam extremely important for T.E.? **[PD/ap/S,PI/ct]**
   - T.E. already has neurologic deficits related to the CVA. It is necessary to precisely document his deficits so that any deterioration or changes in symptoms can be immediately reported to the physicians.

5. T.E.'s current VS are 128/78, 88 (irregularly irregular), 18, 35.8°C (O), and SaO_2 of 96% on 6 L O_2/nc. Are you concerned about any of these numbers and if so why? **[PD/ap/S,PI/ct,ni]**
   - His HR is irregularly irregular. T.E. has a PMH of cardiac dysrhythmias and sudden death. It would be important to find out if this is a new finding.
   - It is also of concern that he is on such a high O_2 flow rate; normal SaO_2 is $\geq$92%.

6. You call the ICU nurse to ask her about the irregular heart rate. She says that he was in a normal sinus rhythm while in the NICU and adds, "It wouldn't be too good if he flipped into A-fib." She suggested calling the physician. What are you going to tell the physician when you call him? What test do you expect him to prescribe? **[PD,P/an/S,PI/ct,ni,tc]**
   - You will identify yourself and that you recently received T.E. as a transfer from NCC. While completing your initial assessment you discovered an irregularly irregular heart rate. Inform him of other VS and T.E.'s current neurologic status. You anticipate that he will order a STAT ECG.

7. Why is atrial fibrillation of concern? **[PD/c/PI/ct]**
   - A-fib results in decreased cardiac output and increases the potential to develop an embolus. T.E. has a PMH of cardiac dysrhythmias, and the development of A-fib could signify a stressed myocardium.

8. Identify 4 nursing interventions that may improve his oxygenation and decrease T.E.'s O_2 requirements. **[I/ap/PI/ct,ni]**
   - Aggressive pulmonary hygiene, including frequent assessment.
   - Encourage deep breathing and coughing.
   - Assist with use of an incentive spirometer (IS).
   - Reposition q2h.
   - Perform NT suctioning prn.
   - Get T.E. out of bed and into a chair as able.
   - Maintain airway and delivery of oxygen.
   - Ensure that T.E. receive his chest physiotherapy and nebulized respiratory treatments as ordered.

9. You wonder if T.E. truly requires 6 L O_2/nc because you continually find his nasal cannula pulled down onto his lip. When you ask him about moving the tubing, he states that it is irritating the inside of his nose. What can you do to decrease the irritability of the high-flow oxygen? **[P/ap/PI/ct,ni]**
   - Add humidification to the oxygen. Respiratory therapists may argue that it does not help but it does.

10. The following is a list of T.E.'s medications. Indicate why he is receiving each. **[PD/ap/PI/ct]**
    - Albuterol 2.5 mg nebulized q4h:
      - Bronchodilator.
    - Heparin sodium 5000 U SQ q12h:
      - DVT prophylaxis.
    - Multivitamin 1 cap PO AM:
      - Improve nutritional status.
    - Nicotine 14 mg top patch qd:
      - Nicotine withdrawal symptoms.
    - Nystatin suspension 4 ml PO tid:
      - Prevention or treatment of oral candidiasis.
    - Psyllium/Sod. Bicarb. 1 packet powder PO tid:
      - Bulk-forming laxative.
    - Ranitidine 150 mg PO bid:
      - Stress ulcer prophylaxis.
    - Ticlopidine 250 mg PO bid:
      - Antihypertensive, beta blockade.

11. Mrs. E. is not coping well with her husband's illness. What measures could be taken to support her? **[P,I/an/PSI/ct,ni,tc]**
    - Be sensitive to her needs and prior experiences that may be feeding into her distress.
    - Assess for the family's knowledge of T.E.'s current status and provide an update or education.
    - Identify an additional family member who can be her support figure.
    - Help the family develop realistic goals, plans, and actions. Include family in T.E.'s plan of care, and provide them opportunities to participate in care (ROM, hygiene, comfort measures).
    - Refer to other health team members as appropriate, such as psychiatric CNS, social worker, clergy, financial counselor, family therapist.
    - Assess previous coping behaviors, and identify both effective and ineffective ones.
    - Identify perceived or actual conflicts.
    - Encourage the family to spend time outside the hospital.
    - Send Mrs. E. home for sleep and a good meal.
    - Give her the direct number to your floor with instructions that if she wakes up during the night and begins to worry about her husband, she can call to check on him.

12. You find yourself speaking very loudly to T.E. due to his expressive aphasia. Your coworker admits she does the same thing when she has patients with expressive aphasia. Why don't you need to speak loudly and what are some ways to enhance communication with this patient? **[P,I/ap/PI,PSI/ct,ni,tc]**
    - Aphasia is the partial or complete inability to use or comprehend language and symbols. This is not the result of impaired hearing or lack of intelligence.
    - To enhance communication, treat the patient as an adult and be respectful; use simple terms and yes/no questions; use gestures, pantomimes, and facial expressions because the patient may respond more easily to nonverbal cues; and give the patient practice with verbal communication, listen carefully, and respond to attempts to communicate.

T.E. was eventually discharged home with some residual expressive aphasia.

Case Study 10: Guillain-Barré Syndrome

Difficulty: ** *Setting:* Extended care facility

Index Words: Guillain-Barré syndrome

You are working at a skilled nursing facility that cares for patients on ventilators. G.W. is your first patient with Guillain-Barré syndrome. G.W. is a divorced, self-supporting 56-year-old woman from a small town who developed a URI after caring for her grandson who had the same. Three weeks later she developed weakness, numbness, and tingling in her feet that progressed up her body. Her physician recognized the seriousness of her condition and transferred her to a tertiary referral center. Within days she became totally paralyzed; she was trached and placed on mechanical ventilation. She spent 1 month in the neuro critical care unit and several months on the floor before being transferred to your facility. Her only inhospital complication was pneumonia, which has totally resolved. The physicians don't know how long the paralysis will last.

1. What adaptations would you or your family have to make if you were paralyzed and unable to perform your normal responsibilities? How would you feel if you were totally dependent on others for your simplest needs? *Use a separate sheet of paper for a detailed response* and include daily care; financial issues, such as who would pay the rent/house note, groceries, utilities, mounting medical bills; social issues, such as who would care for your children, see to their education, meet their emotional needs; self-perception; emotions; etc. **[I/an/S,PI,PSI,HP/ct]**

2. Is G.W.'s case typical? **[A/k/PI/ct]**
   - Yes. The syndrome is characterized by a rapidly progressing symmetrical ascending flaccid paralysis usually following a viral illness. Recovery is usually complete; however, it can take months to years if there is extensive involvement.

3. Why does potentially fatal respiratory dysfunction occur? **[A/k/PI/ct]**
   - The nerves innervating the intercostals and diaphragm are compressed and demyelinated along with all the nerves in the body.

4. Describe a plan for pulmonary hygiene for G.W. **[P/ap/PI/ct,ni]**
   - Using sterile technique, suction the tracheostomy tube when she needs to be suctioned. Trach care per agency policy, usually q12h with inner cannula change at least qd. Get G.W. OOB into a sitting position using assistive devices, such as Hoyer lift or total lift chair at least bid. Use postural drainage positioning while in bed. Monitor for signs and symptoms of respiratory tract infection and report promptly. Have a bag-valve device and suction at the bedside and available for immediate use at all times.

   Instructor Note: Aseptic technique may be used for patients in their home environment.

5. How do you anticipate that G.W.'s nutritional needs are being met? **[I/ap/PI/ct,ni]**
   - She is on strict NPO due to total lack of swallowing ability. She will have a feeding tube in place and will receive tube feeding by continuous drip or intermittent bolus. She will require strict I&O and daily weights.

6. Describe nursing interventions to manage bladder and bowel elimination for G.W. **[I/an/PI/ct,ni]**
   - Urinary: G.W. will either have an indwelling Foley catheter and will require meticulous catheter care to prevent UTI or incontinence pads/adult diapers that need to be checked and changed frequently to prevent skin breakdown.
   - Bowel: you will need to assess G.W.'s abdomen and bowel sounds; accurately record BMs; and initiate a bowel program including digital stimulation, stool softeners, and/or laxatives as prescribed.

7. What are some things you can do to decrease G.W.'s fear and anxiety? **[P,I/ap/PSI/ct,ni,tc]**
   - Because she is totally unable to summon help, place her in a room close to the desk, provide for frequent observation, maintain a routine and schedule, maintain consistency of caregivers, develop rapport and a trust relationships, provide G.W. with frequent updates on condition and plan of care, anticipate needs, develop a communication system using eye movements and blinks, provide for diversional activities, and allow and encourage family and outside support systems to be present as much as possible.

8. You are using your expert nursing skills to avoid complications. List 4 potential complications. **[PD,c,PI,ct]**
   - Infections of any system, thrombophlebitis, muscle atrophy and contractures, GI hemorrhage r/t stress ulcers, malnutrition, constipation, depression.

9. What measures can be taken to prevent pressure ulcers? **[I/ap/PI/ct,ni]**
   - Use an established risk assessment tool to monitor G.W.'s risk factors.
   - Frequently check and remove moisture on the skin from perspiration, wound drainage, and/or fecal or urinary incontinence.
   - Apply protective barriers such as creams or moisture-absorbing pads that wick wetness away from the skin.
   - Apply transparent film occlusive dressings to areas at risk to protect skin from wetness.
   - Turn q1-2h as appropriate.
   - Position prone as appropriate.
   - Exercise caution while turning to prevent injury to fragile tissue.
   - Post the positioning schedule at the bedside.
   - Inspect skin over bony prominences and other pressure points when repositioning at least daily.
   - Position with pillows to elevate pressure points off the bed.
   - Keep linen clean, dry, and wrinkle free.
   - Make bed with toe pleats.
   - Avoid massaging pressure points.
   - Moisturize dry, unbroken skin.
   - Monitor reddened areas closely.
   - Apply elbow and heel protectors as appropriate.
   - Facilitate small shifts in body weight frequently.
   - Once G.W. regains the use of her hands, provide a trapeze to help shift weight frequently.
   - Ensure adequate nutrition, especially protein, vitamins B and C, iron, and calories, using supplements as appropriate (Iowa Intervention Project, 1992).

An additional 3 weeks have passed. G.W. has recovered gross movement of her arms and some respiratory effort. She is still on a ventilator but she has gone from controlled to assisted breathing. This morning G.W. receives a letter from her health insurance company informing her that she has exceeded her lifetime limit and has been dropped from their plan. She is crying hysterically and is choking because of the increased mucous production in her sinuses. Remember that she cannot wipe her eyes or blow her nose to clear it.

10. What can be done for her? **[P/an/S,PI,PSI/ct,ni,tc]**
    - First suction her airway to clear the mucous.
    - Call the physician or practitioner and get a STAT order for an anxiolytic medication to ease her distress. This is especially critical because it appears to be interfering with her breathing.
    - Contact the facility's social service department immediately. They will work with the family or a significant other to identify legal and financial issues that need to be addressed. They can also suggest legal recourse that might be taken based on their experiences with other patients in similar situations.
    - Ask G.W. if she would like to communicate with someone (for example, a friend, clergy person, nurse, social worker, or others) about how she feels, and facilitate this connection.
    - Keep G.W. informed about measures taken on her behalf to minimize the sense of helplessness and despair that she may feel. Watch for depression. As she continues improving physical functioning, watch for indications of suicidal ideation if the financial situation is not resolved.

It took G.W. almost 11 months to recover enough to be discharged to home with the assistance of a home health aide.

Case Study 11: Spinal Cord Injury

Difficulty: **	*Setting:* Rehabilitation facility
Index Words: Spinal cord injury, paraplegia	

T.W. is a 22-year-old man who fell 50 feet from a chairlift while skiing and landed on hard-packed snow. He was found to have a T10-11 fracture with paraplegia. He was initially admitted to the SICU and placed on high-dose steroids for 24 hours. He was taken to surgery 48 hours postaccident for spinal stabilization. He spent 2 additional days in the SICU, 5 days on the floor, and now is ready to be transferred to your rehab unit. He continues to have no movement of his lower extremities.

1. The goal of treatment in the acute phase of spinal cord injury (SCI) is to help T.W. survive the injury and maintain physiologic stability through the period of spinal shock. Once the acute phase is over, T.W. moves into the postacute and early rehab phases. What are the treatment goals for T.W. in these phases? **[P/c/S,PI,PSI/ct,ni]**
   - To ensure continued stability, maintain body function, prevent complications, begin the process of identifying T.W.'s specific needs, and begin teaching T.W. how to complete his ADL.

2. Considering a hierarchy of rehabilitative needs for patients like T.W., number the following from highest (1) to lowest (5) priority. **[P/c/S,PI,PSI,HP/ct]**
   - 4 Community integration and employment.
   - 2 Accomplishment of self-care and ADLs.
   - 5 Self-actualization.
   - 1 Stabilization of the physiologic systems.
   - 3 Adjustment to living at home.

3. T.W. received high-dose steroid therapy every 24 hours then he was placed on a smaller maintenance dose. What effect will steroids have on T.W.? **[AN/ap/PI/ct]**
   - It will decrease inflammation by suppressing his immune system. Although the antiinflammatory effect is desired for his neurologic status, it will render him more vulnerable to nosocomial acquired infections.

4. List 3 critical potential infections that T.W. should be monitored for throughout his hospitalization? **[PD/ap/PI/ct]**
   - Pulmonary.
   - Urinary tract.
   - Wound infection.

A person with an SCI at the T2-12 level should be independent in a wheelchair and able to manage ADL, including bowel and bladder care.

5. T.W. is on vitamin C 1 g PO qid. What is the purpose of this? **[PD/ap/PI/ct]**
   - To acidify the urine and prevent the formation of renal calculi. T.W. is at-risk for renal calculi because of demineralization of bones caused by the nonweightbearing condition and incomplete emptying of the bladder; stone formation is enhanced by alkaline urine.

You request a consultation with a registered dietitian because you realize that T.W. needs proteins for healing; however, too much can stress his kidneys. The RD will adjust his diet to ensure adequate amount of protein, carbohydrates, calcium, magnesium, and zinc.

6. Rehabilitation teaching includes teaching T.W. how to manage his urinary drainage system. What would this teaching include? **[P,I/an/S,PI,PSI/ct,ni,tc]**
   - Maintaining a closed urinary drainage system (UDS).
   - Maintaining patency of the UDS.
   - Irrigation of the UDS using sterile technique.
   - Cleansing the genital skin area at regular intervals.
   - Changing the urinary catheter at regular intervals.
   - Changing the UDS at regular intervals.
   - Cleaning the urinary catheter externally at the meatus.
   - Noting the urinary drainage characteristics.
   - Positioning to promote urinary drainage.
   - Emptying the UDS at regular intervals.
   - Disconnecting the leg bag at night and connecting to a bedside drainage bag.
   - Checking the leg bag straps for constriction at regular intervals.
   - Maintaining meticulous skin care.
   - Cleansing the leg bag daily.
   - Monitoring for bladder distention (Iowa Intervention Project, 1992).

7. What is the usual amount of time for the return of reflex function of the bladder? **[A/k/PI/ct]**
   - 4 to 6 weeks.

8. The large bowel musculature has its own neural center that can directly respond to distention caused by fecal material. This is what allows most SCI patients to regain bowel control. What dietary instructions are important for T.W.? **[P/c/PI/ct]**
   - Increased fluid, high fiber, increase roughage, and warm fluids may stimulate the gastrocolic reflex, which increases peristalsis and contractions of the GI tract.

9. T.W. should also be taught bowel training techniques. What would this teaching include? **[P,I/an/S,PI,PSI/ct,ni,tc]**
   - Instruct T.W. about which foods are high in bulk.
   - Importance of adequate fluid intake.
   - Ensure adequate exercise.
   - Initiate an uninterrupted, consistent time for defecation.
   - Ensure privacy.
   - Administer suppository as appropriate.
   - Perform digital stimulation.
   - Evaluate bowel status regularly (Iowa Intervention Project, 1992).

10. What medications can assist with a bowel program? **[PD/c/PI/ct]**
    - Stool softeners, bulk producers, lubricants, mild cathartics, suppositories.

11. Describe digital stimulation. **[PD/c/PI/ct]**
    - Digital stimulation is used to elicit reflex elimination to evacuate the lower bowel. A well-lubricated finger is inserted into the rectum approximately 1 ½ inches and pointed posteriorly to avoid pushing against the bladder. The finger is then gently rotated for 30 seconds or longer. This can be repeated 3 or 4 times every 10 minutes. Digital stimulation may be used alone or in conjunction with suppositories.

12. T.W. asks you if he'll ever be able to have sex again. What do you tell him and what are some possible referrals? **[P/ap/PSI,HP/ct,ni]**
    - Sexual function is controlled by spinal levels S2-4. Seventy percent of male patients with complete lesions can have erections and coitus; however, they are unable to have an orgasm or ejaculate and, therefore, are infertile. Information about methods other than intercourse should be offered. Sex counseling is an appropriate referral for information, assistance, and support, and all health team members act as secondary (or primary) sources of information and support.
    - Birth control counseling should also be provided. A woman with any SCI lacks sensation during intercourse, but her fertility is not affected and vaginal delivery is possible if pelvic measurements are adequate.

For patients with lesions at T6 or above, there is the potential for autonomic dysreflexia (AD) in response to noxious stimulation of the sympathetic nervous system. The patient develops severe hypertension (as high as 240-300/150 mm Hg), pounding headache, bradycardia, blurred vision, nausea, nasal congestion, and flushing and sweating above the level of the injury and goose bumps or pallor below the level of the injury. Potential causes include bladder distention, obstruction, infection, spasms, catheterization, and bladder irrigations done too fast or with cold fluid; bowel constipation, impaction, or rectal stimulation; and alterations in skin integrity including pressure, infection, injury, and cold or hot. This can cause retinal hemorrhage, CVA, and seizure activity.

13. What are nursing interventions r/t AD? **[P,I/ap/PI/ct/ni]**
    - Prevention of precipitating causes, early recognition, removal of noxious stimuli, call for help but stay with the patient, raise HOB to decrease BP and other measures to control the BP, anticipate administering adrenergic blockers, vasodilators, and/or ganglionic blockers.

For additional information contact:

National Spinal Cord Injury Association
545 Concord Ave, Suite 29
Cambridge, MA 02138
1-800-962-9629

Case Study 12: Aneurysm

Difficulty: *** *Setting:* Hospital

Index Words: Aneurysm, cerebrovascular accident

R.P. is 72 years old, retired, and in good health. His only medication is an aspirin a day. While bending over to tie his shoes, R.P. developed a severe headache, muscle rigidity, slurred speech, confusion, and nausea. He was taken to the ED, where it was discovered that he had a subarachnoid hemorrhage from a ruptured grade III cerebral aneurysm. The aneurysm was surgically repaired 15 days ago, and R.P. is now being transferred to your unit.

In addition, you receive the following report. R.P. is alert and maintains eye contact but is aphasic. He does withdraw from painful stimuli and plantar reflexes bilaterally. His cardiovascular system is stable, and he has a L peripheral IV that is heparin-locked and bilateral TED hose. He is on 2 L O_2/nc and has scattered coarse breath sounds with a weak cough effort. His abdomen is distended but he does have bowel sounds in all 4 quadrants; his tube feeding is at 80 ml/h. Last bowel movement (BM) is unknown. He has a Foley to down drain and his groin skin folds are a little reddened. There is no other skin breakdown. He gets out of bed (OOB) to the total lift chair bid and tolerates it well.

1. What other information would you like to have? **[PD/ap/PI/ct,tc]**
   - Current VS and VS trends, medications, lab and ABG values, family situation including education level, and discharge planning.

2. R.P.'s medications are listed below. Explain why he is getting each. **[PD/ap/PI/ct]**
   - Heparin 5000 Units SC q12h:
     - DVT prophylaxis.
   - Metoprolol (Lopressor) 50 mg per feeding tube bid:
     - Antihypertensive.
   - Clonidine 0.2 mg topical patch q week:
     - Antihypertensive.
   - Tylenol 650 mg per feeding tube q4h prn:
     - Antipyretic, analgesic.
   - Temazepam (Restoril) 15 mg per feeding tube q hs prn:
     - Sleep aid.
   - MOM 30 ml per feeding tube prn:
     - Laxative.

3. Current VS are 150/85, 82, 18, 37.8°C (ear), and reported as stable. Do any of the VS concern you? **[PD/an/PI/ct]**
   - Yes, the BP is high despite the administration of antihypertensives. After vascular surgery, it is especially important to keep the BP under control so as not to cause rebleeding because the aneurysmal pressure is determined by the central BP. Of vascular surgery patients, 35% to 40% rebleed postoperatively, and of these, approximately 40% die.

4. What laboratory tests would be indicated for the daily draw? **[P/ap/S,PI/ct]**
   - CBC, Chem 7 (serum electrolytes, BUN, creatinine, glucose), Mg, calcium.
   - The PT and PTT would also be drawn if R.P. were unstable.

5. What are nursing interventions related to R.P.'s pulmonary hygiene? **[P,I/ap/PI/ct,ni]**
   - Frequent lung assessment, monitor oxygen saturation, encourage CDB, and, if he is uncooperative, you may have to NT suction him to help clear secretions, turn every 2 hour, get him OOB.
   - See that respiratory therapy performs postural drainage and chest percussion therapy (CPT) if ordered.

6. What additional information given in or omitted from report is of concern to you? **[PD/an/PI,PSI/ct]**
   - Neuro status and his rehab potential, abdominal distention and unknown BM, groin skin folds reddened, and family situation.

7. If R.P.'s neurologic status started to deteriorate, what test would you anticipate the physician ordering? **[PD/ap/PI,ct]**
   - CT scan of the brain.

8. Lab results the next morning are: Na 140 mEq/L, K 4.2 mEq/L, Cl 100 mEq/L, CO_2 26 mEq/L, BUN 20 mg/dl, creatinine 1.2 mg/dl, glucose 107 mg/dl, WBC 12 mm^3, Hgb 13.4 g/dl, Hct 37.6%, platelets 184 mm^3. Do these concern you, and what might it indicate? **[PD/an/PI/ct]**
   - All are within normal except the WBC count, which could indicate an infection.

9. What are potential sites of infection for R.P.? **[PD/ap/S,PI/ct]**
   - Respiratory tract, urinary tract r/t Foley, CSF, surgical wound, blood, IV site, and other invasive sites.

10. Identify 2 nursing interventions that address R.P.'s groin redness. **[P,I/ap/PI/ct,ni]**
    - Wash the area with soap and water, rinse well, and dry thoroughly.
    - Increase the air circulation to the area, assess for *Candida* infection, and report if found (anticipate treatment with a topical antiyeast agent).

Case Study 13: Closed Head Injury

Difficulty: ***	*Setting:* Hospital
Index Words: Closed head injury	

Y.W. is a 23-year-old male student from Thailand studying electrical engineering at the university. He was ejected from a moving vehicle which was traveling 70 mph. His injuries included a severe closed head injury with an occipital hematoma, bilateral wrist fractures, and a R pneumothorax. During his NICU stay, Y.W. was intubated and placed on mechanical ventilation, had a feeding tube inserted and was placed on tube feedings, had a Foley catheter to down drain, and multiple IVs inserted. He developed pneumonia 1 month after admission.

1. Describe the term *primary head injury.* **[A/k/Pl/ct]**
   - The initial tissue damage resulting from the traumatic impact. A primary head injury can include the scalp, skull, or brain tissue itself. Hemorrhage or hematoma, brain tissue ischemia, cerebral edema, and/or infection can begin almost immediately in response to the primary injury and can cause increased intracranial pressure (IICP) or herniation.

2. Describe *secondary head injury.* **[A/k/Pl/ct]**
   - This is an event that complicates the primary injury and causes further damage. Secondary damage may increase the risk for death or may result in a worse outcome. Events precipitating a secondary head injury may include systemic hypotension, hypoxemia, hypercapnia, sustained IICP, respiratory complications, and infections, among others.

3. Why is increased intracranial pressure (IICP) so clinically important, and what are 5 signs and symptoms? **[A/c/Pl/ct]**
   - IICP has a negative effect on cerebral blood flow and, therefore, on the amount of O_2 available to the neurons. Signs and symptoms include altered or decreased LOC; worsening headache; pupillary dysfunction; blurred vision; weakness or sensorimotor changes; nausea or vomiting; alterations in VS such as a widened pulse pressure or bradycardia; and impaired reflexes such as corneal, gag, swallow, and posturing.

4. List 4 medication classifications and 8 nursing measures that the ICU nurses could use to control or decrease the ICP? **[PD/c/PI/ct,ni]**
   - Medication classifications include osmotic diuretics (mannitol) to reduce cerebral edema, loop diuretics to excrete fluids, corticosteroids to stabilize the cell membrane and reduce cerebral edema, antipyretics to reduce metabolic needs, mild sedatives, BP control for either hypertension or hypotension.
   - Nursing measures include elevate HOB 15 to 30 degrees, maintain head and neck in neutral position (no flexion of neck), maintain a patent airway and hyperventilate to maintain $PaCO_2$ 25 to 35 mm Hg as prescribed, limit endotracheal suctioning to no longer than 15 seconds, reposition patient at regular intervals (avoid extreme flexion at the hip or knees and isometric exercises such as the Valsalva maneuver), keep the environment cool or apply hypothermia blanket to maintain body temperature within normal limits, minimize or eliminate stress situations (counsel families to avoid emotionally stimulating the patient), control environmental stimuli (noise, temperature, light, odors), initiate pain management, initiate comfort measures, space patient care activities to allow for periods of rest.

5. Y.W.'s medication list included clindamycin 150 mg per feeding tube q6h, ranitidine (Zantac Elixir) 150 mg per feeding tube bid, and phenytoin (Dilantin) 100 mg IVPB tid. Indicate why he is on each. **[PD/c/S,PI/ct]**
   - Clindamycin for pneumonia.
   - Zantac Elixir for stress ulcer prevention.
   - Dilantin for prevention/control of posttraumatic seizures.

6. A STAT portable CXR was ordered after each central venous catheter (CVC) was inserted. According to hospital protocol, no one is permitted to infuse anything through the catheter until the CXR has been read by the physician or radiologist. What is the purpose of the CXR, and why isn't fluid infused through the catheter until after the CXR is read? **[PD/k/S,PI/ct]**
   - The CXR is taken to (1) determine if the physician inserting the catheter has created a pneumothorax or hemothorax, and (2) confirm that the tip of the catheter has been correctly placed in the superior vena cave or R atrium and not in the head or neck.

Yin spent 2 months in acute care and is now on your rehab unit. He follows commands but tends to get very agitated with too much stimulation. His trach site is well healed and the pneumonia is finally resolving. He is still receiving supplemental tube feeding and has some continued incontinence of both bowel and bladder. Y.W. has a very supportive group of friends who are students at the University, several of them are also from Thailand.

7. Y.W.'s latest lab results are as follows, Na 149 mEq/L, K 4.2 mEq/L, Cl 119 mEq/L, CO_2 21 mEq/L, BUN 12 mg/dl, creatinine 1.2 mg/dl, glucose 123 mg/dl, WBC 15.4 mm^3, Hgb 14.9 g/dl, Hct 36.4%, platelets 140 mm^3. Are any of these of concern to you, and what would you suggest to correct them? **[E/an/S,PI/ct]**
   - Elevated Na: Y.W. needs increased amounts of free water (administer per feeding tube).
   - Elevated Cl: follows the Na and is treated the same way.
   - Slightly decreased CO_2: probably from tachypnea, which is typical of head injured patients, no specific treatment.
   - Slightly elevated glucose: possibly because of tube feeding, no specific treatment, monitor; and probably r/t corticosteroids.
   - Increased WBC: probably r/t known pneumonia, continue antibiotics, monitor for signs of worsening pneumonia or new infection

8. Are you surprised by Y.W.'s agitated behavior? Explain. **[PD/c/PI,PSI/ct]**
   - After severe head injury, patients frequently get a postconcussion syndrome, in which they have headaches, dizziness, intolerance to stress, noise, or emotional excitement, easy fatigability, apprehension, inability to concentrate, poor memory, and mood or behavior fluctuations.

9. Outline a general rehabilitation plan for Y.W. based on the above data. **[P/an/S,PI,PSI/ct,ni]**
   - Set realistic goals and maintain a consistent approach. Prevent further complications (skin, infections, DVTs, safety, nutrition deficits); maximize cognitive function; maximize communication; help Y.W. relearn ADL, bowel, and bladder retraining; have Y.W. plan an exercise program to regain balance and muscle strength; and provide psychologic support through friends and others.

10. Y.W.'s mother has just arrived in the U.S. and speaks no English. What measures can be taken to facilitate communication between medical personnel and his mother? **[P,I/an/PSI/ni,tc]**
    - Contact Y.W.'s Thai friends at the university and ask them to serve as interpreters between the mother and the medical staff.
    - Ask the Thai friends to help develop a communications board with English words under each Thai word.

11. Y.W.'s mother will need a place to stay while in the U.S. What can you do to facilitate the initial contact with the Thai community? **[P/ap/PSI/ni,tc]**
    - Again, ask the Thai students if they could make initial contact for Mrs. W. to stay with a Thai family. That family may be able to help interpret for Mrs. W.

12. What special discharge planning considerations are there in this case? **[P/an/S,PI,PSI/ct]**
    - Y.W. is a foreign student whose mother is present but speaks no English. He is going to require long-term rehabilitation and it will have to be decided whether he will stay in the U.S. or return to Thailand. If it is decided he will return to his native country, he will have to be stable enough for an international flight and arrangements will have to be made for his care in Thailand. Diplomatic consulates or embassies can be very helpful in communicating with the mother, investigating resources, and making the necessary arrangements.

For additional information contact:

Brain Injury Association Help Line
1776 Massachusetts Ave. N.W., Suite 100
Washington, DC 20036
1-800-444-6443

Case Study 14: Epidural Abscess

Difficulty: ***	*Setting:* Hospital
Index Words: Epidural abscess	

G.B.'s family reports that he has had progressive back pain since his decompression laminectomy 4 months ago and is now unable to walk. He has become increasingly confused over the past 2 weeks, is occasionally SOB, and is now unable to care for himself. He looks dehydrated and possibly septic. G.B. is very angry at being brought to the hospital and states, "I had this back worked on 4 months ago and I don't intend to have it done again!!" G.B. is 72 years old and had multiple health problems including GI hemorrhages, hypertension (HTN), elevated glucose, chronic lymphocytic leukemia (CLL), a remote history of kidney stones, an appendectomy, shrapnel from WW II, and a fx R femur from a mining accident. His family reports that G.B. was allergic to penicillin as a child but cannot remember what reaction he experienced.

1. Based on the information given above, review the following list of admission orders. Place an "I" by each inappropriate order and state why it is inappropriate. **[E/an/S,Pl/ct]**
   ___ Routine VS.
   ___ Routine neuro checks.
   ___ Up ad lib.
   ___ CBC, Chem 7, urinalysis, ABG, PT, PTT.
   ___ O_2 to keep SaO_2 greater than 90%.
   ___ IV D_5½ NS with 20 mEq of KCl/L at 100 ml/h.
   ___ NPO.
   ___ Cefazolin (Kefzol) 1 g IV q8h.
   ___ Ranitidine (Zantac) 50 mg IV q8h.
   ___ Codeine 30 mg IM q4-6h prn for pain.
   ___ Droperidol (Inapsine) 0.25 ml IV q8h prn for nausea.
   ___ Acetaminophen (Tylenol) 650 mg PO q4-6h prn for fever.

   <u>Inappropriate Orders</u>
   - VS should be taken at least q4h until stable.
   - Neuro checks should be completed at least q4h until stable.
   - G.B. should be on bed rest until a specific diagnosis made.
   - The IV order may be changed when the lab results return.
   - G.B. may be allergic to penicillin; cefazolin may cause an allergic reaction.
   - Acetaminophen should be ordered as a suppository.

2. Admission VS are 165/85, 76, 20, 36.7°C. Do any of the VS concern you? Explain. **[PD/an/Pl/ct]**
   - BP is elevated; he has a PMH of HTN and he is agitated. Before treating the BP, G.B.'s BP should be repeated when he is less agitated. If the BP remains elevated, he may need an IV or SL form of BP medication until he can resume PO intake.
   - If G.B. is septic, you would expect him to have a fever. With a history of CLL, immunosuppression or lack of ability to mount a febrile response is a concern.

3. You get the following lab results, Na 132 mEq/L, K 3.7 mEq/L, Cl 98 mEq/L, CO_2 27 mEq/L, BUN 13 mg/dl, creatinine 0.6 mg/dl, glucose 138 mg/dl, WBC 36 mm^3, Hgb 10.8 g/dl, Hct 31.3%, platelets 130 mm^3. You call the physician to report them. What orders do you anticipate in regard to a change in IV solution? **[E/an/Pl/ct]**
   - Change the IV to D_5½ NS with 20 mEq of KCl/L.

4. What part of G.B.'s PMH is consistent with the CBC results? **[PD/an/Pl/ct]**
   - CLL.

5. What noninvasive diagnostic test might be done to determine G.B.'s problem? **[A/an/Pl/ct]**
   - CT scan of spine.

6. Why would an MRI be contraindicated in G.B.'s case? **[A/c/S,Pl/ct]**
   - During magnetic resonance imaging, G.B. will be subjected to a strong magnetic field. The shrapnel fragments could be shifted or pulled out of his body and lacerate everything in their paths.

7. G.B.'s family had to leave the hospital for a short time. When you enter his room, you find him trying to climb over the siderails. What should you consider before applying a vest (Posey) or wrist restraints? **[P/c/S,Pl/ct,ni]**
   - You first must know your institution's policy. Most institutions require a physician's order and very frequent checks on the patient so that the restraints do not cause further harm. A vest restraint may be effective in keeping G.B. in bed while not restricting limb movements. Wrist or limb restraints may be necessary to protect lines (IVs, monitoring equipment, drains). Placing patients in restraints often makes them more agitated. Proper application of restrains is imperative so that the circulation or innervation of a limb is not compromised. Consider someone (nursing assistant or volunteer) who may be available to stay with G.B. until his family returns.

8. As the afternoon progresses, G.B.'s oxygen saturation decreases from 96% on 2 L O_2/nc to 88%. The physician orders oxygen by mask at 6 L. What are 4 nursing interventions that can help improve his oxygenation status? **[P,I/c/Pl/ct,ni]**
   - Make sure G.B. is turned q2h, have him cough and deep breathe at least q2h, obtain an incentive spirometer and help G.B. use it, and elevate HOB if medically cleared.

9. Diagnostic tests reveal that G.B. has an epidural abscess near his laminectomy incision, and he is scheduled for surgery. G.B. has already stated he does not plan to have any more surgery. Do you feel he is competent to make the decision? How would you proceed with obtaining consent? **[P,I/an/Pl/ct]**
   - Determine if G.B. has a Living Will or has designated a Health Care Power-of-Attorney. With the individual named on the Health Care Power-of-Attorney present, the surgeon should explain, in detail, the planned procedure along with risks, benefits, and consequences of not proceeding. Because G.B. has been confused, the Health Care Power-of-Attorney agent should be asked to sign the surgical consent form.
   - If no Health Care Power-of-Attorney has been named, the family should be present and a family member sign the consent form for G.B.
   - The main focus of all this must be respecting G.B.'s wishes, *not* the wishes of health care professionals or family members.

The family tells the surgeon to go ahead with the surgery, against G.B.'s wishes. It was decided that he is not competent to make the decision for himself at this time.

Instructor Note: You may wish to discuss the ethical issues this presents with your group, since this is a common ethical problem.

10. What are considerations for discharge planning? **[P/an/S,Pl,PSl/ct]**
    - Is his family willing to consider managing G.B. at home with home health nurses, or will he need ECF placement?
    - Is there someone to be with him 24 hours/day?
    - Does G.B. or his family need the assistance of a financial counselor?
    - Get Social Services involved.
    - What is the physical layout of the home, and would it be possible for G.B. to go home in a wheelchair, if necessary?
    - Begin teaching the family ASAP specifics related to his care.
    - Provide ongoing family support as they make difficult decisions.

Case Study 15: Meningitis

Difficulty: ***	*Setting:* Hospital
Index Words: Meningitis, hyperglycemia	

D.H., a 54-year-old resort owner, has multiple chronic medical problems including type II DM for 25 years, IDDM for the past 10 years, a renal transplant 5 years ago with no signs of rejection at last biopsy, HTN, and remote peptic ulcer disease (PUD). His medications include insulin, his immunosuppressives, and 2 antihypertensives. He visited his local physician with c/o L ear, mastoid, and sinus pain. He was diagnosed with sinusitis and *Candida albicans* (thrush); cephalexin (Keflex) and nystatin (Mycostatin) were prescribed. Later that evening he developed N/V, hematemesis, and weakness, and was taken to the ED. He was admitted and started on IV antibiotics, but his condition worsened throughout the night; his dyspnea increased and he developed difficulty speaking. He was flown to your tertiary referral center and was intubated en route. On arrival, D.H. had decreased LOC with periods of total unresponsiveness, weakness, and cranial nerve deficits. His diagnosis is meningitis complicated by an aspiration pneumonia and atrial fibrillation. D.H. has continued fevers and leukocytosis despite aggressive antibiotic therapy.

1. Why is D.H. at particular risk for infection? **[PD/c/S,PI/ct]**
   - He is on immunosuppressive therapy for his kidney transplant.
   - His diabetes also places him at risk for infection.

2. Describe bacterial meningitis. **[PD/k/PI/ct]**
   - It is an infection that results in inflammation of the meningeal membranes covering the brain and spinal cord. It is a pyogenic infection, and the purulent material spreads quickly through the CSF. The bacteria and exudate create vascular congestion, and the arachnoid villi can become obstructed. This leads to IICP, which can cause brain herniation and death.

3. What is the probable route of entry of bacteria into D.H.'s brain? **[PD/c/PI/ct]**
   - The ear or sinuses. Bacteria can also enter by way of the bloodstream or a penetrating head wound.

4. How do you think D.H. might have developed an aspiration pneumonia? **[A/k/S,PI/ct]**
   - It is possible that D.H. aspirated when he developed N/V and hematemesis before his transport. It is also likely that he aspirated during emergent intubation en route.

5. What factors influenced the physicians' decision to transport D.H. from a smaller hospital to a tertiary referral center? **[PD/c/S,PI/ct]**
   - His history of renal transplant, immunosuppression, and IDDM.
   - His diagnosis of sinusitis provides a route of entry to the brain and increases his potential for meningitis
   - He displayed signs of meningitis with IICP through the night.
   - The physician believed that D.H.'s chances of survival would be improved if he had the advantage of the resources at a large tertiary referral center.

6. Name 4 tests that could be used in the diagnosis of meningitis. **[PD/k/PI/ct]**
   - Lumbar puncture with CSF analysis and culture.
   - CT scan with contrast.
   - Skull, sinus, and CXR to help rule out or establish other diagnoses.
   - Blood, urine, and sputum C&S to identify specific causative organisms.
   - Latex antigen test for detection of bacterial antigens in the blood, urine, or CSF.

7. The following is a list of D.H's medications. Indicate next to each why he is receiving it. **[PD/ap/S,PI/ct]**
   - Sliding-scale regular insulin SC.
     - For known type I type I DM.
   - Sucralfate (Carafate) 1 g per NGT q6h.
     - A stress ulcer prophylaxis.
   - Azathioprine 100 mg in 100 ml D_5W IVPB qd.
     - An immunosuppressant given to kidney transplant recipients.
   - Imipenem/cilastatin (Primaxin) 500 mg IVPB q6h.
     - A broad-spectrum antibiotic.
   - Methylprednisolone (Solu-Medrol) 125 mg IV q8h.
     - Has immunosuppression and antiinflammatory action.
   - Digoxin 0.125 IV qd.
     - For atrial fibrillation, to slow ventricular rate.
   - Metronidazole (Flagyl) 500 mg IV q6h.
     - An antibiotic for anaerobic coverage.
   - Sulfamethoxazole 800 mg/trimethoprim (Septra) 160 mg IV q12h x 15 days.
     - A fixed combination antibiotic.

   Instructor Note: Antibiotics should be based on culture and sensitivity results as well as coverage for known opportunists in immunosuppressed patients.

8. The lab just called you with a glucose result of 350 mg/dl. Identify 3 factors that could contribute to D.H.'s elevated glucose level. **[PD/ap/PI/ct]**
   - He is diabetic.
   - It could be exacerbated by stress, infection, steroids, and, possibly, IV fluids with dextrose.

9. List 7 nursing interventions for management of D.H.'s current problems. **[P,I/an/S,PI,PSI/ct,ni,tc]**
   - Make sure everyone performs good handwashing technique on entering and leaving D.H.'s room (physicians, nurses, family, laboratory technicians).
   - Monitor VS and immediately notify the physician if D.H. spikes a fever. Obtain cultures before giving antipyretics or antibiotics.
   - Monitor and maintain adequate oxygenation.
   - Administer medications on time (antibiotics, immunosuppressants, digoxin, pain medications).
   - Monitor glucose and give insulin as prescribed.
   - Maintain sterile technique when performing dressing changes and endotracheal suctioning, and immediately report abnormalities.
   - Monitor and report abnormalities in laboratory values.
   - Obtain daily weights as requested.
   - Keep siderails up.
   - Closely observe his emotional status.

10. List 6 nursing interventions to prevent complications. **[P,I/an/S,PI,PSI/ct,ni,tc]**
    - Everyone should perform good handwashing technique on entering and leaving D.H.'s room (physicians, nurses, family, laboratory technicians).
    - Hang a sign over D.H.'s bed with instructions "No BPs or needle sticks in *(specify which arm has the shunt; R or L)* arm." Check the shunt for bruits.
    - Maintain the integrity of the Foley catheter and drainage bag.
    - Turn D.H. regularly, apply skin lotion, and inspect pressure areas.
    - Obtain consultation for registered dietitian to calculate nutritional requirements.
    - Obtain a PT consultation to maintain mobility.
    - Encourage family members to participate in D.H.'s care.
    - Educate family about preventing infections when D.H. goes home.

11. D.H.'s family is staying at a nearby motel. His adult son brings his mother to the hospital. Mrs. H. says she just wants to stay with her husband around the clock. She states, "I took care of him for 35 years now, and I'm not going to abandon him now when he needs me the most." How would you respond? **[P,I/an/PSI/ct,ni,tc]**
    - Acknowledge the legitimacy of her fear.
    - Work out a schedule with the family so she can stay with him and still get adequate food and rest. Stick to the plan.
    - Ask her to always let you know where she can be found. If she is financially able, she might rent a pager.
    - Promise you will contact her if he "takes a turn for the worse."
    - Make sure that the plan is posted for other nurses and physicians to see.
    - Be sure to discuss advanced directives and Health Care Power-of-Attorney with Mrs. H.

D.H.'s infection destroyed his cadaver kidney. He developed multiple system organ failure and died 7 weeks later.

Case Study 16: Parkinson's Disease

Difficulty: ***	*Setting:* Outpatient clinic
Index Words: Parkinson's disease	

T.S. is a 76-year-old widower being seen in your outpatient clinic for a medication refill for his Parkinson's disease. He is a retired railroad engineer who derives great pleasure from his daily walks with his dog around his neighborhood and collecting railroad memorabilia. T.S. was diagnosed with moderate (stage III) Parkinson's disease 2 years ago. He does not smoke cigarettes or drink alcohol. His PMH includes a femur fx at age 22, a cholecystectomy at age 47, and a transurethral resection of the prostate (TURP) at age 72.

1. Because of the interference of normal muscle tone and control of smooth muscle, patients with Parkinson's disease exhibit a classic triad of symptoms. Name them. **[PD/k/PE/ct]**
   - Tremors, rigidity, and akinesia (complete or partial loss of muscle movement).

2. Parkinson's is a disease of the elderly with symptoms usually first noted bxt 60-70 year olds. Why are we seeing a growing number of people with Parkinson's disease? **[PD/c/PI/ct]**
   - There is a growing number of elderly and elderly people are living longer; therefore, more people will develop the disease.

3. Symptoms vary and are highly individualized. List 8 symptoms associated with Parkinson's. **[PD/k/C/ct]**
   - Increased muscle rigidity, jerky "cogwheel" motions.
   - Masklike face, blank facial expression, unblinking "stare."
   - Drooling r/t increased difficulty chewing and swallowing.
   - Weak monotone voice, slow and slurred speech.
   - Unintentional tremors: "pill-rolling" which stops during intentional movements.
   - Rapid, severe fatigue.
   - Restlessness, compelling need to walk.
   - Loss of postural reflexes, stooped, shuffling gait, propulsive gait.
   - General weakness and muscle fatigue.
   - Muscle cramping.
   - Autonomic manifestations, diaphoresis, seborrhea, postural hypotension, decreased libido, GI hypomotility, urinary hesitancy.

Medical management of the patient with Parkinson's is usually directed toward control of symptoms with drug therapy, supportive therapy, physiotherapy, and possibly psychotherapy. Pharmacotherapy can be fairly complex in these patients because there are several types of antiparkinson drugs with different mechanisms of action. The physician works with the patient to achieve the most effective regimen and often involves trial-and-error periods.

4. Why can't we just give oral dopamine as replacement therapy, and what medication do we give instead? **[PD/c/PI/ct]**
   - Dopamine can't be given orally because it is metabolized before reaching the brain. Levodopa is given instead and is the metabolic precursor of dopamine. It crosses the blood-brain barrier and restores dopamine levels.

5. Levodopa is often given in combination with carbidopa. Why? **[PD/c/PI/ct]**
   - Carbidopa prevents the peripheral metabolism of levodopa and, therefore, less levodopa is needed and side effects are diminished. Side effects can be severe and can include N/V, postural hypotension, dizziness, dry mouth, choreiform movement, cardiac dysrhythmias, GI bleeding, urinary retention, depression, hallucinations, and confusion.

6. What are 5 nursing interventions to decrease the number or severity of side effects of antiparkinson medications? **[P,I/ap/S,PI,PSI/ct,ni]**
   - Take medication with meals to decrease GI upset.
   - Change positions slowly to avoid postural hypotension; may need elastic hose.
   - Give sugar-free candy, rinse mouth frequently with water, and/or use artificial saliva products to reduce dry mouth.
   - Begin on a bowel regimen to prevent constipation.
   - Report unusual or new symptoms, especially spasmodic winking, twitching, facial grimace, or tongue protrusion. The medication dosage may need to be adjusted.

7. What advice will the registered dietitian give T.S. about his diet? **[I/ap/S,PI/ct]**
   - Avoid vitamin B_6 and decrease protein intake as both of these interfere with the effectiveness of levodopa. CHO:protein ratio should be 7:1.
   - Frequent small meals to help avoid nausea and stomach upset. Take meals shortly after taking medication.
   - Eat soft, ground food if dysphagia is present.
   - Increase fluids and high dietary fiber to prevent constipation.
   - Avoid alcohol because it decreases levodopa's effectiveness.

8. T.S. asks you to explain "Parkinsonian crisis." Describe it in a way he can understand, and describe what someone should do if it occurs. **[P/ap/S,PI,PSI/ct,tc]**
   - It is a sudden and severe increase in the tremors, rigidity, and slowness of movement (the triad) that can lead to a fast or irregular heart beat and paralysis of muscles. The muscle paralysis can make him stop breathing. If this happens, his family needs to immediately call 911 and get him to the hospital.

9. If you were a home health nurse, list 6 things that you would assess to determine if T.S.'s care can be managed in his home. **[P,I/an/S,PI,PSI/ct,ni]**
   - Are there a telephone and a list of emergency numbers by the phone?
   - Number of stairs and presence of handrails.
   - Layout of home and lighting.
   - Are there throw rugs, loose carpeting, or other items on the floor that he could trip over?
   - Location of bathroom, tub and/or shower. Are there safety devices in the bathroom?
   - The meal situation.
   - Transportation.
   - Social support system.

10. How might T.S's PMH affect his symptoms? **[PD/ap/S,PI/ct]**
    - A previous fx femur could cause stiffness or arthritic changes complicating T.S.'s gait, a previous cholecystectomy could affect the GI tract, and an enlarged prostate (despite the TURP) could enhance urinary symptoms.

For additional information, contact:

Parkinson's Disease Foundation, Inc.
650 West 168th St. or 710 W. 168th St.
New York, NY 10032
1-800-457-6676 (Toll Free)
1-212-923-4700

Case Study 17: Subarachnoid Hemorrhage

Difficulty: ***	*Setting:* Hospital
Index Words: Subarachnoid hemorrhage	

R.G. is a 50-year-old woman who was being arrested by the police when she collapsed and had a seizure. She was transported by ambulance to the ED where a CT scan revealed a grade II subarachnoid hemorrhage (SAH). Her urine and toxicology screen were positive for cocaine, opiates, barbiturates, and benzodiazepines. The ED nurse was able to contact a son from a phone number in her purse. You are caring for R.G. 2 days postadmission. The neurosurgeons have decided to postpone surgery for 5 to 10 days because this is the time when most rebleeds occur. In the meantime, they have ordered "subarachnoid precautions."

1. What is the purpose of subarachnoid precautions, and list 9 nursing interventions you would initiate. **[P,I/ap/S,PI,PSI/ct,ni]**
   - Subarachnoid precautions are aimed at preventing IICP and reducing environmental stimuli.
   - Private room, dimmed light with blinds drawn, HOB elevated 30 to 45 degrees.
   - Complete bed rest.
   - Turn q2h with deep breathing only.
   - Provide all nursing care for R.G.
   - R.G. is to avoid any exertion.
   - Caution R.G. against coughing, sneezing, or straining, avoid valsalva maneuver.
   - Administer stool softeners and/or mild laxatives but avoid enemas.
   - No TV, radio, or reading.
   - Limit visitors and caution them to be quiet and not excite her.
   - Treat headache.
   - Initiate DVT prophylaxis.

2. Describe the 5 grades of cerebral aneurysms and their criteria. **[PD/k/PI/ct]**
   - Grade I: minimal bleeding, asymptomatic.
   - Grade II: mild bleeding, alert, headache, nuchal rigidity, minimal neurologic deficit.
   - Grade III: moderate bleed, drowsy or confused, nuchal rigidity, some focal deficit.
   - Grade IV: moderate to severe bleed, stupor, hemiparesis, nuchal rigidity, decerebration.
   - Grade V: severe bleed, deep coma, decerebrate rigidity, moribund.

3. Why is cerebral angiography helpful in cerebral aneurysms? **[PD/c/PI/ct]**
   - Cerebral angiography provides a definitive diagnosis. It shows the exact structure, size, and site of aneurysm. It will also show the presence of vasospasm.

4. R.G. is very uncooperative. What psychosocial issues may be contributing to her behavior? **[PD/an/PI,PSI/ct]**
    - She is under arrest and will go to jail after discharge.
    - Her drug screen was positive for multiple drugs.
    - She may be having withdrawal symptoms.
    - R.G. probably has little to no family support.
    - She may have difficulty comprehending instructions due to the brain lesion.
    - She may have an altered perception of her situation.
    - She may believe that the police are behind her imposed bed rest.

5. Identify 6 nursing interventions that address R.G.'s fear and anxiety. **[PD/an/S,PI,PSI/ct,ni,tc]**
    - Develop a trust relationship with R.G. and become familiar to her.
    - Try to maintain the same caregivers each shift.
    - Frequently orient her to time, place, and situation.
    - Obtain pharmacologic support for withdrawal symptoms.
    - Try to establish family contact and assess family situation; if appropriate, allow family to visit.
    - Obtain a social work referral.
    - Explain all procedures and rationales to R.G. before doing them.
    - Involve R.G. in planning her care.

6. The physician prescribes folic acid 0.2 ml IV qd for R.G. Why? **[PD/c/PI/ct]**
    - Folic acid is a supplemental vitamin to prevent macrocytic anemia in alcoholic and malnourished people.

7. R.G. is on phenytoin (Dilantin) 100 mg PO tid and her serum Dilantin level is 7.2 μg/ml. Why is she on Dilantin, and what dose adjustment do you anticipate? **[PD/k/PI/ct]**
    - Dilantin is prophylaxis to decrease the seizure threshold which may be increased because of the brain injury. Therapeutic blood levels are 10 to 20 μg/ml. R.G.'s level is low, and you should anticipate a dose increase.

8. R.G. will be discharged with a prescription for phenytoin. In view of her previous lifestyle, list 3 main concerns with respect to this prescription. Explain. **[I/an/S,PI,PSI,ct]**
    - She may not have financial means or motivation to refill her prescription.
    - She may not want to take her phenytoin as ordered.
    - If she resumes her polypharmacy substance abuse pattern, she may experience profound and unpredictable drug-drug interactions.

The city released R.G. when she was admitted so the "taxpayers" wouldn't have to pay for her hospitalization. She will be transferred to a rehabilitation facility for further treatment. Her medical care will be complicated by her psychosocial and drug history.

9. List 6 essential members of the rehabilitation team who will be involved in R.G.'s care. **[P/ap/PI,PSI/ct]**
    - R.G., her son, nurse, physician, physical therapist, drug counselor/social worker, psychiatrist.

10. What 2 measures would be essential to include in R.G.'s discharge planning? **[P/an/S,PSI,PI/ct]**
    - Refer R.G. to Narcotic's Anonymous (NA), a support group for recovering addicts. There is also a Cocaine Anonymous.
    - The social worker will find a halfway house, or R.G. can stay with friends or relatives to get away from her previous toxic living environment. If she goes back to her old neighborhood she is more likely to have access to drugs and fall back into her old pattern of behavior.

CHAPTER 7. ENDOCRINE DISORDERS

Case Study 1: Type II Diabetes Mellitus

Difficulty: *	*Setting:* Outpatient clinic
Index Words: Type II diabetes mellitus	

You are volunteering at a Health Fair being conducted at a local community health clinic in a large metropolitan area. You are assigned to work with an advanced practice nurse in diabetes management and are assisting in the screening process for hyperglycemia and high WHR (waist-hip ratio). During the course of the day you meet M.M., a 42-year-old African American woman, whom you suspect has some type of diabetes mellitus. A nursing history reveals the following findings: Ht 5′6", Wt 210 lb, WHR = 0.96. M.M.'s mother, age 72, and two maternal aunts have type II diabetes mellitus (DM). M.M. has smoked 1½ packs/day of cigarettes for over 25 years and admits she should get more exercise. Screening glucose level (finger stick) is 310 mg/dl. On interview, M.M.'s only complaint is increasing fatigue over the past month and mild nocturia.

1. List the major risk factors for type II DM. Place a check mark (✓) next to the risk factors that M.M. has. **[A/k,c/PI,HP/ct]**
   - ✓ Age.
   - ✓ Family history.
   - ✓ Male pattern obesity (waist-hip ratio [WHR] >1.0 for men and 0.8 for women).
   - ✓ Hispanic, African American, or Native American.

2. What is the manifestation of type II DM that M.M. has (above). **[A/c/PI/ct]**
   - Screening plasma glucose of 310 mg/dl.

3. Identify additional data that would be necessary to arrive at a definitive diagnosis. **[A/k/PI/ct]**
   - Three-hour glucose tolerance levels, fasting plasma glucose, complete drug history to rule out drug reactions that may affect blood glucose (e.g., thiazides or beta-blockers), and a thorough health history to distinguish diabetes from other disorders, such as Cushing's syndrome. Additional information should include a dietary history and further questions regarding other possible signs/symptoms of diabetes, such as gestational weight of children.
   - Glycosylated hemoglobin test (written as GHb or HbA_{1c}) indicates the degree of irreversible glycosylation in RBCs (filling red blood cells' receptors with glucose), and shows the measure of glucose control up to 100 to 120 days before the test. The test is not affected by time of day, fasting, or any of the variables that normally cause fluctuations in serum glucose levels. This test is becoming invaluable in monitoring glucose control over an extended period of time.

   Instructor note: Tell students to watch for HbA_{1c} to be used more frequently to monitor overall control. Remind the students it is *not* the same as the more commonly used hemoglobin test.

4. During a brief physical assessment, the practitioner checks M.M.'s eyes with an ophthalmoscope. Why? **[A/c/Pl/ct]**
   - Because of glycosylation, DM patients tend to develop coronary artery disease (CAD). This problem is made worse by poor glucose control. The retinal arteries are the smallest visible arteries in the body; hence, they act as early indicators for CAD as well as retinal damage. Frequent and thorough eye examinations are essential for diabetics.

5. M.M. tells you she has a neighbor who had to start taking insulin for diabetes after she had "bad pneumonia." Her neighbor is very thin. M.M. asks if she will need insulin and if she will lose weight like her neighbor. How would you respond to her (in plain English)? **[I/c/Pl/ct,ni,tc]**
   - There are different types of diabetes (also called "sugar" by some folks). Some people get diabetes after they are sick and something happens to wipe out their insulin. They lose weight because the cells are starving—insulin isn't there to help food go into the cells. Your diabetes is different. In people like you (M.M.), there is plenty of insulin but it doesn't work right. It doesn't help your body make energy. In your kind of diabetes, diet and exercise help because they help insulin work better. Some people with your kind of diabetes also take special pills to help their own insulin work better.

6. M.M. tells you that she knows if she would just stop eating "sweet things" she would not have diabetes. How would you correct her understanding of the disease using understandable terminology? **[P,I/ap/Pl/ct,tc]**
   - Diabetes is not just a problem of sugar. Although glucose ("blood sugar") levels are important for the diagnosis and control of the disease, diabetes affects how the body uses all types of foods, including carbohydrates, fats, and proteins.

7. During the interview, the nurse takes M.M.'s blood pressure and asks whether she's ever been told she has heart trouble (coronary artery disease). Explain why. **[A/c/Pl/ct]**
   - There is a strong association between diabetes and hypertension, atherosclerotic heart disease, renal disease, cerebrovascular disease, and peripheral vascular disease. The high levels of circulating glucose contribute to glycosylation of many types of cell receptors (the cell receptors plug up with glucose). This has a powerful effect on lipid metabolism and contributes to atherosclerotic plaque development in cerebral, peripheral, renal, and coronary arteries. The effect on the kidneys also contributes to hypertension.

   Instructor note: Recent research about glycosylation is very exciting; it goes a long way toward clarifying the relationship between Type II DM and associated vascular disease that features prominently in the disastrous consequences of DM (American Diabetes Association, 1993; Brown, 1994).

8. Discuss 2 modifiable behaviors M.M. engages in that will aggravate the pathologic effects of her type II DM. **[A/c/PI/ct]**
   - M.M.'s smoking history means that the atherosclerotic disease process will be accelerated. In addition, it is highly likely that she either has or will develop chronic obstructive pulmonary disease as a complicating factor to development of CAD.
   - M.M. is admittedly sedentary. There is evidence that moderate aerobic exercise, over time, helps reduce some of the complications of Type II DM and helps control hyperglycemia.
   - The sedentarism and smoking together is a time bomb, especially since women tend to be more susceptible to the harmful effects of smoking than men. Finally, smoking tends to promote male-pattern abdominal obesity, which is associated with increased risk of type II DM.

9. M.M. agreed to come to the clinic for help; her GHb was 13%. What does this tell you about M.M.'s glucose control in the past few months? **[A,PD/c/PI/ct]**
   - Normal GHb for adults is 4% to 8%; 13% indicates poor glucose control during the 3 months before detection of her type II DM.

10. Identify 3 content areas of diabetes education that are important for newly-diagnosed diabetics. Identify 3 important learning objectives for each content area. **[PI/k/S,PI,PSI,HP/ct,ni]**
    - *Nutrition:*
      Individualize meal plan; describe the appropriate carbohydrate, protein, fat composition of the diet using 1994 American Diabetes Association standards; describe the importance of even small amounts of sustained weight loss, avoiding weight gain, losing abdominal fat; identify nutritional resources appropriate to the individual's ethnicity and income; refer to a Registered Dietician for special needs or dietary problems.
      Instructor's note: Recent dietary recommendations for type II DM have changed. Food exchanges or calorie counts have been replaced by an emphasis on the carbohydrate, protein, fat ratio in the diet. Moreover, studies have shown that a loss of just 10 pounds can result in very positive changes in blood lipids. Finally, the recommended order in which goals should be set in getting the disease under control is (1) get glucose within normal limits (maximum 140 mg/dl), (2) get blood pressure under control, and (3) work on longer-term diet and weight control issues.
    - *Psychologic adjustment:*
      Express feelings of anxiety openly; identify support groups and resources; identify coping strategies for adapting to a chronic disease.
    - *Medications:*
      Discuss purpose and use of oral hypoglycemics; discuss goals of insulin preparations if required; describe signs/symptoms of hypoglycemia; identify treatment measures for hypoglycemia; discuss how to buy, store, and use insulin preparations if required.
      Instructor note: Emphasize the need to keep all medications in a safe place. Oral hypoglycemics can be particularly lethal and are a common source of toxicity in children.
    - *Special problems related to illness and stress:*
      Wound care; foot care; signs/symptoms of infections; who to contact in emergency.

11. Discuss 2 recommendations that you would make to individuals at the Health Fair regarding primary prevention of diabetes. **[P/k/HP/ct,ni]**
    - Primary prevention should be directed toward encouraging lifestyle changes, including exercise, weight control or weight loss, and knowledge of risk factors such as age, heredity, and body fat pattern ("beer belly").

12. Explain why blood glucose testing is recommended to monitor glucose rather than urine dipstick testing. **[A/c/PI/ct]**
    - Although dipstick urine testing is commonly used to identify glucose "spilling over" from the kidney, it is highly inaccurate; the renal "spill" threshold for glucose can be affected by many factors and is widely variable between individuals.
    - Urine testing cannot detect hypoglycemia; however, laboratory-based urine testing is important to check for protein-related pathologic changes in renal function.
    - Blood glucose testing devices now commonly in use offer more accurate and reliable measurement on which to base treatment; the primary objection is the expense of monitoring materials and the invasive nature of the procedure.

    Instructor Note: Recent studies have shown the cost/benefit advantage of early detection and effective management of type II DM. Unfortunately, the estimated $350/month cost required for good glucose management is rarely covered by third-party health plans.

Case Study 2: Iatrogenic Cushing's Syndrome

Difficulty: *	*Setting:* Home care
Index Words: Cushing's syndrome, chronic obstructive pulmonary disease	

You graduated 3 months ago and are working with a home care nursing agency. Included in your caseload is J.S., a 60-year-old man suffering from chronic obstructive pulmonary disease (COPD). He has been on home oxygen, 2 L O_2/nc, for several years. Approximately 2 months ago, he was started on steroid therapy. Medications include metaproterenol (Alupent) inhaler, theophylline (Theo-Dur), terbutaline, dexamethasone, digoxin, and furosemide (Lasix). Not surprisingly, he also has a 50-pack-year history of cigarette smoking. On the way to visit J.S., you remember he has been progressively exhibiting signs/symptoms of Cushing's syndrome. You suspect J.S occasionally forgets to take his medication because he always seems to have "extra" pills in the bottle at the end of the month.

1. After you meet J.S. you begin an assessment and note the following findings. Place a check mark (✓) in the blank next to the signs/symptoms that characterize Cushing's syndrome. **[A/c/Pl/ct]**
   ___ Barrel chest.
   ✓ Full-looking face ("moon facies").
   ✓ BP 180/94.
   ___ Pursed-lip breathing.
   ✓ Thin arms and legs.
   ✓ Bruising on both arms.
   ✓ Acne.
   ___ Diminished breath sounds.
   ✓ Truncal obesity with fat around clavicles and the neck.
   ✓ Weakness and fatigue.
   ✓ Impaired glucose tolerance.

2. Differentiate between the cause of Cushing's syndrome and Cushing's disease. **[D/k/Pl/ct]**
   - The most common cause of Cushing's syndrome is iatrogenic due to long-term therapy with synthetic glucocorticoids; Cushing's disease is a result of excess ACTH production from a pituitary tumor called an adenoma.

3. Identify 3 to 4 general topics to be included in a teaching plan for J.S. **[P/ap/S,Pl/ct,ni,tc]**
   - Promote self-care through good nutrition and maintaining fluid balance.
   - Increase J.S.'s awareness of home safety issues.
   - Prevent infection through attention to skin integrity and handwashing.
   - Check blood pressure regularly and take blood pressure medications.
   - Take medications as scheduled.

4. Identify possible consequences of suddenly stopping the dexamethasone therapy. **[PD/c/S,PI/ct]**
   - During exogenous steroid therapy, the feedback system between and among the hypothalamus, pituitary, and adrenal gland(s) is/are suppressed; if steroids are stopped suddenly, the patient develops signs/symptoms of adrenal insufficiency. Return of normal adrenal function can take as long as 9 months, so steroids must be withdrawn slowly. It is essential that patients understand they must not stop taking dexamethasone abruptly.

5. The home care nurse informs the physician of the patient's signs/symptoms. The physician decides to change J.S.'s prescription to prednisone given on alternate days. Explain the rationale for this change. **[P/c/PI/ct]**
   - Administering steroids on alternate days may decrease side effects and diminish the degree of hypothalamic-pituitary-adrenal suppression. In addition, prednisone is shorter acting with adrenal suppression lasting 1 ¼ to 1 ½ days. In contrast, dexamethasone causes adrenal suppression lasting 2 ¾ days and would not be suitable for alternate-day therapy.

6. It is easy to forget what medications have been taken when, especially when there are several different drugs and times involved. List at least 3 ways you can help J.S. remember to take his pills as prescribed. **[P,I/ap/PI/ct,ni,tc]**
   - Help him develop a checklist—perhaps a pocket-calendar—to monitor his medications; this could also be useful in weight, blood pressure, glucose, and symptom monitoring.
   - Recommend a divided container in which pills can be placed in advance; this way, J.S. can immediately see if he has forgotten to take the pills assigned for a specific time.
   - Help him develop a plan where he takes his pills at times of the day related to other activities, such as with meals or when he brushes his teeth at night.
   - Suggest he purchase a pocket container for his pills that can provide an emergency dose if he is traveling or caught away from home (remind him to compensate for this in his "pill-count" at home).

7. J.S. states that his appetite has increased but he is unable to satiate his appetite because of shortness of breath and he has been losing weight. How would you address this problem? How might his diet be modified? **[P/an/Pl/ct,ni]**
   - Before anything is changed, you need to perform a thorough assessment that includes an evaluation of his shortness of breath, weight and body fat distribution, and current dietary patterns. Be especially aware of male-pattern body fat and upper back and neck fat distribution contributing to shortness of breath.
   - Dietary management of glucose and fat intake with Cushing's syndrome is advised because of altered carbohydrate and fat metabolism. When weight gain is evident, a calorie-restricted diet is advised. However, because this patient is having difficulty eating due to dyspnea, dietary management should be oriented toward calorie-rich foods and frequent, smaller portions. (This is what the books say; in reality, however, COPD patients often forget to eat more frequently or may not be aware of how little they are actually taking in.)
   - Do not use expectorants or bronchodilators immediately before meals; expectorating mucous and the taste of inhaled medication is not conducive to eating. Have J.S. do his breathing treatments from ½ to 1 hour before eating, then rest to help minimize his dyspnea as well as his anorexia. Meals should be taken with a minimum of distraction.
   - Avoid a big carbohydrate load at any meal; carbohydrates produce increased CO_2 that contributes to increased respiratory fatigue. _Instructor note:_ Because carbohydrates are usually easier to eat, COPD patients tend to eat mashed potatoes, pasta, rice, and bread first. The effort to expire the increased CO_2 contributes to fatigue, and the person does not eat a full meal.
   - Meal planning for patients with multiple chronic conditions can be difficult and often requires the help of a registered dietitian (RD).
   - Energy conservation techniques should be discussed in relation to meal preparation and consumption.

8. You advise J.S. to take his prednisone with food and then ask him a series of questions related to his vision. Discuss the rationale behind these nursing care actions. **[P,I/c/Pl/ct,ni,tc]**
   - Patients taking glucocorticoid therapy are more susceptible to peptic ulcers and cataract formation.

9. Differentiate between the glucocorticoid and mineralocorticoid effects of prednisone. **[A/k/Pl/ct]**
   - Prednisone is an intermediate-acting glucocorticoid that has minimal mineralocorticoid activity. Suppression of inflammatory and immune response is the primary effect of prednisone. There should be minimal sodium and water retention if any. Synthetic glucocorticoids possess less mineralocorticoid activity than natural glucocorticoids.

10. How would your assessment change if J.S. were taking a glucocorticoid that also has significant mineralocorticoid activity? **[A/c/Pl/ct,ni]**
    - You would pay greater attention to assessing for signs/symptoms of fluid excess, such as neck vein distention; decreased urinary output; peripheral edema; increase in respiratory difficulty; crackles; weight gain; and signs/symptoms of potassium deficit (don't forget to check magnesium along with potassium).

11. Review J.S.'s list of medications. Based on what you know about the side effects of loop diuretics and steroids, discuss the potential problem of administering these in combination with digoxin. **[A/c/Pl/ct]**
    - Although prednisone has less mineralocorticoid activity than other steroids, the combination of prednisone and Lasix could lead to hypokalemia, as well as hypomagnesemia. Hypokalemia increases the risk of digoxin toxicity.

12. Realizing that patients like J.S. are susceptible to all types of infections, you write guidelines to prevent infections. Identify 4 major points that these guidelines will include. **[P/c/S,Pl/ct,ni]**
    - Avoid people with infections, especially children, and avoid crowds.
    - Wash hands frequently (teach appropriate hand washing).
    - Maintain a nutritious diet.
    - Take meticulous care of any open wound, and report any signs/symptoms of infection (fever, increased weakness, aching, redness around a wound).

Case Study 3: Addison's Disease (Adrenal Hypoplasia)

Difficulty: *	*Setting:* Outpatient clinic
Index Words: Addison's disease, adrenal hypoplasia	

E.H. is a 60-year-old woman who has rheumatoid arthritis. For the past 12 years she has been taking prednisone 60 mg daily (40 mg in the AM, 20 mg in the PM), and nonsteroidal antiinflammatory drugs (NSAIDS) to control her disease and symptoms. As a result of her autoimmune disorder and/or long-term steroid use, E.H. has adrenal insufficiency. The physician adjusts her steroid dosage for replacement therapy. In your nursing role, you are asked to conduct educational sessions designed to teach E.H. about her condition and the treatment she needs.

1. E.H. states she doesn't understand how her taking steroids has caused her body to lose it's ability to produce the "the real thing." How would you explain this paradox in terms she can understand? **[A,P/c/Pl/ct,ni,tc]**
   - The paradox can be explained to the lay person by using the phrase, "If you don't use it, you lose it." Because she has been taking an external steroid that the adrenal gland normally produces, the brain doesn't have to tell the adrenal gland to keep working. The adrenal gland takes a "vacation," gets lazy, and decreases in size. When you stop taking external steroids, the adrenal gland either takes awhile to get back to work or may not be able to resume its normal function.

2. People receiving steroid replacement should be taught signs/symptoms that signal the dosage is too low. What are the signs/symptoms of inadequate steroid replacement? **[A/k/Pl/ni,tc]**
   - Inadequate steroid replacement can be characterized by a wide variety of symptoms. Mental changes can include lethargy, depressed feelings, and decreased concentration. Other symptoms can include weakness, fatigue, anorexia, nausea, vomiting, weight loss, salt craving, muscle weakness (related to hyponatremia, hyperkalemia, and hypercalcemia), menstrual changes, and dizziness (low blood pressure).

3. What would you teach someone like E.H. about the nutritional implications of adrenal insufficiency? **[P/c/Pl/ct]**
   - Avoid periods of fasting because the body does not function normally in protecting itself during hypoglycemic episodes. Use more frequent fruit and vegetable snacks to maintain optimal glucose levels. Her diet needs to be especially high in protein, calcium, and magnesium and low in sodium and carbohydrates.

4. Explain why the AM dosage of prednisone is higher. **[PD/c/Pl/ct]**
   - Higher prednisone doses are given in the morning to mimic the normal variation of adrenocortical hormone levels in the body: higher in the AM and lower in the PM.

5. E.H. confides in you that she is afraid of taking steroids any longer because she has read about the deleterious effects of steroid abuse by athletes. How would you counter this misconception and alleviate E.H.'s concern? **[A/an/PI.PSI/ni,tc]**
   - Do not "rush in" to correct E.H.'s misconceptions right away. First ask her what else she knows or has heard. This will give you hints about the level at which to aim your explanation.
   - Explain to E.H. that "steroids" includes a broad classification of many different hormones.
   - It will help E.H. to understand the difference between anabolic steroids and glucocorticoids. Androgens are strong anabolic agents; that is, they stimulate formation and growth of muscular and skeletal protein. Athletes have been known to use androgens to increase weight, musculature, and muscle strength. E.H. should be assured that she is not taking androgens and is not at risk for the side effects associated with their abuse.

6. How would teaching differ for this patient (on replacement therapy) as compared with teaching required for the patient taking therapeutic doses of glucocorticoids? **[P/c/PI/S,PI,PSI,HP/ni,tc]**
   - Many aspects of teaching would be similar. The primary difference would be the focus on stress management since stress might precipitate an adrenal crisis in the individual with adrenal insufficiency. For the patient taking steroids for conditions unrelated to adrenal function, the risk of a stress-induced crisis is far less. However, adrenal insufficiency can occur in persons taking long-term steroids if they are suddenly discontinued.

7. The patient states she is under a lot of stress because of her son's recent diagnosis of cancer and her husband's upcoming retirement. What are the teaching implications of this information? **[PD,P/c/S,PI,PSI/ct]**
   - Because E.H. cannot increase her body's cortisol production during stress, small stressors such as a cold, tooth extraction, emotional tension, or changes in environmental temperature can be life-threatening. Therefore, E.H. will need to understand the relationship between increased periods of stress and the risk for insufficient levels of cortisol. She should be taught to recognize stressful situations, to eliminate as many stressors as possible, and to wear an identification bracelet or tag stating she has Addison's disease. *She should know that a physician should be consulted regarding adjustment of steroid doses when she is under unavoidable stress.*

8. You realize that taking exogenous cortisol can result in a variety of pathophysiologic alterations often described as Cushing's syndrome. Since E.H. will be taking lifelong steroids, would you expect to see the signs/symptoms associated with Cushing's syndrome in this individual? Explain your answer. **[PD/c/PI/ct]**
   - Since this patient is receiving life-long steroids for adrenal atrophy, she should not demonstrate signs/symptoms of excess cortisol or Cushing's syndrome. This would occur only if the steroid dosage were too high and she were receiving too much prednisone.

9. What signs/symptoms should you teach E.H. to monitor that would indicate excessive drug therapy? **[P/c/PI/ct,ni]**
    - Rapid weight gain, including truncal fat accumulation.
    - Change in facial appearance (rounding).
    - Peripheral edema.
    - Hypertension.
    - Signs of immunosuppression (colds, flu, infections).
    - Fever.

10. You instruct E.H. on administration of a parenteral form of hydrocortisone. Under what circumstances should she take the parenteral form of the drug? **[P/c/S,PI/ct,ni]**
    - If she cannot retain the oral form because of nausea/vomiting.

11. What measures should E.H. take to prevent an acute episode of adrenal insufficiency? **[P,I,E/k/PI,HP/ct]**
    - Do not omit a drug dose; keep sufficient medication on hand.
    - When she travels, teach her traveling companion how to give the injectable form.
    - Monitor herself for presence of increased stressors (fever, infection, dental work, personal or family crises).
    - Monitor herself daily for weight changes.
    - Watch herself for indications of insufficient glucocorticoid levels and report immediately.
    - Maintain a regular daily schedule with regard to sleep patterns, meals, and exercise.

12. E.H. tells you she never used to take pills at all. She says she hates to be "addicted to a drug." What will you tell her? **[P/c/PI,PSI/ct,ni,tc]**
    - Acknowledge that it must be frustrating to need to take medication on a daily basis for life.
    - Explain the difference between being addicted to a drug and requiring that drug to replace something your body needs but no longer normally manufactures.
    - Emphasize the importance of taking her medication faithfully so her body maintains its "normal" patterns.

Case Study 4: Hypothyroidism

Difficulty: **	*Setting:* Outpatient clinic
Index Words: Hypothyroidism	

You are working in a community outpatient clinic where you perform the intake assessment on R.M., a 38-year-old woman who is attending graduate school. Her chief complaint is overwhelming fatigue that is not relieved by rest. She is so exhausted she has difficulty walking to classes and studying. She has coarse, sparse scalp hair; scaly skin; slightly slurred speech; thick tongue; a hoarse voice; puffiness around the eyes; yellowish-colored skin and nails; and swollen neck. Initial VS were 92/64, 56, 12, 96.8°F (rectal).

1. Compare her VS with those of a healthy person her same age. **[A/c/PI/ct]**
   - The pulse is bradycardic; bradycardia may be normal in athletes, but it is abnormal for nonexercisers.
   - Temperature is lower than expected, indicating decreased metabolism and heat production.

2. List 8 general questions you might ask R.M. to get a "ball park" idea of what is going on with her. **[A/c/PI,PSI/ct,tc]**
   - Describe the fatigue. Is it relieved by rest?
   - When did you first notice the fatigue?
   - What makes it better? What makes it worse?
   - Any recent changes in appetite or fluctuations in weight?
   - How do temperature changes affect you?
   - Any changes in bowel elimination?
   - Any chest pain? Any swelling or edema in extremities?
   - Does she have a family history of thyroid problems?
   - Any recent changes in her life, her family, her job?
   - Have there been any other changes in her health?
   - Describe her menstrual cycle.

3. You know that *some* of R.M.'s symptoms could be caused by depression, hypothyroidism, anemia, cardiac disease, fluid and electrolyte imbalance, or allergies. As part of your screening procedures, how would you begin to investigate which of these conditions probably *do not* account for R.M.'s symptoms? **[A/an/PI/ct,ni]**
   - Conduct a thorough health history and physical assessment. Focus on a good assessment of the cardiopulmonary system, listening to heart and lung sounds, and checking for peripheral edema.

You found no obvious irregularities in R.M.'s cardiopulmonary assessment.

4. Unnecessary diagnostic tests are expensive. What tests would you think would be the most important to be obtained on R.M. and why? **[A/c/Pl/ct]**
   - CBC with differential to evaluate possibility of anemia, infection, and allergies.
   - Chem 20 to evaluate fluid and electrolyte status.
   - T_3, T_4, and TSH (thyroid stimulating hormone); TSH regulates the secretion of T_3 and T_4, circulating levels of T_3 and T_4 serve as a feedback mechanism to turn-off TSH.

After reviewing the laboratory results, the family nurse practitioner diagnoses R.M. with hypothyroidism and places her on thyroid replacement therapy.

5. The practitioner prescribes levothyroxine (Synthroid) 1.7 μg/kg body weight/day. R.M. weighs 130 lb. What should be her daily dose of Synthroid in milligrams? How would her prescription read? **[P/k/S/ct]**
   - 130 lbs = 59.1 kg; 59.1 kg x 1.7 μg = 100.5 μg = *0.1 mg.*
     <u>*Note:*</u> Micrograms are alternately written μg or mcg.
   - Her prescription reads: levothyroxine (Synthroid) 0.1 mg PO qd.

6. R.M.'s T_3 and T_4 levels were decreased and the TSH level was increased. Explain the relationship between these lab results and hypothyroidism. **[PD/c/Pl/ct]**
   - A decrease in T_3 and T_4 levels results in the release of TSH from the pituitary. TSH, in turn, stimulates the manufacture and secretion of T_3 and T_4. In hypothyroidism, the gland is unable to produce T_3 and T_4 despite increases in TSH.

7. What patient teaching needs will you review with R.M. before she leaves? Remember medication issues. **[P/ap/Pl,PSl/ct,ni,tc]**
   - Take 1 pill every AM before breakfast; preferably the same time every day. If a dose is missed, take it as soon as you remember it, unless it is almost time for the next dose.
   - This drug should not be discontinued without consulting the practitioner.
   - Report an increase in presenting symptoms to the clinic immediately. Write the clinic telephone number down for her.
   - Report side effects of medication such as heat intolerance, nervousness, excitability, profound weight loss, chest pain, irritability, fast or irregular pulse, diarrhea, weight loss.

8. Why would you want to obtain a complete drug history on R.M.? **[A/c/Pl/ct]**
   - Synthroid can interact with a few medications, such as anticoagulants. Instruct her to call and check before she takes any other medications, including over-the-counter products.

9. What general teaching issues would you address with R.M.? **[P/ap/S,PI,PSI,HP/ct,ni,tc]**
   - Do not change brands or use generic substitutions for levothyroxine—bioequivalence problems have been observed.
   - Maintain a well-balanced diet; follow prescribed caloric intake to promote weight loss. Avoid salty foods because of the potential for CHF (congestive heart failure) and myxedema.
   - Encourage moderate exercise, but prevent overexertion. A walking program several days per week starting at 10 to 15 minutes per day would be a good start for her; increase walking time by 1 to 2 minutes per week until she reaches 20 to 30 minutes per day. Drink plenty of fluids.
   - Plan frequent rest periods until her dosage is established.
   - Establish regular sleep patterns (7 to 8 hours of sleep/night)
   - Prevent skin breakdown with good hygiene and application of unscented lotions/creams to replace lubrication. Even though skin breakdown may be microscopic, the small lesions can be sources of infection.
   - Prevent heat loss by layering clothing.
   - Prevent or treat constipation with adequate fluid intake and high-fiber diet.
   - Teach her how to take her pulse accurately.

10. R.M. wonders if she should take iodine supplements if she decreases her salt intake. She recognizes that salt is a significant source of iodine in her part of the country. What would you explain to her? **[A,P/an/ct,tc]**
    - R.M.'s question is very insightful. If iodized salt is her major source of iodine, eliminating table salt from her diet may jeopardize her iodine levels. Ask her about other sources of iodine in her everyday diet, such as ocean seafood. If she eats a balanced diet, she probably will have enough iodine in her diet. Reassure her that you will be expecting her to return to the clinic for follow-up visits to monitor her progress.

11. What should you teach her regarding prevention of myxedema coma? **[P/c/S,PI,PSI/ct,tc]**
    - Caution R.M. to
      - Take prescribed medication exactly as directed at the same time each day.
      - Not change brands of medication without consulting her physician.
      - Avoid stressful events such as infection, trauma, exposure to cold, which could cause an exaggerated form of hypothyroidism.
      - Wear an identification bracelet or necklace indicating she is hypothyroid, name and dosage of medication, name and phone number of physician.
      - Avoid over-the-counter drugs such as sedatives or analgesics; explain that medication does not cure hypothyroidism, and she will be required to take it for the rest of her life.

12. Before R.M. leaves the clinic, she asks how she will know if the medication is "doing its job." Outline simple expected outcomes for R.M. **[E/c/PI/ct,tc]**
    - Gradually increases her activity tolerance over 2 to 3 months, achieves bowel pattern that was typical before onset of illness, maintains body temperature of 98.6°F, gradually decreases body weight, improves mental function, improves skin color, and lessens dryness.

13. Several weeks later, R.M. calls the clinic stating she can't remember if she took her thyroid medication. What additional data should you obtain, and how would you advise her? **[A,P,I/an/PI/ct,ni,tc]**
    - Suggest that R.M. obtain a daily pill dispenser. Instruct her to fill the container at the beginning of each week so that she will know if she accidently omits a dose.
    - Ask her about the time/day of last pill, if she's missed any other doses recently, and her current pulse rate.
    - Advising R.M. would be based on knowledge that Synthroid has a half-life of 6 to 7 days, thus missing a dose would not place her at risk for complications such as might be experienced in patients missing a dose of, for example, glucocorticoids. If R.M. has only missed one dose and it is still early in the day, advise her to take the prescribed dosage.

14. Under what circumstances should R.M. hold the drug or call the clinic? **[P/k/S,PI/ct,ni,tc]**
    - Hold dose if resting pulse is >100 beats per minute.
    - Notify physician if 2 to 3 doses are missed.

R.M. comes in 2 months later for a follow-up visit. You can't believe she is the same person. She looks and walks 10 years younger. Her skin appears more moist and her hair is beginning to come in with its normal feel. "You can't believe how much different I'm feeling," she says. "I'm discovering what it's like to live again."

Case Study 5: Multinodular Goiter with Primary Hyperparathyroidism

Difficulty: **	*Setting:* Hospital
Index Words: Thyroid, parathyroid, goiter	

You are working on an oncology unit and will be receiving a client from the recovery room. The PACU (post-anesthesia care unit) nurse calls and gives the following report. C.P., a 50-year-old woman, had a total thyroidectomy (multinodular goiter), left superior and right inferior parathyroidectomy due to adenoma; the EBL (estimated blood loss) was 25 ml. VS are 130/82, 80-90, 20. She has a peripheral IV of $D_5 \frac{1}{2}$ NS with 20 mEq KCl and 10 mEq calcium gluconate infusing at 100 ml/h. She has received a total of 50 mg meperidine (Demerol) IVP and she remains alert and oriented. C.P.'s PMH includes TAH (total abdominal hysterectomy) for fibroids, and low-level radiation treatments to the neck 38 years ago for eczema. Her medications include estradiol (Estrace), lovastatin (Mecavor), and levothyroxine (Synthroid). Both parents are living; her father had an MI at 70 years old, her mother has hypothyroidism but never had thyroid tumors. Preoperative laboratory findings: calcium 11.2 mg/dl, phosphorus 2.4 mg/dl, Cl 106 mEq/L, alkaline phosphatase 112 U/L, elevated parahormone and TSH levels, creatinine 1.4 mg/dl.

1. What additional data should you obtain from the recovery room nurse? **[A/ap/Pl/ct]**
   - When was the preoperative Ca level drawn? What is C.P.'s postoperative calcium level? Any signs/symptoms of tetany or respiratory distress (e.g., stridor)?

2. What preparations will you take before C.P. arrives? **[P/c/Pl/ct,ni]**
   - C.P.'s airway may become compromised because of edema from the surgery or internal hemorrhage at the surgical site. You should make sure there is a tracheostomy tray or intubation tray at the bedside.
   - Humidified oxygen and suction equipment should be at the bedside and operational.
   - Place a suture removal set in the room (to relieve respiratory obstruction from internal hemorrhage).
   - Place an IV pole in the room.
   - Place an ampule of calcium gluconate at the bedside (in the event tetany develops).

3. You receive C.P. from the recovery room. How will you focus your initial assessment and why? **[P/c/S,PI/ct,ni]**
   - Your assessment should begin with the ABC. Airway: hoarseness, weak voice because of edema or damage to the recurrent laryngeal nerve; ask C.P. to immediately report any sensation of swelling or tightening in her airway (laryngeal spasm). Breathing: assess V_T, ask C.P to immediately report any choking sensation or difficulty swallowing. Circulation: assess for hemorrhage into the neck tissues, check the surgical site and dressing, monitor VS.
   - Check for tetany (calcium deficiency secondary to parathyroid tissue removal).
   - Raise the siderails.
   - Check to see if the ice bag needs to be refilled.

4. During your initial assessment you document negative Chvostek's and Trousseau's signs. Describe data that would support this conclusion. **[PD/k/PI/ct]**
   - Negative Chvostek sign: no contraction of the upper lip, nose, or side of the face when the facial nerve is tapped adjacent to the ear.
   - Negative Trousseau's sign: no sign of carpopedal spasm, marked by adduction of the thumb and extension of the fingers, when you inflate a BP cuff and occlude the arterial blood flow for 1 to 4 minutes.

5. Explain why C.P. would have been taking Synthroid preoperatively. **[PD/c/PI/ct]**
   - The aim of exogenous hormones, such as Synthroid, is to inhibit TSH (thyroid-stimulating hormone) secretion and suppress the goiter.

6. Identify the major risk factor that may have contributed to the development of parathyroid adenoma in C.P. **[PD/k/PI/ct]**
   - A history of radiation therapy to the neck.

   Instructor's note: Estrace and birth control pills may alter thyroid hormone assays and may have led to early detection.

7. Identify 4 nursing diagnoses for C.P. **[PD/an/S,PI,PSI/ct]**
   - Risk for ineffective breathing pattern r/t airway obstruction associated with hemorrhage and laryngeal stridor.
   - Risk for physical injury r/t increased neuromuscular excitability associated with hypocalcemia.
   - Risk for laryngeal nerve injury r/t surgery.
   - Risk for decreased cardiac output r/t dysrhythmias associated with hypocalcemia and altered electrical conduction.
   - Knowledge deficit r/t surgical treatment, follow-up, long-term treatment.
   - Fear r/t outcome of surgery and possible diagnosis of cancer.

8. Identify 4 nursing measures that you should include in the postoperative care of C.P. **[P/ap/PI,PSI/ct,ni,tc]**
   Anticipate and monitor for signs of:
   - Respiratory distress: advise C.P. to talk as little as possible to prevent swelling; keep head of her bed elevated and apply ice bag to her throat; instruct C.P. to notify you if she experiences any signs or symptoms of airway obstruction (swelling or difficulty breathing).
   - Hypocalcemia (tetany or convulsions): monitor Ca levels; keep an ampule of calcium gluconate at the bedside to be used as prescribed; keep side rails up while in bed; note any muscular irritability; test for tetany.
   - Hemorrhage at the surgical site: visualize her neck and incision site when you take her VS and have her report any pressure sensation in her neck/throat.
   - Injury to the laryngeal nerve: when C.P. does speak, you should note any voice changes that may indicate injury to the laryngeal nerve.
   - Keep C.P. informed of her progress (including lab value trends).

9. Identify nursing care measures that reduce the risk for postoperative swelling. **[P/ap/PI/ct,ni]**
   - Semi-Fowler's position, prevent hyperextension or flexion of the head/neck, position sandbags at both sides of the neck to limit movement, teach C.P. to support her neck with her hands while getting out of bed, apply ice as directed.

10. The next day, 24 hours after surgery, C.P. calls you into her room complaining of numbness around her mouth and tingling at the tips of her fingers. She appears restless but is alert and oriented. Realizing that C.P. may be experiencing hypocalcemia, you decide to notify the physician. What should you do in the interim before the physician returns your call? **[P,I/ap/S,PI,PSI/ct,ni,tc]**
    - Raise the head of the bed.
    - Stay with C.P. and thank her for reporting the change in status to you.
    - Closely monitor for wheezing or dyspnea and cardiac dysrhythmias.
    - Reassess Chvostek's and Trousseau's signs.
    - Check the patency of the IV, and prepare for calcium gluconate infusion.

11. What emergency equipment should you gather? **[P/c/S,PI/ct,ni]**
    - The tracheostomy tray, endotracheal tube, and an ampule of calcium gluconate should already be at the bedside.
    - Obtain anticonvulsant medications and materials for padding the siderails.

C.P. is given supplemental calcium gluconate and recovers without further complications. C.P. is being discharged 48 hours postoperatively. She states that she can't wait until she can stop taking the Synthroid.

12. How would you respond to her statement? **[PD/k/PI/ct,ni,tc]**
    - Inform C.P. that she has had a total thyroidectomy and will require lifelong thyroid replacement therapy.

Case Study 6: Hyperthyroidism

Difficulty: **	*Setting:* Hospital
Index Words: Hyperthyroidism	

K.B. is an 80-year-old woman admitted to the hospital following a 5-day episode of the "flu" with c/o DOE (dyspnea on exertion), palpitations, chest pain, insomnia, and fatigue. Her PMH includes CHF (congestive heart failure) and HTN (hypertension) requiring antihypertensive medications (she states that she has not been taking these medications on a regular basis). K.B. was diagnosed with Graves' disease 6 months ago and was placed on propylthiouracil (PTU) 100 mg PO q6h. Assessment findings are as follows: Ht 62", Wt 100 lb. Appears anxious and restless. Loud heart sounds; VS are 150/90, 104 irregular, 20, 100.2°F; 1+ pitting edema noted in lower extremities. Diminished breath sounds with fine crackles in the posterior bases. K.B. states she recently lost her husband. Laboratory findings: Hgb 11.8 g/dl, Hct 36%, ESR (erythrocyte sedimentation rate) 48 mm/h, Na 141 mEq/L, K 4.7 mEq/L, Cl 101 mEq/L, BUN 33 mg/dl, creatinine 1.9 mg/dl, T_4 RIA 14.0 μg/dl, T_3 230 ng/dl.

1. Of the physical assessment and laboratory findings, which represent manifestations of hypermetabolism? **[PD/k/Pl/ct]**
   - Anxiety, restlessness, insomnia, increased SBP (systolic blood pressure), palpitations, dysrhythmias, tachycardia, dyspnea, elevated temperature, low weight-to-height ratio (Ht 5'2", Wt 100 lb).

2. What additional subjective and objective data would you gather for someone with Graves' disease? **[E/c/Pl/ct]**
   - Additional signs/symptoms of adrenergic stimulation: depression, irritability, tremor, ocular stare, lid lag, wide pulse pressure.
   - Additional signs/symptoms of excess thyroid hormone: hyperphagia, myopia, cardiac hypertrophy.
   - Additional signs/symptoms of immunologic component: diffuse goiter, ophthalmopathy (exophthalmos, periorbital edema, periorbital and conjunctival inflammation, decreased extraocular muscle movement, corneal injury, blurred vision, eye pain, photophobia, and diplopia).
   - Changes in hair, skin, nails.
   - Ability to complete ADL (suffers from fatigue).
   - Changes in bowel pattern: increased frequency or diarrhea.

3. Following AM rounds, the physician leaves the following orders. Which of the orders would you question and why? **[E/an/PI/ct]**

    Propranolol (Inderal) 20 mg PO q6h.
    Dexamethasone (Decadron) 10 mg IV q6h.
    Verapamil (Calan SR) 120 mg PO qd.
    Diet as tolerated, high-protein.
    STAT ECG.
    Up ad lib.

    - The beta-adrenergic blocker Inderal should not be prescribed for patients with a history of CHF; the negative inotropic side effects could diminish cardiac output and worsen the CHF.
    - Given K.B.'s history of hyperthyroidism, irregular heart rate, elevated temperature, chest pain, and history of CHF, the activity order should be questioned; decreased activity would decrease myocardial oxygen consumption and metabolic activity.

4. Develop 4 priority nursing diagnoses for K.B. **[PD/an/PI,PSI/ct]**
    - Decreased cardiac output r/t dysrhythmias associated with increased SNS (sympathetic nervous system) activity.
    - Hyperthermia r/t hypermetabolism (increased heat production).
    - Inadequate oxygenation r/t hypermetabolism.
    - Altered nutrition, less than body requirements r/t increased metabolic needs.
    - Risk for activity intolerance r/t altered metabolism, fatigue, weakness.
    - Knowledge deficit r/t taking prescribed medications.
    - Body image disturbance r/t physical manifestations of Graves' disease.

5. Later on your shift, you note that K.B. is extremely restless and is disoriented to person, place, and time. VS are 104/62, 180 and irregular, 32 and labored, 103°F. Her ECG shows atrial fibrillation. What do these findings indicate? **[PD/c/PI/ct]**
    - K.B. is in thyroid storm or thyrotoxic crisis.

6. What would you do *first*? **[P,I/ap/PI/ct,ni]**
    - Call a CODE! Thyroid storm constitutes a medical emergency.

K.B. is in thyroid crisis. The physician orders the following: STAT ABG; digoxin (Lanoxin) 0.125 mg IVP q8h x 3 doses; IV of D_5W at 100 ml/h; Lugol's solution (strong iodine) 10 drops PO tid; increase propylthiouracil (PTU) to 200 mg PO qid; hydrocortisone (Hydro-Cort) 100 mg IVP q8h; cardiac monitor; absolute bed rest; cooling blanket for temp >102°F; acetaminophen (Tylenol) 650 mg PO prn temp >100°F.

7. Why did the physician order acetaminophen instead of salicylates? **[PD/k/PI/ct]**
    - Salicylates should be avoided in patients with hyperthyroidism because they compete with thyroid hormone for protein-binding sites, thereby increasing free thyroid hormone levels.

8. Identify 4 nursing measures that would be essential in caring for K.B. **[P/ap/PI/ct,ni]**
   - Promote the reduction of thyroid hormones, reduce heart rate, and reduce hypermetabolic state by administering antithyroid and iodine medications, digoxin, and glucocorticoids as prescribed. Monitor for a reduction in dysrhythmias, pulse and respiratory rate, temperature, diaphoresis, tremors, and thyroid hormone levels.
   - Promote reduction in body temperature by administering Tylenol as prescribed, applying the cooling blanket, and maintaining a cool environmental temperature.
   - Monitor for fluid volume deficit: monitor neurologic status; I&O; change in electrolytes; increased H&H, serum osmolality, and urine specific gravity.
   - Monitor for fluid volume overload: assess for increased BP, JVD (jugular vein distention), dyspnea, crackles, edema.
   - Monitor for signs/symptoms of hypercalcemia: assess c/o headache, altered LOC, arrhythmias, shortened QT interval on ECG, weak or flaccid muscles, N/V; increased urine output; monitor serum Ca levels.
   - Monitor for signs/symptoms of hypokalemia.

9. Identify 2 possible contributing factors that may have precipitated K.B.'s thyroid storm. **[PD/c/PI/ct]**
   - Thyroid crisis may be precipitated by a major stressor such as an infection (K.B. had the "flu") and the recent loss of her husband.
   - Although not substantiated in the history, K.B. may have stopped taking her antithyroid therapy (the history indicates she does not take antihypertensive medication regularly).

10. Before discharge, the physician discusses 2 treatment options with K.B. and her family: radioactive iodine therapy (RAI) using ^{131}I, and subtotal thyroidectomy. K.B. is fearful of radiation treatment and asks you for your opinion. How would you respond? **[P,I/ap/PI,PSI/ct,ni,tc]**
    - Ask K.B. and her family to explain their "fears" related to radiation therapy. Clarify any misconceptions, and provide accurate information regarding radiation. Facilitate the decision-making process, but do not influence their decision.

11. K.B. decides to receive ^{131}I. During pretreatment instructions, the family asks if she will be radioactive and what precautions they should take. Outline important guidelines for instructing K.B. and her family on home precautions. **[P,I/c/S,PI,PSI/ct,ni,tc]**
    - Precautions are dose dependent, but the usual dose used to treat hyperthyroidism is generally low enough to allow for outpatient administration.
    - Urine, saliva, sweat, and feces will contain radioactive iodine, but K.B. will not be "radioactive."
    - Home instructions should include increased oral intake to enhance excretion; flush the toilet 2 to 3 times after each stool and thoroughly wash hands after using the bathroom; wash towels, undergarments and bed linens separately; rinse the sink and clean the tub after each use; use individual eating utensils.
    - Even though the amount of radiation in K.B.'s body is minimal, she should be instructed to avoid kissing, intercourse, or holding a child or baby.

12. Discuss how your discharge teaching instructions will differ from those you would give to someone following a subtotal thyroidectomy. **[P,I/c/PI/ct,tc]**
    - Subtotal thyroidectomy involves removal of one lobe (75% to 80%); therefore, hypothyroidism does not occur as often as following radioactive iodine therapy. However, because the remaining tissue may hypertrophy over time, hyperthyroidism can develop again. Therefore, teaching for K.B. should include a discussion of the major side effect of RAI (hypothyroidism). She should be informed of the signs and symptoms and importance of reporting them to the physician.

Case Study 7: Type II Diabetes Mellitus

Difficulty: **	*Setting:* Hospital
Index Words: Type II diabetes mellitus	

A.R. is a 50-year-old Native American college professor (medical anthropology) with a history of Type II diabetes mellitus (NIDDM) for the past 10 years. He has been controlling his glucose by taking glyburide (Diabeta, Micronase) and using a 2000 calorie ADA (American Diabetes Association) diet. He is aware of the higher incidence of type II DM in his people and is open to anything he can learn about it. His blood glucose level had been fairly consistent with an average AM reading of 200 mg/dl. He is 74" and weighs 220 lb, having lost 10 lb over the past month. Six months after hospitalization for viral pneumonia, A.R. is readmitted for hyperglycemia. He has been running higher blood glucose levels (280 to 300 mg/dl) and has lost 10 lb. He is currently on a medical leave of absence from work. His medical history includes a myocardial infarction, hypertension, and renal insufficiency.

1. Dr. J., A.R.'s physician, determines that A.R. requires insulin for glucose control and orders regular human insulin per sliding scale before breakfast and supper; NPH human insulin 20 Units before breakfast and supper. When would you expect the regular insulin to have its peak effect compared with NPH? **[PD/k/PI/ct]**
   - Regular human insulin peaks in 2 to 3 hours, whereas NPH human insulin peaks in 4 to 10 hours. Note the difference between these peak action times and those for the animal insulin. With animal insulins, regular insulin peaks in 2 to 4 hours, whereas NPH insulin peaks in 6 to 12 hours.

   Instructor Note: The treatment of diabetes has changed rapidly in recent years. Unfortunately, many current drug guides have failed to keep up with the pace. The pharmacokinetics of human insulin, both regular and NPH, are faster than animal insulin (pork and beef), but most references still list them as the same.

2. You are aware of the new American Diabetic Association (ADA) (1994) nutrition recommendations and principles for people with diabetes mellitus (ADA, 1994). A.R.'s physician does not appear aware of these guidelines. You would like to try these guidelines on A.R. to see if he can obtain better glucose control. You know A.R.'s physician has been open to new ideas in the past as long as they have a sound, scientific basis. What collegial strategy might you use to approach him about a change in A.R.'s treatment plan? **[P/ap/PI/ct,ni,tc]**
   - Go to the library and obtain a copy of the ADA (1994) nutrition recommendations and principles to share with Dr. J. Run a search over the past 2 years and pick out several research-based articles and any consensus statements about nutrition, pharmacologic intervention, exercise, and prevention programs for type II DM. Tell him you're interested in A.R.'s progress and you thought he might be interested in some articles you gathered that may be helpful. Ask if he thinks the contents may help in the management of A.R.'s diabetes.

   Instructor Note: If teamwork in the current health care environment is to be effective, it is critical that nurses treat one another, as well as other health care workers, with professional respect and courtesy. They also need to feel confident in the scientific basis for their practice strategies. It is critical as well as professional behavior for us to acknowledge our limitations, be willing to learn from others, and identify those members of the team who can bring their expertise "to the table" in each particular situation.

3. What other health care professionals may be helpful to you in working out a strategy for A.R.'s care? **[P,I/c/PI,PSI/ct]**
   - Endocrinologist or diabetologist (physician who specializes in working with diabetes).
   - A Certified Diabetes Educator (CDE) (usually a registered nurse or registered dietitian), who usually knows "the latest" in diabetes management techniques.
   - A dietitian to help with nutrition management.
   - An exercise physiologist or physical therapist to help develop an activity/exercise program.
   - A pharmacist who can help all concerned understand drug types and metabolism, and who can help with drug-drug interaction issues.

4. None of the other nurses on your unit knows about the more recent developments in diabetes management. Many of the patients on your floor are diabetics. What are 3 activities you can undertake to promote professional growth and development on your unit? (Be creative!) **[P/an/S,PI,PSI,HP/ct,ni,tc]**
   - Work with the CDE, pharmacist, Dr. J., and others to develop an inservice on "new developments in type II DM management" for nurses on your unit.
   - Assemble a notebook with recent articles and references (including the ADA [1994] nutrition recommendations and principles) that can be made available.
   - Develop 1-page "news flashes," each about one aspect of diabetes management and leave them in the employee lounge, on the back of doors in restrooms, etc. Key information should be placed in a box in larger print for "quick reference."
   - Offer to help assemble a committee on your unit to revise the standards of care for diabetic patients.

5. A.R. says he isn't too keen on "jabbing himself with a needle a couple times a day." He wants to know why he can't keep on taking the oral insulin he has been using (glyburide). What is the basis for your response? **[P/c/PI,PSI/ct,tc]**
   - Oral hypoglycemia agents are not insulin preparations. The glyburide helps control high blood glucose by stimulating the pancreas to increase insulin output; it also may help by increasing insulin receptor sensitivity to insulin. This is quite different from giving insulin to patients who have little or no pancreatic insulin production.

A.R.'s revised care plan calls for tighter glucose control with glucose levels of 80 to 120 mg/dl being the recommended range. Dr. J. has discussed with him the importance and benefit of keeping his glucose below 140 mg/dl, and you are going to talk to him about administering his insulin.

6. While you are teaching A.R. how to administer the insulin, he asks why it is necessary to prepare the regular insulin first. Offer a meaningful reason for this procedural step. **[PD,P/c/S/ct,ni,tc]**
   - The old rule "clear before cloudy" is a useful guide. Regular insulin should be clear; if regular insulin in the bottle is not clear, it has a contaminant. There is no way of knowing what that contaminant is. Hence, that insulin must be disposed of. By following the "clear before cloudy" rule, one can be more certain that the regular insulin is uncontaminated. This is particularly important because you are counting on the regular insulin to be more rapidly available.

7. At 0300 A.R. calls you into his room c/o of sweating, nausea, and "shakiness." What would you do first? **[A,PD,P,I/ap/PI/ct,ni]**
   - Check fingerstick blood glucose; if BG <70 mg/dl, treat with fast-acting CHO.
   - If the above is not available, call the lab for a blood glucose. In the meanwhile, based on his diagnosis and the timing of his insulin, treat A.R. with the assumption he is hypoglycemic.

   Instructor Note: In many places, nurses no longer have access to blood glucose monitoring devices. This may result in a delay of several minutes. The rule of thumb is: when in doubt, treat for hypoglycemia.

It is determined that A.R.'s blood glucose is 65 mg/dl.

8. Of the following choices, indicate which item(s) would be appropriate to give A.R. to immediately treat hypoglycemia. **[P/ap/PI/ct,ni]**
   ✓ ½ cup pure orange juice.
   ___ 1 slice of bread.
   ✓ 2 graham cracker squares.
   ___ 1 glass of milk.
   ___ Half a bagel.
   ✓ ½ cup soda pop (not diet or sugar-free).

9. Of the following statements, which one(s) indicate that A.R. requires further teaching regarding self-care? **[A/an/S,PI/ct]**
   - ✓ My wife and I enjoy soaking in our hot tub.
   - ✓ My feet get cold, and the heating pad I use sure helps.
   - ___ I'll have to have my wife help me look at my feet since I can't see as well as I used to.
   - ✓ Sometimes I can't even feel my feet, especially if I've been sitting for a long time.
   - ___ These thick toenails should probably be cut by a doctor.
   - ✓ This file I have works great for these calluses on my feet.

10. A.R. says he has read that exercise can help people with diabetes. Outline the benefits and risks of exercise for the diabetic patient in general. State how the risks can be minimized. **[P,I,E/an/S,PI,HP/ct]**
    - Benefits: improves receptor sensitivity to insulin, lowers blood glucose, assists with weight loss, reduces abdominal body fat deposition, promotes CV fitness, helps regulate blood pressure, improves lipid profile, improves peripheral circulation, promotes positive mood states, improves functional capacity.
    - Risks: can precipitate angina, MI, or sudden death if precautions and guidelines are not observed; can precipitate exercise-related hypoglycemia if activity and food intake are not coordinated.

    Instructor Note: Exercise, like medications, should be prescribed for individuals with special health problems. In the case of those with existing cardiovascular disease, it should be undertaken with guidelines and supervision. Diabetics often are eligible for existing cardiac rehabilitation programs.

11. Develop a teaching plan that addresses the special needs of A.R. as he embarks on an exercise program. Include at least 8 points. **[P/ap/S,Pl/ct,ni]**
    - Obtain clearance from the physician responsible for A.R.'s care.
    - Begin with light-level aerobic activity, particularly walking.
    - Start slowly and increase the length of the exercise session gradually; for example, start at 5 minutes per day and increase by 1 to 2 minutes per week. Never exercise to the point of exhaustion; if a person is out of breath, tell him or her to *slow down*.
    - Drink plenty of fluids.
    - Teach A.R. to monitor his pulse and regulate his activity so he doesn't "overdo it." Discourage competitiveness in exercise.
    - Each session of activity should include a warm-up and cool-down period when the muscles are prepared for activity.
    - Eat 1 to 3 hours before exercise; check blood glucose level before, during, and after exercise to establish a baseline and evaluate response (may need to adjust insulin, increase carbohydrate intake, or both).
    - The onset of chest discomfort, sudden onset of extreme fatigue or weakness, and dizziness or nausea means stop the exercise immediately and get help.
    - Carry a diabetes ID card.
    - Carry an emergency glucose supply.
    - Inspect feet before and after activity, paying special attention to "hot spots," toenails, and blisters.

12. The dietitian evaluates A.R.'s eating pattern and determines his frequent hyperglycemic episodes are related to eating candy or sweet rolls during these periods and lack of knowledge regarding the difference between simple and complex carbohydrates. Offer an analogy that would help A.R. comprehend this concept. **[I/c/Pl/ct,tc]**
    - Simple glucoses can be viewed as a piece of paper thrown onto a fire; the paper burns quickly and vanishes. In contrast, a log thrown on the fire (complex carbohydrate) lasts a long time. A "Twinkie," for example, can be likened to a piece of paper, whereas a slice of bread or glass of milk parallels the longer action of the log for fueling the fire. (Any appropriate analogy is acceptable.)

Case Study 8: Pituitary Macroadenoma with Diabetes Insipidus

Difficulty: ***	*Setting:* Outpatient clinic, hospital
Index Words: Pituitary macroadenoma, diabetes insipidus	

W.V., a 40-year-old woman, has been referred to the endocrine clinic of a large metropolitan medical center by her primary care physician. She presents with a history of bilateral hemianopsia, headaches, menstrual disturbances (amenorrhea), dyspareunia, and lethargy. An extensive history reveals polyuria and polydipsia. Her family physician suspects an anterior pituitary tumor. GH, prolactin, TSH, LH, and FSH levels are unremarkable. A dexamethasone suppression test (or cortisol/ACTH challenge test) and 24-hour urine for 17-hydroxysteroids (17-OHCS) are planned.

1. W.V. is aware of the high probability of a pituitary tumor but she doesn't understand why the physician wants to test her kidneys. How would you explain the relationship between the pituitary and adrenal glands and the need for adrenal function studies to her? **[P,I/ap/PSI/ct,ni,tc]**
    - Your symptoms could be due to a number of different pathologic processes. Your physician has already narrowed the list of possible causes by checking the hormone levels from your pituitary gland, which is located in your head. The pituitary gland and the adrenal glands, located on top of your kidneys, work closely together to release or inhibit the release of their respective hormones. This process is similar to a thermostat that turns off the furnace when room temperature rises. Because the adrenal glands can affect the pituitary gland and your pituitary can affect your kidneys, your doctor wants to check all three.

    Instructor Note: Nearly 30% of macroadenomas do not produce excess hormone.

2. Identify 4 nursing diagnoses for W.V. **[PD/an/S,PI,PSI/ct]**
    - Anxiety r/t uncertainty about problem cause and outcomes of treatment.
    - Pain: headache r/t brain tumor.
    - Risk for self-esteem disturbance r/t changes in body characteristics associated with hormonal excess.
    - Sexual dysfunction r/t alteration in menstrual cycle, dyspareunia.
    - Risk for activity intolerance r/t fatigue.

The dexamethasone suppression test was normal but the 24-hour urine for 17-OHCS was elevated. An MRI (magnetic resonance imaging) was ordered.

3. The MRI confirms a macroadenoma of the anterior pituitary. The physician advises a transsphenoidal hypophysectomy. What questions would you anticipate W.V. might have? **[P/an/PI,PSI/ct]**
    - Does this mean I have cancer? What is the treatment for this anterior pituitary tumor? Will the treatment reverse the symptoms I've been having? Are they going to have to cut a big hole in my head? Will there be a scar? Will I look like a monster? Will there be hormonal problems without the pituitary? Will I have to take medications for the rest of my life?

4. While W.V.'s physician arranges for her admission to the hospital and schedules her transsphenoidal hypophysectomy, you enter her examining room to conduct preop teaching. You find W.V. crying. She says she is embarrassed by the hormonal changes and states, "I'm afraid my husband won't love me anymore." What approaches would be appropriate for addressing the patient's fear? **[P/an/PSI/ct]**
   - Clarify knowledge about disease and anticipated effects on body appearance after surgery; provide an environment that encourages questions and information seeking; enable W.V. to maintain optimal level of independence and personal control; assess factors affecting self-esteem and negative self-appraisal (including possible abusive relationship); encourage W.V. to identify positive attributes that she possesses; encourage W.V. to recognize self-enhancement activities.
   - Ask if she would like to invite her husband to join you in discussing these issues; it may help break the ice in letting them talk about her disorder and coming surgery.

5. During preop teaching, W.V. states she is fearful of the procedure. She says she doesn't understand how a tumor in the brain can be removed through the nose. How would you explain the procedure to minimize her fear? **[P,I/an/PSI/ct,ni,tc]**
   - Using a model/picture, explain that a small incision is made under the upper lip, where the inner lip meets the gums. The physicians use a flexible scope to see and remove the tumor. Care should be taken to assure W.V. that this approach is a successful method for removing these types of tumors, and point out the advantages of such an approach (e.g., no obvious incision scar).

6. Identify 2 major teaching needs for postop care based on the transsphenoidal approach. Outline important educational points for each area to address during preop teaching with W.V. **[P,I/an/PI,PSI/ct,ni,tc]**
   - Prevent increased intracranial pressure: W.V. will be kept in a semi-Fowler's position to decrease intracranial pressure; teach her she must not cough, sneeze, or blow her nose.
   - Prevent infection: drink plenty of fluids; encourage frequent, gentle mouth rinsing, use of soft sponges or toothettes for oral and dental care; teach proper handwashing and instruct W.V. to keep hands away from suture line; immediately report runny nose, postnasal drip, stiff neck, persistent headache.
   - Prevent atelectasis: encourage to turn q2h; teach deep breathing, sighing, and mouth breathing.

7. W.V. is admitted and undergoes a successful transsphenoidal hypophysectomy. Ten hours postop, W.V. calls her nurse into her room complaining of postnasal drip. She is frequently swallowing. What 5 actions should the nurse take and give your rationale. **[P,I/an/PI/ct,ni,tc]**
   - Using a penlight, illuminate the back of W.V.'s throat to observe the color (frank blood, mucous, clear fluid) and quantity of the drainage.
   - Check the external nasal dressing (nasal drip pad) for signs of a "halo" ring which would indicate a cerebrospinal fluid leak.
   - Take VS.
   - Keep W.V. on bed rest and elevate the HOB.
   - Assess for early signs of infection, such as meningitis (e.g., temperature elevation, nuchal rigidity, headache, change in quality and location of pain).
   - Save the nasal dressing in case the physician wants it sent to the laboratory for an accurate assessment of glucose content (test-tape assessment is often unreliable).

8. The nurse notes the following assessment findings: VS 100/66, 98, 16; W.V. c/o thirst; her skin is flushed; her urine output 300 ml/h with a specific gravity of 1.003, and she is flaccid (e.g., no muscle tone). What additional information should you gather before calling the physician? **[A/an/PI,PSI/ct]**
   - Take her temperature (may be elevated in dehydration or infection).
   - Assess neurologic status: note signs/symptoms of dehydration (hyperosmolality), such as restlessness and irritability.
   - Assess for other signs/symptoms of hypovolemia, such as dry and sticky mucous membranes; O >1, dry skin with poor turgor.

9. The nurse suspects fluid volume deficit related to inadequate release of ADH. While waiting for the surgeon to return her call, what should the nurse's priority intervention(s) be? **[P,I/an/S,PI/ct,ni]**
   - Calculate I&O for net gain or loss; document any change in appearance and specific gravity of urine; ensure safety precautions; monitor neurologic status, and observe for signs of hypernatremia.

10. The surgeon orders a serum and urine osmolality and electrolytes. The lab reports a urine osmolality of 95 mOsm/kg, serum osmolality of 315 mOsm/kg, and sodium level of 146 mEq/L. Discuss the significance of each. **[PD/an/PI/ct]**
   - Insufficient ADH (antidiuretic hormone) secretion from the anterior pituitary causes immediate excretion of large volume of dilute urine, leading to increased plasma osmolality; dehydration develops rapidly without ongoing fluid replacement.
   - The serum osmolality and sodium are only slightly elevated; indicating that W.V.'s fluid replacement is adequate (intake matches her urinary output).

11. Replacement therapy for diabetes insipidus includes administration of aqueous vasopressin (Pitressin) or the synthetic vasopressin analog desmopressin (DDAVP). Compare the advantage(s) and disadvantage(s) of using desmopressin versus aqueous Pitressin in this situation. **[E/ap/PI/ct]**
    - Vasopressin is given IM; DDAVP is given intranasally by nasal spray or intranasal pipet.
    - Vasopressin directly stimulates the musculature of the GI tract; DDAVP does not.
    - DDAVP is more potent, longer-acting, and more appropriate for chronic diabetes insidipus.
    - W.V. has nasal packing; therefore, desmopressin could not be given until the packing is removed. Vasopressin will probably be administered until the nasal packing is removed.

12. How will the nurse evaluate the effectiveness of drug and fluid therapy? **[E/an/PI/ct,ni]**
    - Stable VS, I&O balance, electrolytes within normal limits, moist mucous membranes, good skin turgor, W.V. will not c/o thirst.

Case Study 9: Pheochromocytoma

Difficulty: ***	*Setting:* Hospital
Index Words: Pheochromocytoma	

You are a nurse on a medical unit. One of your patients, T.L., a 40-year-old man who works as a communications supervisor, is being evaluated for uncontrolled HTN. He c/o frequent episodes of chest pain and palpitations, diaphoresis, job stress, nervousness, epigastric distress after eating, and pounding migraine headaches that leave him exhausted. He states that these episodes have increased in frequency and duration; he now experiences several episodes a week, and each episode lasts 1 to 3 days. He has taken a variety of antihypertensive medications, none of which have successfully controlled his HTN. His blood pressure is labile; sometimes it is normal and other times it is 220/120. Cardiac workup reveals no significant cardiovascular abnormalities. He has a 27-pack year smoking history. T.L.'s 24-hour urine analysis reveals: vanillylmandelic acid (VMA) 12 mg/24h; epinephrine 45 ng/24h, and norepinephrine 100 ng/24h; CT scan reveals a single adrenomedullary tumor. T.L. is diagnosed with pheochromocytoma and scheduled for an adrenalectomy.

1. The physician informs T.L. that an adrenal tumor is causing his symptoms. T.L. is obviously upset with his diagnosis. He states he doesn't understand how a tumor on top of his kidney can cause high blood pressure. He asks if this means he has cancer. How would you respond? **[PD/ap/PSI/ct,ni,tc]**
   - This type of tumor is usually benign; the tumor releases substances called catecholamines (epinephrine and norepinephrine) that are responsible for his high blood pressure and all the other symptoms that he has been experiencing.

2. The physician advises T.L. to undergo an adrenalectomy. He is immediately started on phenoxybenzamine (Dibenzyline) 20 mg PO q8h, and propranolol (Inderal) 40 mg PO bid. What is the connection between these two drugs and the diagnosis? **[PD/c/PI/ct]**
   - Pheochromocytoma is a catecholamine-producing tumor. Smaller tumors produce norepinephrine; larger tumors tend to produce both norepinephrine and epinephrine.
   - Phenoxybenzamine is a long-lasting, alpha-adrenergic blocker; it blocks epinephrine- and norepinephrine-induced vasoconstriction and results in decreased BP and tachycardia.
   - Propranolol blocks stimulation of $beta_1$ receptors, resulting in decreased heart rate and decreased AV conduction.

3. Some people experience paroxysmal, or sudden, periodic attacks of HTN that correspond to the release of epinephrine and/or norepinephrine. Under what circumstances would T.L. most likely experience a paroxysmal hypertensive event? **[PD/c/PI/ct]**
   - A paroxysm may be precipitated by any activity that compressed the tumor, such as heavy lifting, exercise, defecation, eating, emotional stress, or changing position.

4. What measures to prevent a paroxysmal hypertensive event should you teach T.L.? **[P,I/ap/PI/ct,tc]**
   - Instruct T.L. to avoid any activity that places pressure on the abdomen (such as heavy lifting, straining at stool, constipation, rubbing or pressing on the abdomen, bending or flexing the body, or sudden position changes) and to reduce caffeine intake.

5. T.L. is given hydrocortisone (Solu-Cortef) 100 mg IV push preoperatively. Discuss the significance of this drug in the preoperative period. **[PD/c/PI/ct]**
   - Because half of the adrenal gland will be removed, T.L. will be at high risk for depletion of both glucocorticoids and mineralocorticoids. Solu-Cortef, having both glucocorticoid and mineralocorticoid activity, is frequently administered.

6. Following the surgery, T.L. is taken directly to the intensive care unit. The anesthesiologist gives the admitting nurse the following report: the surgery went well, and T.L. should wake up shortly; his VS have been running 180/90, 88, 16, 96.1 °F; he's got a left subclavian Swan-Ganz catheter and 2 large-bore peripheral IVs with D_5W running at a total of 125 ml/h; urine output during OR was 200 ml. What additional data should the ICU nurse elicit from the anesthesiologist? **[E/an/PI/ct]**
   - What were T.L.'s CVP (central venous pressure) readings during surgery? Did he have any electrolytes drawn (particularly Na, K)? What was his glucose? What was his cardiac rhythm? Did T.L. receive any cortisol during surgery?

7. Identify 3 postoperative nursing diagnoses for T.L. **[PD/an/S,PI,PSI/ct]**
   - Risk for fluid volume deficit r/t sodium and water loss associated with deficiency of adrenal cortex hormones.
   - Risk for injury r/t weakness and electrolyte imbalance.
   - Ineffective individual coping r/t abnormal response to stressors.
   - Risk for infection r/t immunosuppressive effects of cortisol therapy.
   - Anxiety r/t surgical outcome.

8. For each nursing diagnoses identified above, outline 2 to 3 nursing measures. **[P/an/S,PI,PSI/ct,ni,tc]**
   - Risk for fluid volume deficit: monitor hourly I&O and VS; monitor hydration parameters including hemoglobin, hematocrit, and BUN; administer IV fluids and cortisol as directed.
   - Risk for injury related to weakness, electrolyte imbalance, and hypoglycemia: monitor electrolytes and serum glucose as directed and report abnormalities; elevate all siderails; assess for signs/symptoms of hypoglycemia, sodium and potassium imbalances; dangle T.L. on the side of the bed before ambulating.
   - Ineffective individual coping related to inability to mount normal response to stressors: maintain quiet environment; educate family about importance of minimizing physical and emotional stressors during postoperative period.
   - Risk for infection: Maintain asepsis during invasive procedures and/or dressing changes; encourage coughing, deep breathing; instruct family to wash their hands on entering and leaving T.L.'s room; educate T.L.'s family about not exposing him to people with known or suspected infections.
   - Anxiety: Keep T.L. informed about his progress; encourage him to ask questions and express his concerns.

Case Study 10: Syndrome of Inappropriate Antidiuretic Hormone Secondary to Bronchogenic Carcinoma (Small Cell)

Difficulty: ***	*Setting:* Hospice care, hospital emergency department
Index Words: Syndrome of inappropriate antidiuretic hormone, oat cell cancer	

You are a hospice nurse caring for G.N., a 40-year-old man diagnosed with oat cell carcinoma of the lung with widespread metastasis. He is receiving morphine sulfate (MS Contin) 30 mg PO q6h for chronic pain management, prednisone (Deltasone) 10 mg PO qd, and is on 2 L O_2/nc. He is currently undergoing radiation treatments for palliative relief of shoulder and chest pain. At the weekly patient care conference, you and the physician discuss the possibility that G.N. is experiencing SIADH (syndrome of inappropriate antidiuretic hormone) related to his tumor. G.N. and his wife desire only comfort measures; they are against hospitalization and all means of artificial life support.

1. How would you differentiate between the onset of SIADH and the side effects of radiation, morphine, or prednisone therapy? **[PD/c/Pl/ct]**
   - The major side effects of radiation therapy are pneumonitis and increased shortness of breath, anorexia, and fatigue (usually increases as week progresses with improvement on the weekend).
   - The major side effects of prednisone are increased susceptibility to infection, adrenal suppression, anorexia, nausea, weight gain, decreased wound healing, muscle wasting, and depression.
   - The major side effects of MS Contin are sedation, confusion, hypotension, and constipation.
   - SIADH is marked by altered LOC, exertional dyspnea, fatigue, anorexia, impaired taste, thirst, N/V, abdominal cramps, decreased urine output, serum hyponatremia and hypoosmolality, increased urine osmolality. Without the benefit of laboratory analysis it would be difficult to definitively detect SIADH. G.N.'s increased weight could be r/t steroid therapy; neurologic changes could be r/t metastatic cancer, morphine administration, or electrolyte imbalance; anorexia, fatigue, and increased shortness of breath could be secondary to radiation treatments. However, SIADH should be suspected if G.N. c/o headache or demonstrates decreased level of consciousness *and* experiences a significant decline in urine output.

During your daily assessment, you note that G.N. is complaining of increased nausea and malaise. He has gained 5 pounds over the last 3 days without signs of edema, and his urine appears to be more concentrated. His wife states he has been sleeping a lot more lately. After consulting with the physician, you draw blood for a serum sodium level and deliver the blood to the laboratory for analysis.

2. The laboratory reports a serum Na of 122 mEq/L. Explain why individuals with SIADH-induced total body water gain generally do not have the hypernatremia and dependent edema that is commonly seen in congestive heart failure and cirrhosis of the liver. **[PD/an/PI/ct]**
   - SIADH-induced increases in extracellular fluid volume result in serum hyponatremia and hypoosmolality; hyponatremia suppresses renin/aldosterone secretion and results in decreased reabsorption of Na in the proximal tubule, resulting in further serum hyponatremia and urinary hyperosmolality.

3. During collaboration, you and the physician discuss the treatment plan of restricting fluids to 500 ml/d and increasing the oral salt intake to raise G.N.'s serum sodium level. As you analyze G.N.'s total clinical picture, is there reason to question this plan of action? **[E/an/PI/ct]**
   - Yes; in SIADH, the fluid is usually restricted to 600 to 800 ml/d. In addition, individuals undergoing radiation therapy are instructed to increase their water intake to facilitate the removal of the products of cellular destruction. The 500 ml/day limitation may be too restrictive.

4. G.N.'s wife asks how she can help her husband adhere to the fluid restriction when he seems to be so thirsty. What strategies can you offer her? **[P/c/PI/ct,ni]**
   - Encourage ice chips and flavored popsicles or hard candy to relieve the sensation of thirst.
   - Provide cold water on a "swish and spit" basis to relieve dry mouth without increasing fluid intake.
   - Teach her how to provide frequent oral hygiene.
   - Space fluids throughout a 24-hour period.
   - Measure urine output (fluid intake should not exceed urine output).

5. Two days later, G.N.'s wife calls to inform you that her husband is vomiting, is disoriented to time and place, and c/o severe headache. What will you do first? **[I/ap/PI/ct]**
   - Immediately notify the physician. G.N. is exhibiting clinical manifestations of severe hyponatremia (<120 mEq/L) and is at high risk for seizures or coma.

6. The physician explains the situation to G.N.'s wife, and she agrees to have her husband transported to the ED for IV administration of sodium chloride and diuretics. You call the ED to inform the staff of G.N.'s arrival. What information should you convey to the triage nurse? **[P,I/an/PI/ct,ni]**
   - The nurse should be informed of a brief history, his current condition, and his most recent serum sodium level. The nurse also should be informed of the physician's plans to administer IV sodium chloride and diuretics.
   - The nurse should be informed of G.N.'s advanced directives about no additional care (e.g., other than palliative).

   Instructors Note: The private physician will convey pertinent information directly to the ED physician.

7. The ED physician prescribed the following: start an IV of 3% sodium chloride and infuse 100 ml over 1 hour; then draw STAT serum Na, Cl, HCO_3, and osmolality and send urine for osmolality. Administer furosemide (Lasix) 40 mg IV push. Discuss the possible consequences of too rapid infusion of the saline solution. **[PD/ap/PI/ct]**
   - Infusion of 3% NS solution can induce severe volume overload and pulmonary edema (100 ml of 3% NS contains 50 mEq Na). G.N. should be closely observed for signs of neurologic deterioration, CHF, and pulmonary edema. The goal of hypertonic NS therapy is to elevate the Na level enough to alleviate signs of neurologic compromise—not to raise the level to "normal."

8. When should the Lasix be given? Explain. **[PD/ap/PI/ct]**
   - Lasix should be given concurrently with sodium chloride infusion. Lasix is administered to prevent circulatory overload as fluid shifts from the intracellular to intravascular compartment.

9. Identify priority assessment parameters the ED nurse should monitor during this acute period. **[A/c/PI/ct]**
   - Neurologic assessment q15 minutes; immediately report any signs of deterioration to the physician.
   - VS q15 minutes; immediately report signs of fluid overload, increased BP, increased pulse, or presence of an S_3 gallop.
   - Monitor signs/symptoms of pulmonary edema; increased respiratory rate, respiratory difficulty, or rales/crackles.
   - Assess for signs/symptoms of potassium deficit related to Lasix therapy. (Don't forget magnesium!)

10. Upon discharge from the ED, the physician orders demeclocycline (Declomycin). Analyze the high-risk side effects of democlocylcine for G.N. **[PD/an/S,PI/ct]**
    - Because demeclocycline is an antibiotic and G.N. is immunosuppressed secondary to radiation treatments and prednisone therapy, he should be closely observed for signs/symptoms of superinfection. The drug can cause rashes and photosensitivity, which is also a concern for individual receiving radiation therapy.
    - The side effects of demeclocycline include increased thirst, increased urination, N/V, weakness and fatigue. Because G.N. recently developed SIADH, it will be especially important for you to monitor urine output and weight.

11. Outline important teaching guidelines r/t demeclocycline therapy that you would address with G.N. and his wife. **[P/an/S,PI/ct]**
    - Instruct G.N. to take medication as prescribed.
    - Carefully monitor urine output and weight.
    - Drink 240 ml fluid when taking demeclocycline, and do not take any other medications at least 1 hour before or after demeclocycline.
    - Avoid milk, other dairy products, and antacids within 1 to 3 hours of medication because calcium decreases absorption.
    - Teach use of sunscreen and protective clothing when outdoors.
    - Report signs/symptoms of infection, such as loose or foul-smelling stools; white, black, or furry patches on the tongue.

Case Study 11: Type I Diabetes Mellitus

Difficulty: ***	*Setting:* Home care, ED, hospital
Index Words: Type I diabetes mellitus, hypoglycemia, hyperglycemia, depression	

P.W. is a 40-year-old disabled man who recently lost his wife to metastatic breast cancer. His brother has taken him into his home. P.W. has a 22-year history of insulin-dependent diabetes mellitus (IDDM, now called type I diabetes mellitus). Until recently, he has taken responsibility for the management of his disease and has been actively involved in the local chapter of the American Diabetic Association. PMH includes 2 amputated toes on his R foot, retinopathy and visual impairment in both eyes, and angina on exertion from coronary artery disease that severely restricts his activity. Since he began treatment with an ace-inhibitor 2 years ago, his blood pressure has gone from 182/128 to 126/78 mm Hg. Currently, he is 71" tall and weighs 135 lb. P.W.'s sister-in-law, who is an LVN/LPN, says P.W. has lost about 12 pounds in the past 3 weeks. Over the past few years, P.W. has been administering a multidose (3 injections) regimen of regular human insulin to himself (1 before each meal and 1 injection of NPH human insulin at bedtime. Recently his blood glucose levels have been increasingly inconsistent and labile, and he has been labeled "noncompliant." It is Monday. You are the home care nurse assigned to visit P.W. 3 times per week for teaching and evaluation. P.W.'s brother and sister-in-law express concern that P.W. seems to be indifferent about his nutritional and pharmacologic regimens.

1. List measures you normally would address in teaching for both hypoglycemia and hyperglycemia (6 each). **[I/k/S,PI/ct]**
   - *Hyperglycemia:*
     Administer the prescribed insulin dose at the proper time.
     Adhere to meal schedules and prescribed snacks.
     Maintain good personal hygiene.
     Adhere to sick-day rules when ill.
     Monitor blood glucose levels.
     Contact physician if blood glucose is beyond the prescribed limit.
     Wear diabetic medical identification.
   - *Hypoglycemia:*
     Take prescribed insulin dose at the proper time.
     Eat meals at proper times.
     Provide compensation for exercise or physical activity.
     Recognize symptoms and treat immediately.
     Carry simple carbohydrate such as glucose tablets at all times.
     Monitor blood glucose levels.
     Wear diabetic medical identification.

<u>Note:</u> Current practice promotes tighter glucose management to prevent long-term complications of DM. In the past, patients' glucose often would be allowed to swing to 180 mg/dl or higher. These are the current recommendations for glucose:

1. Blood glucose levels of 60-120 mg/dl preprandial and 180 mg/dl 1 hour postprandial (Hollander, Castle, Joynes, & Nelson, p. 11, 1990).
2. The general goal is 70-120 mg/dl (as close to "normal" as possible). At this level, HbA_{1c} should be about 6% over time. Normal values for adults/elderly should be about 4% to 8%. For rough estimates of glucose levels over a period of weeks, consider an HbA_{1c} of 6% to be equal to 110 mg/dl and an HbA_{1c} of 10% to be about 250 mg/dl (Hollander et al., p. 11, 1990).
3. It may take weeks, months, or even more than a year to reach these goals safely, but it can be done (Hollander et al., p. 12, 1990). To try to reduce blood glucose levels too quickly, risks repeated hypoglycemic reactions and the frustration (as well as danger) of the Somogyi phenomenon.
4. HbA_{1c} should be done at the beginning of a risk modification program and repeated on a 4 to 8 week basis until the value is stable. Note that this value will change more slowly and be more stable, over time, than blood glucose levels.

Also note that the new 1995 American Diabetic Association guidelines are more flexible than the former guidelines and accommodate carbohydrate counting or exchanges. Current exchange lists have been published by the American Diabetes Association and the American Dietetic Association, under the title *Exchange Lists for Meal Planning*. This and other information may be obtained from the American Dietetic Association, Chicago, IL, Products and Services Division, 1-800-877-1600x5000, FAX 1-312-899-4899.

In the past, some urinary glucose and ketones often were tested at home by dipstick. Although some adults still use this method of "controlling" their disease because of habit or limited financial resources, it is grossly inaccurate. Blood glucose monitoring is the recommended method for controlling type I DM. For gestational diabetes management, consult recent authoritative sources.

As you start to review the above measures with P.W., you notice he already seems aware of what he should do to control his blood glucose. You also are concerned that he seems to be distracted and "drifts off" in the middle of a discussion; his affect also appears flat.

2. You take P.W.'s resting vital signs and get the following: 174/108, 82, 20, 98.4°F (oral). Are these values acceptable? If not, indicate which one(s) are not and what you think is happening. **[A,PD/an/ct]**
   - P.W.'s blood pressure is 174/108, both systolic and diastolic are far too high and should be reported immediately.
   - Based on the above information, you suspect P.W.'s problem is depression, not lack of education.
   - You think he has not been taking his ace-inhibitor as prescribed.

You ask P.W. if he has been taking all his medications. He says "Yes" but adds that he discovers "extra" blood pressure pills left over at the end of each week. He seems to be confused about the reason for the "leftover" pills. You decide to do a glucose stick. He registers 348 mg/dl.

3. Based on all the above information, what 2 other assessments will you want to perform on P.W.? **[A,PD/an/PSI/ct,ni]**
   - The confusion, flat affect, distractibility, in addition to his "forgetting" measures of self-care, lead you to be concerned about his mental status. You would want to (1) perform a brief neurologic assessment and (2) assess his emotional status relating to clinical signs/symptoms of depression. *Be sure to question about suicidal ideation!*

4. You decide to call P.W.'s physician. Specifically, what information are you going to give her? **[P/an/S,PI,PSI/ct,tc]**
   - Introduce yourself and briefly relate P.W.'s history. Report vital signs, his current glucose level, and your assessment of his mental/emotional status giving her specific behaviors you have observed. Tell her about his weight loss, skipped meals, inability to keep track of his medications, and his wife's recent death.

P.W.'s physician says she wants to hospitalize him for evaluation and stabilization; this also would give the opportunity for a psychiatric consult. P.W. says he refuses to go to "that hospital where my wife died." In discussion with P.W. and the physician, it is decided that you will check on his progress daily; someone from the home care agency will call q8h for a progress report. P.W.'s sister-in-law agrees to monitor his blood glucose and vital signs and see that he takes all his medications. If P.W.'s condition does not improve or becomes worse, he must enter the hospital for treatment. The physician agrees with you about his being depressed and starts P.W. on sertraline (Zoloft) 50 mg qd to be taken with his bedtime snack for his depression.

5. The next day, during your midafternoon visit to P.W.'s home, he tells you he has a headache and is feeling "fidgety." His pulse is 124, his gait is unsteady, speech is slightly slurred, and blood glucose is 48 mg/dl. What will you do? **[A,PD,P/ap/S,PI/ct,ni]**
   - Have him drink a glass of juice immediately. Follow this by a small snack. Stay with him and recheck his blood glucose in 20 to 30 minutes. If his glucose does not improve or if he becomes unconscious, dial 911 for emergency treatment and have him transported to the hospital. You will remain with him until the paramedics arrive.

6. In an effort to determine the cause of this hypoglycemic reaction, what questions should you ask his sister-in-law? **[A/an/PI/ct,tc]**
   - What did he eat for lunch?
   - Did he eat at his usual time in relation to the insulin injection?
   - Did he have his normal insulin dose?
   - Has he been doing anything like heavy work or exercising?
   - Has he had any alcohol today?

7. You ask the sister-in-law who gave him his insulin injections today: did he administer it himself, or did she? You also ask her to check the insulin vial to see if some insulin appears to be unaccounted for. Explain your rationale. **[A/an/S,PI,PSI/ct,ni,tc]**
   - An insulin reaction could be the result of an accidental "overdose" because of P.W.'s confusion.
   - An insulin "overdose" also may reflect a suicide attempt.
   - Both P.W. and his sister-in-law may have administered insulin before lunch.

8. If P.W. were to become unconscious during a hypoglycemic episode, how would you revise nursing management of his condition in this setting? **[P/ap/Pl/ct,ni]**
   - Clients who are unable to ingest quick-acting carbohydrates will require SC or IM glucagon (1 mg), generally followed by administration of 50 ml 50% IV glucose. If P.W. has a glucagon syringe, use it as an emergency measure. You are authorized only to follow your agency protocol for emergency management. Administering care outside or beyond this coverage means you are functioning beyond your scope of practice.
   - Dial 911 for emergency support, and stay with P.W. until help arrives. Then notify the physician what happened and which hospital P.W. is being taken to. Chart precise notes on the sequence of events, individuals notified, and actions taken.

9. P.W.'s sister-in-law phones you on Sunday morning stating that P.W. is "very sick." What questions would you ask her to help you decide the best course of action? **[A/an/Pl/ct,tc]**
   - Describe what she means by "very sick."
   - Has she performed a blood glucose test on him? If so, when and what was the reading?
   - What are his vital signs?
   - When did he last eat, and what time did he take his last insulin injection? How much insulin did he take? Is he experiencing thirst, abdominal pain, vomiting, confusion, foul breath, labored breathing? Is he fully alert?

10. Under what circumstances is P.W. likely to experience diabetic ketoacidosis? **[PD/k/Pl,PSl/ct]**
    - Too little insulin in conjunction with increased calorie intake.
    - Periods of physical or emotional stress.

P.W.'s sister-in-law informs you that his blood glucose is too high for the machine to read. You tell her to dial 911 immediately; advise her to tell them P.W. is diabetic and his blood glucose is over 400 mg/dl.

11. What can the ED nurse do to prepare for P.W.'s arrival? **[P/c/Pl/ct,ni]**
    - Have a glucose meter calibrated and ready.
    - Be prepared to draw blood for stat blood glucose level and electrolytes.
    - Prepare to do VS.
    - IV setup to administer regular human insulin in NS.
    - Prepare a separate IV setup with NS that can run at 150 ml/h.
    - Connect to cardiac monitor.

12. The nurse does a quick assessment upon arrival. Outline essential components of an abbreviated assessment specific for this situation. **[A,P/ap/Pl/ct,ni]**
    - Airway, breathing, circulation.
    - VS.
    - Assess for Kussmaul's respirations characteristic of DKA.
    - Assess for foul (acetone) breath, altered level of consciousness, flushed appearance, dry mucous membranes, hypotension, tachycardia.
    - Assess for signs/symptoms of dehydration, hypovolemic shock.

13. Laboratory tests reveal the following: Na 135 mEq/L, K 5.6 mEq/L, Cl 92 mEq/L, BUN 38 mg/dl, glucose 682 mg/dl, WBC 15.7 mm^3, Hct 53%, pH 7.30, $PaCO_2$ 36 mm Hg, PaO_2 86 mm Hg, and HCO_3 18 mEq/L. Interpret the lab values in relation to this situation. **[A,PD/an/PI/ct,ni]**
    - The glucose obviously is very high; the sodium and chloride are low-normal which suggests an osmotic diuresis from hyperglycemia.
    - The ABGs indicate metabolic acidosis.
    - The acidotic state alters cellular membrane permeability and allows Na ions, normally most abundant outside the cell, to diffuse inward, and K ions, most abundant inside the cell, to diffuse outward. This is a very dangerous situation. The underlying condition must be corrected, and insulin must be administered to temporarily drive K back into the cell.
    - BUN is elevated to reflect protein breakdown and urea formation.
    - Hct is slightly elevated, suggesting hemoconcentration.

14. Write 3 nursing diagnoses that depict the care priorities for this situation. **[PD/c/S,PI,PSI/ct]**
    - Risk for injury: DKA secondary to insufficient insulin or possible infection.
    - Altered tissue perfusion r/t altered fluid and electrolyte balance.
    - Risk for injury r/t altered level of consciousness.
    - Risk for decreased cardiac output: cardiac arrest r/t elevated K.

15. The physician prescribes an IV drip per infusion pump of regular human insulin 100 units in 100 ml NS at 6 U/h for blood glucose >300 mg/dl, hourly glucose check, repeat electrolytes and serum glucose in 2 hours. What effect should the insulin infusion have on the client's physical condition and how should the nurse revise the physical assessment plan? **[A,P/an/PI/ct,ni]**
    - As insulin is administered, K will be driven back inside the cell. The nurse should closely watch the cardiac monitor and assess for signs/symptoms of hypokalemia. As the plasma glucose levels fall, the patient should be monitored for hypoglycemia and cerebral edema that may accompany a rapid insulin-induced drop in blood glucose levels. Glucose levels, neurologic assessments, VS, and urine volume should be monitored closely.

16. Following the DKA episode, for which P.W. was hospitalized, P.W. shares with his nurse, "I don't have the will to go on living without my wife...I wish everyone would just let me die." How should the nurse respond? **[A,PD,E/an/PSI/ct,ni,tc]**
    - Keep in mind that he has only been taking the antidepressant for several days and it may not have taken effect yet.
    - Ensure that he receive a psychiatric consult ASAP.
    - Directly question him about suicidal ideation; institute suicide precautions if necessary to ensure his safety.
    - Request a psychiatric nurse specialist consult for evaluation and support.

A few days later, when you visit P.W. to facilitate his discharge, you find the combination of antidepressant and improved health status has contributed to an improvement in P.W.'s mental status. He impresses you as being alert and intelligent. Although he verbalizes a sense of great loss and sadness about his wife's death, he no longer seems to be so overwhelmed. He says he has not heard about the 1994 American Diabetes Association nutrition recommendations and principles for people with diabetes mellitus and expresses interest in learning "as much as he can." You chart that he appears to be open and receptive to teaching about management of his condition. You make a mental note to yourself that a "noncompliant" patient often is a person in trouble who needs help, not a label.

CHAPTER 8. IMMUNOLOGIC DISORDERS

Case Study 1: Primary Immunodeficiency Disease

Difficulty:[1] **	*Setting:* Student health center
Index Words: Primary immunodeficiency disease	

You are a nurse at the student health center (SHC) at a local university. T.Q., a 19-year-old male student, visits the clinic the first day of Autumn Quarter to inform you of his immunodeficiency problem. He gives you a letter from his attending physician, a vial of gamma globulin, and asks you if you would give him his "shot." The letter, written by T.Q.'s physician, states that he was diagnosed with primary immunodeficiency disease 4 years ago. He has an adequate number of B-cells but inadequate numbers of immunoglobulin. T.Q. has a history of chronic sinus and upper respiratory tract infections and occasional GI tract infections. He is maintained on 0.66 ml/kg gamma globulin IM every 3 weeks. T.Q. responds well to his treatment and has suffered no side effects from gamma globulin other than occasional redness at the injection site. T.Q. has no other known illnesses or allergies and is on tetracycline for acne. T.Q. is 5′11′, weights 190 lb, has several pustular lesions on his face and neck, and his VS are 134/78, 84, 20, 98.8°F.

1. What actions will you take first? **[A/an/PI/ct,ni,tc]**
    - Determine if T.Q.'s physician resides in your state; a prescription from another state may not be honored across state lines.
    - If T.Q. is from out of state, inform the student health center physician; s/he should call T.Q.'s physician to obtain a copy of T.Q.'s medical records and medical treatment plan (if a FAX is available, this can be accomplished in a matter of minutes). The SHC physician can then prescribe the appropriate drug, dose, and frequency of injection for T.Q.

2. What should you do while the physician is verifying information? **[P,I/ap/PI/ct,ni]**
    - Place T.Q. in a treatment room and assess his physical status to obtain a baseline for future reference.
    - Place the written documentation from T.Q.'s physician in his health record.
    - Consult with the health services physician about giving T.Q. an IM injection of gamma globulin.

3. Would you give T.Q. his own medication? **[PD/an/PI/ct,ni]**
    - Inquire about the proper handling and storage of the gamma globulin. This drug must be stored between 35°C and 46°C and *not* frozen; if it has been stored at the proper temperature, go ahead and use it. Each dose costs approximately $300.

[1] Please note: there are *no beginner* (*) case studies in this chapter.

4. What other assessments should you make before T.Q. leaves? **[I,E/an/PI/ct,ni,tc]**
   - T.Q.'s knowledge base pertaining to signs and symptoms of impending infection; side effects of gamma globulin; importance of student health monitoring. Although T.Q. is likely very knowledgeable about his condition, you should determine his level of understanding.

5. You note on T.Q.'s health record that he has not received his polio, measles, mumps, or rubella vaccines. What explanation can be given for the lack of these vaccinations? **[PD/c/PI/ct]**
   - Immunization should not be given to immunosuppressed patients, because they are produced from live viruses. T.Q. is protected from these viruses as long as he is receiving gamma globulin.

T.Q. is very knowledgeable about his condition. After receiving his injection, he makes an appointment to return to student health in 3 weeks. T.Q. complains of a stuffy nose on his next appointment.

6. How should you respond to T.Q.'s complaints? **[P,I/an/PI/ct,ni]**
   - T.Q. has a PMH of chronic sinus and upper respiratory tract infections and occasional GI tract infections. Focus your assessment on signs/symptoms of infections in these areas first.

7. If T.Q. is developing a sinus infection, what signs are you likely to encounter upon examining T.Q.? **[PD/c/PI/ct]**
   - Reddened nasal mucosa with thick, purulent drainage; elevated temperature.

T.Q.'s nares do not appear swollen or red, although he does have some clear mucus drainage. His temperature is normal at 98.4°F. T.Q. is due for his next injection of gamma globulin.

8. Should you give the medication or ask him to return when he is no longer having nasal stuffiness? Why or why not? **[P,I/an/PI/ct,ni]**
   - Give the gamma globulin: at present, T.Q. does not have an infection; however, he needs the gamma globulin to provide him with protection from developing a sinus infection.

9. Should any adjustments be made in T.Q.'s class schedule or activities because of his condition? **[PD/ap/PI,PSI/ct,ni,tc]**
   - No: T.Q. should be encouraged to eat a well-balanced diet, get adequate rest, and maintain a normal schedule.

10. How do primary immunodeficiencies differ from secondary immunodeficiencies? **[PD/k/PI/ct]**
    - "Primary" involves components of the immune system itself, such as hypogammaglobulinemia; whereas "secondary" immunodeficiencies are due to disease or its treatment. Persons with primary disease are immunodeficient; persons with secondary disease are immunocompromised.

11. Explain why T.Q. is at greater risk for the development of infections than his classmates. **[PD/c/PI/ct]**
    - Immunoglobulin are necessary to fight off invading antigens and prevent disease development. T.Q.'s B cells are either unable to synthesize or release adequate numbers of immunoglobulin in response to foreign antigen. This places him at greater risk to develop disease than normal persons.

12. How do injections of gamma globulin help T.Q. fight off infections? **[PD/ap/PI/ct]**
    - Gamma globulin replaces the immunoglobulins that T.Q. is unable to produce; they attack foreign antigens and prevent disease from occurring.

13. What are the major side effects that could occur from injections of gamma globulin? **[PD/k/PI/ct]**
    - Pain or tenderness at injection site; urticaria; angioedema; anaphylaxis; wheezing; difficulty breathing; hives; chest tightness; fever; chills; swelling of the tongue or lips; N/V; headache; back, hip, or joint pain; and tiredness.

14. Given the nature of and side effects associated with gamma globulin, how long should T.Q. wait at the health center before leaving? **[PD/k/PI/ct]**
    - At least a half hour.

Case Study 2: Human Immunodeficiency Virus

Difficulty: **	*Setting:* Physician's Office
Index Words: Human immunodeficiency virus	

You are working at a physician's office where you have just taken C.Q., a 38-year-old woman, into the consultation room. C.Q. has been divorced for 5 years, has 2 daughters (ages 14 and 16), and works full-time as a legal secretary. Two weeks ago she visited her doctor for a routine physical examination and requested that an HIV (human immunodeficiency virus) test be performed. C.Q. stated that she was in a serious relationship, is contemplating marriage, and just wanted to make certain she was "Okay." No abnormalities were noted during C.Q.'s physical examination and blood was drawn for routine blood chemistries, hematology studies, and an ELISA (enzyme-linked immunosorbent assay) test, also knows as the EIA (enzyme immunoassay) test. C.Q. is at the office to receive her lab results. The physician informs you that C.Q.'s EIA was positive.

1. What is an EIA test? Does a positive EIA mean that C.Q. definitely has HIV? **[A,PD/c/PI/ct]**
   - No: the EIA, or ELISA, is a common test performed to screen for HIV-1 virus antibodies. Because any screening test can result in a false-positive, the ELISA would have to be repeatedly positive and a second blood test, such as a Western blot test, would be used to confirm the diagnosis.

2. You explain to C.Q. that one of her tests needs to be repeated and you need to draw another blood sample. Why wouldn't you tell C.Q. that her first test result was positive and that another test is needed before the diagnosis can be confirmed? **[PD/c/PI,PSI/ct]**
   - Because of the medical and social significance of a positive HIV test, test results must be accurate and correctly interpreted. The U.S. Public Health Service states that an individual can be said to be HIV positive *only after* the EIA test is active and another test, such as the Western blot test, is positive. C.Q. has had only one positive test and does not meet the criteria for confirmatory HIV positive results. She should not be subjected to the emotional stress of a false-positive result.

The physician informs you that C.Q.'s Western blot test results confirm that she is HIV positive and requests that you be present when he talks to her. Before leaving C.Q.'s room, the physician requests that you obtain another blood sample for further testing, give C.Q. verbal and written information about local AIDS support groups, and help C.Q. call a friend to accompany her home this evening. She looks at you through her tears and states, "I can't believe it. J. is the only man I've had sex with since my divorce. He told me I had nothing to worry about. I can't believe he would do this to me."

3. C.Q.'s statement is based on 3 assumptions: that J. is HIV-positive, that he intentionally withheld that information from her, and that he intentionally transmitted the HIV to her through unprotected sex. Based on your knowledge of HIV infection, how would you counsel C.Q.? **[P/ap/PI,PSI/ct,ni,tc]**
   - First ask C.Q. if she received a blood transfusion between 1978 and 1985; if she had dental work, surgery, or trauma within the last several years; if she ever used a needle to inject drugs into her body (even once); or if she ever had sex with someone who later learned he was HIV-infected.
   - Suggest that C.Q. talk to J. about undergoing HIV testing; there is a possibility that J. is not infected or that he is unaware that he has HIV infection.
   - Have C.Q. make another appointment soon to talk about her disease.

4. In addition to offering alternative explanations and exploring alternatives, what is your most important role at this time? **[I/an/PSI/ct,ni,tc]**
   - Stay with C.Q. and offer emotional support. Allow her to cry and ventilate her frustration, demonstrate compassion toward her, and remain nonjudgmental.

5. Identify 4 nursing diagnoses for C.Q. **[PD/an/PI,PSI/ct]**
   - Anxiety r/t diagnosis.
   - Powerlessness r/t diagnosis.
   - Potential for ineffective individual coping r/t diagnosis.
   - Risk for injury to self or others r/t shock of diagnosis.
   - Risk for infection r/t immunocompromise.

6. C.Q. had a positive EIA test and is seropositive for HIV, why doesn't she have signs or symptoms of infection of AIDS? **[PD/k/PI/ct]**
   - C.Q. has been exposed to HIV and has produced antibodies to the virus. The median duration between development of HIV antibodies and the onset of clinical disease may be several years; the detection of antibodies can occur any time between when they are produced to when she develops clinical disease.

7. What assessment findings would support a diagnoses of AIDS? **[A,PD/k/PI/ct]**
   - Recurrent vaginal infections, lymphadenopathy, fever, fatigue, weight loss, chronic diarrhea.

   Instructor Note: Women tend to develop AIDS sooner than men, usually presenting with vaginal infections first.

8. Why is it a good idea that someone C.Q. trusts escort her home this evening? **[A,P/ap/PI,PSI/ct]**
   - C.Q. has just received very disturbing news and is distraught. She is at increased risk of injury if she attempts to drive home by herself and needs the emotional support of someone who cares about her.

C.Q. gives you the name and phone number of a relative she wants you to call. You remain with her until she leaves with her relative.

9. Has C.Q.'s right to privacy been violated? Explain why or why not? **[A/c/PSI/ct]**
   - No: you have not divulged C.Q.'s HIV status, C.Q. also gave implied permission to contact the relative when she supplied the name and phone number.

10. C.Q. returns to the office 4 days later to discuss her diagnosis. What issues will you discuss with her at this time? **[P,I/an/S,PI,PSI/ct,ni,tc]**
    - Who should be told about the positive result; if C.Q. has not done so, suggest that she talk to J. about undergoing HIV testing because there is a possibility that J. is not infected or is unaware that he has HIV infection.
    - Inform her what is entailed in a medical evaluation.
    - How to reduce risk of transmission.
    - Implications for pregnancy.
    - Importance of influenza vaccine yearly, and pneumococcal and hepatitis vaccine.
    - Provide C.Q. with information about social services, financial assistance programs, and any clinical trials that she could become involved in.
    - Signs and symptoms of infection and to notify the physician at the first sign of infection.
    - Importance of maintaining a well-balanced diet and activity schedule.
    - Staging of the disease is based on clinical findings and CD4 cell count; CD4 cell count is the best available marker for differential diagnosis, prognosis, and need for prophylaxis against HIV-related infections; when C.Q. becomes symptomatic, blood will be drawn for a CD4 cell count.

11. Does C.Q. have a legal responsibility to inform J. of her HIV status? **[PD/c/PSI/ct]**
    - C.Q. does not have a legal responsibility; however, she has a moral responsibility to inform him in case he is unaware of his own HIV status.

Two weeks later C.Q. visits the office and asks to speak to you in private. She thanks you for talking to her the day she received the news of her diagnosis. She pulls a gun from her purse and states, "I was going to go out into the waiting room and blow J. away, because I thought he was cheating on me." She tells you that J. confessed to her he was afraid to tell her about his hemophilia because she might leave him. J. is HIV tested at regular intervals and his last HIV test, 6 months ago, had been negative. J. was retested and was positive for HIV. J.'s doctor discussed the possibility of transmission through recombinant factor VIII products. C.Q. tells you that they are going to get married and invites you to the wedding. She stops at the door and says, "At least we won't have to worry about 'safe sex' with each other!"

Case Study 3: Human Immunodeficiency Virus/ Acquired Immune Deficiency Syndromes

Difficulty: **	*Setting:* Hospital
Index Words: Human immunodeficiency virus, acquired immune deficiency syndrome	

K.D. is a 36-year-old gay professional man who has been HIV positive for 6 years. Until recently, he demonstrated no signs or symptoms of AIDS. The appearance of purplish spots on his neck and arms persuaded him to make an appointment with his physician. Upon arrival at the doctor's office, the nurse performed a brief assessment. His VS were 138/86, 100, 30, 100.8°F. K.D. stated that he had been feeling fatigued for several months and is experiencing occasional night sweats but he had been working long hours, was skipping meals, and had been particularly stressed over a project at work. K.D.'s physical was within normal limits except for his low-grade fever and skin lesions. The doctor ordered a CBC, lymphocyte studies, and a PPD. K.D. made an appointment to return in 5 days to discuss the results of his tests.

Over the next 2 weeks, K.D. developed a fever of 101°F, nonproductive cough, and increasing shortness of breath. At midnight he became acutely SOB, so his roommate, J.F., took K.D. to the ED where he was subsequently admitted to the hospital with probable *Pneumocystis carinii* pneumonia. Bronchoalveolar lavage examined under light microscopy confirmed the diagnosis. K.D.'s admission WBC and lymphocyte studies demonstrated a increased pattern of immunodeficiency from earlier studies. K.D. was placed on nasal oxygen, IV fluids, and IV trimethoprim/sulfamethazine (Septra).

1. What is *Pneumocystis carinii* pneumonia (PCP)? **[PD/k/PI/ct]**
   - *Pneumocystis carinii* is like a fungus that is normally found in the human lung, but it does not cause disease in healthy individuals; it develops when the host's immune systems are critically impaired.

2. What is the significance of the purplish spots over K.D.'s neck and arms? **[PD/ap/PI/ct]**
   - This is indicative of Kaposi's sarcoma, a neoplasm that begins in the skin but involves other organs; the malignancy is believed to be endothelial in origin.

3. Identify 4 nursing diagnoses for K.D. **[PD/an/PI,PSI/ct]**
   - Impaired gas exchange r/t PCP infection.
   - Risk for respiratory failure r/t PCP.
   - Risk for infection r/t immunosuppression.
   - Anxiety r/t PCP complication.
   - Fear r/t diagnosis of AIDS.

4. What precautions will you need to use when caring for K.D.? **[PI/ap/P,I/ct,ni]**
   - Universal blood and body fluid precautions.

5. What will be the focus of your ongoing assessment (list 5)? **[P,I/an/PI,ct,ni]**
   - Lung sounds, oxygenation status, vital signs (e.g., indications of infection such as fever, chills); fluid and electrolyte status; laboratory values.

6. What major side effects of the drug Septra should you monitor K.D. for? **[P/c/S/PI/ct]**
   - Rashes, N/V, severe diarrhea, phlebitis at IV site, aplastic anemia, agranulocytosis, anaphylaxis.

7. Compare and contrast HIV positive status with AIDS. **[PD/c/PI/ct]**
   - HIV-positive status indicates that the person has become infected with the virus and has produced antibodies to HIV; HIV positive individuals are not necessarily sick and may not know they are infected; people with AIDS are HIV positive and also have signs and symptoms of immune deficiency and/or opportunistic infections.

8. Why is K.D.'s development of PCP of particular importance in light of his HIV status? **[PD/k/PI/ct]**
   - It indicates that he has developed the disease, AIDS, and is no longer immunocompetent enough to fight off infections that do not generally cause disease.

9. K.D. has been seropositive for several years, yet has been asymptomatic for AIDS. What factors may have influenced K.D.'s development of pneumocystis? **[PD/c/PI/ct]**
   - He had been under considerable pressure at work, has been working long hours, and not maintaining good eating habits; such "cofactors" may have triggered activation of the virus-producing immunodeficiency and allowing opportunity for *pneumocystis* to cause illness.

K.D. is responding well to treatment and plans are being made for discharge. He will be started on AZT therapy and inhaled pentamidine, and followed on an outpatient basis.

10. K.D. was taught about disease transmission and safe sex, as well as encouraged to maintain good exercise, rest, and dietary habits when he was diagnosed as HIV positive. Give at least 4 additional topics that should be discussed with K.D. before he goes home. **[P,I/an/S,PI,PSI/ct,ni,tc]**
    - He should avoid persons with infections.
    - He should understand the signs/symptoms of infections.
    - He should understand the importance of follow-up care.
    - He should be given written information about area support services.

11. What laboratory data will most likely be monitored on K.D. in the future? **[PD/c/S,PI/ct]**
    - Total lymphocyte count, absolute B and T cell counts and helper/suppressor cell ratios, CBC, platelets, and routine blood chemistries.

12. List at least 5 other opportunistic infections that K.D. is at risk for developing. **[PD/c/PI/ct]**
    - *Candida albicans*, *cryptosporidium*, toxoplasmosis, *Mycobacterium pneumonia*, cytomegalovirus (CMV); herpes simplex, histoplasmosis, tuberculosis.

Case Study 4: Cardiomyopathy/Heart Transplant

Difficulty: **	*Setting:* Hospital
Index Words: Cardiomyopathy, cardiac transplant	

J.P., a 56-year-old man, developed a severe viral infection and suffered fatigue, fever, and myalgia. Although he recovered from the acute episode, J.P. never quite regained normal activity level. Six months later, J.P. continued to find it difficult to work a 10-hour day as a brick mason so he returned to his physician. Diagnostic studies revealed CHF r/t postviral cardiomyopathy. Following medical management with digoxin (Lanoxin) and furosemide (Lasix), his condition stabilized and he returned to work, but his attendance was erratic. J.P.'s condition gradually deteriorated, and he was readmitted to the hospital 16 months later with complaints of dyspnea with minimal exertion, fatigue, orthopnea, chest pain, anorexia, and feelings of abdominal fullness. He had 1 + peripheral edema and was diaphoretic. Further studies revealed that J.P. had cardiac dilation, moderate to gross ventricular hypertrophy, and poor systolic ejection fraction, consistent with severe congestive cardiomyopathy. Because J.P.'s only other health problem is mild hypertension, heart transplant evaluation was recommended. J.P. and his wife discussed his prognosis and agreed to an evaluation for possible heart transplantation.

1. If J.P. is accepted for cardiac transplantation, what data will be collected in addition to his past medical history, current diagnostic findings, and cardiac evaluation? **[P/an/PI,PSI/ct]**
   - Pulmonary, renal, and infectious disease evaluation; laboratory data including hematologic, immunologic, biochemical, virologic, and microbiologic evaluation; evaluation for other chronic illnesses; psychologic evaluation; and potential for compliance.

2. What criteria for heart transplantation does J.P. meet that will make him eligible for cardiac transplantation? **[PD/ap/PI,PSI/ct]**
   - He is only 56 years old, he has severe heart disease despite medical therapy, he is psychologically stable, he is capable of understanding the procedure and compliance requirements, and he is a nonsmoker.

3. Cite 5 contraindications for cardiac transplant. **[PD/k/PI/ct]**
   - Active infection; active ulcer disease; pulmonary hypertension; pulmonary function less than 60% of predicted or history of chronic bronchitis; severe peripheral vascular disease, irreversible organ dysfunction; malignancy; or high risk for life-threatening noncompliance (cognitively impaired, psychologic instability, recent history of drug or alcohol abuse, smoker, no established address, previous demonstration of repeated noncompliance).

4. J.P. is accepted for cardiac transplant and placed on the waiting list. What fears or concerns may J.P. experience during this waiting period? **[PD/ap/PSI/ct]**
   - Fear that his condition may worsen and he could die before a suitable donor is found; guilt/concern that another person must die in order for him to receive a heart; dependency on medication for survival; not knowing when or where the transplant will take place; fears regarding recovery and survival of the graft.

J.P. received a phone call to report to the hospital immediately because a donor heart had become available.

5. What compatibility tests are preformed to determine eligibility for transplantation and to ensure as close a match as possible? **[PD/k/PI/ct]**
   - Identical ABO blood groups and body size and weight.
   - A Panel Reactive Antibody (PRA) testing is done to ensure relative immunologic compatibility between the donor and recipient; the recipient's serum is incubated with a random pool of lymphocytes. The crossmatch is negative if no lymphocytes are destroyed, and the recipient has no preformed antibodies. This means the transplant can be performed. The crossmatch is positive if lymphocytes are destroyed, and indicates the recipient has preformed antibodies. This means the transplant cannot be performed because the recipient is likely to reject.
   - Donor-specific crossmatching is usually not done because of time limitations.

6. As the nurse on the transplant unit, how can you best help J.P. prepare for his heart transplant? **[P,I/an/PI/ct]**
   - Establish a trusting relationship with J.P. and his wife; answer their questions honestly; encourage them to express their fears and concerns; allow them time together when possible; explain all care, procedures, and ICU routines; inform them about where his wife may wait during the surgery and about visitation following the surgery; ask J.P. and his wife if he has given advanced directives and made out a will.

J.P.'s surgery and recovery were uncomplicated and he was sent home and referred to cardiac rehabilitation after adjustment of his immunosuppression therapy and appropriate teaching. J.P. was readmitted for low grade fever and dyspnea 6 weeks after surgery. Cardiac biopsies demonstrated moderate acute rejection.

7. What is the etiology of acute rejection and how does it differ from chronic rejection? **[PD/k/PI/ct]**
   - Acute rejection occurs within the first 3 months after transplantation and is cell mediated; an antigen on the transplanted heart prompts lymphocytes to mature into helper T cells that, in turn, increase the production of killer T cells. Killer T cells attack the transplanted heart and cause rejection. Unfortunately, patients remain asymptomatic because they are on immunosuppression drugs; therefore, rejection must be diagnosed by endocardial biopsy.
   - Chronic rejection occurs 3 months or more following transplantation and is mediated by both T and B cells that cause progressive CAD (coronary artery disease) and limits long-term survival. Also, because the transplanted heart lacks nervous connection with the rest of the body, the patient will not experience angina to warn of CAD; prognosis depends on severity of the reaction.

8. The nurse can anticipate that prompt immunosuppressive therapy will be instituted using what drug? How does this drug alter the rejection process? **[PD/k/PI/ct]**
   - The standard immunosuppressive therapy used for organ rejection is Solumedrol IV bolus, then taper down to a maintenance dose of prednisone; steroids prevent antigen recognition, thereby reducing lymphocyte migration to the donor organ.
   - If the patient does not respond to the increased dose of steroids, muromonab-CD3 (Orthoclone OKT-3) is tried; this drug reverses acute rejection by blocking the maturation and function of T cells.

9. What is the most important nursing intervention for J.P. at this time and why? **[P,I/ap/PSI/ct,ni]**
   - Providing emotional support; J.P. will be very fearful about the possible loss of the transplanted heart.

J.P. responded positively to steroid therapy and was released to home after 5 days. J.P. was again admitted to the hospital with renewed complaints of dyspnea, low-grade fever, and ankle swelling 7 months later. Both J.P. and his wife are anxious and fearful.

10. Explain what may be happening to J.P. physiologically. **[PD/c/PI/ct]**
    - J.P. is likely experiencing chronic graft rejection; due either to an ongoing, low-grade, immunologic injury to the heart muscle, or accelerated graft atherosclerosis involving diffuse disease.

11. How will treatment for this episode of graft rejection differ from treatment for his earlier episode of rejection? **[PD/k/PI/ct]**
    - Treatment will be the same, IV Solumedrol and prednisone; adjustments may be made to his oral immunosuppressant drugs.

12. J.P.'s prognosis for the future will depend on what factors? **[PD/c/PI/ct]**
    - His response to IV steroids, the extent of tissue damage that is currently present, the degree of rejection persistence, his attitude and compliance to the posttransplant regimen, and his psychologic status.

Case Study 5: Cadaveric Kidney Transplant

Difficulty: **	*Setting:* Hospital
Index Words: Cadaveric kidney transplant, chronic renal failure	

W.V. is a 47-year-old man who lives with his wife and 2 teen-aged sons. W.V. developed chronic renal failure 12 years ago after acute renal failure due to phenacetin use. W.V. has taken phenacetin since his early 20s for migraine headaches. Large doses of phenacetin over the years can cause analgesic-induced nephropathy. This drug was subsequently removed from the market. W.V. was initially placed on hemodialysis but was switched to peritoneal dialysis so he could remain employed as an auto mechanic. Three months ago W.V. received a cadaveric transplant, or cadaver kidney. He recovered without complications and his serum laboratory values returned to normal. He was placed on immunosuppressive therapy, including cyclosporine (Sandimmune), and prednisone (Orasone) and was discharged to home. W.V. returned to work 3 weeks later.

Today W.V. reported to his physician for routine follow-up. His VS are 148/92, 88, 24, 99.2°F. His lab data revealed a serum creatinine 1.2 mg/dl and BUN 22 mg/dl, with normal serum electrolytes. W.V. has gained 5 pounds since discharge from the hospital.

1. What histocompatibility studies are generally performed before renal transplant and why are they important? **[PD/k/PI/ct]**
   - ABO compatibility: compatibility for red cell ABO antigens; incompatibility would result in the occurrence of hyperacute organ rejection.
   - HLA (human leukocyte antigen): individuals presensitized to major human HLA, through multiple pregnancies or frequent transfusions, are at high risk for harboring such "preformed" antibodies; a positive crossmatch indicates the presence of preformed antibodies that would result in early rejection; tissue matching is used to provide the closest possible match to decrease the possibility of organ rejection.

2. By what criteria was W.V. considered a good candidate for renal transplantation? **[PD/c/PI/ct]**
   - Younger than age 70, absence of chronic illnesses, potential for increased quality of life, history of compliance with required restrictions.

3. If W.V.'s kidney is producing sufficient urine and he is feeling well, why is it necessary to monitor his laboratory data? **[A/c/PI/ct]**
   - To detect impending disease or rejection of his transplanted kidney.

4. What is the possible significance of W.V.'s current blood pressure? **[PD/an/PI/ct]**
   - One blood pressure reading is not necessarily significant, but because it is above the 140/90 standard for a "normal" blood pressure, it should be compared with baseline studies to determine if this is normal for him or represents a change in BP status.

5. How does the drug cyclosporine (Sandimmune) protect W.V.'s kidney from rejection, and what are the most important side effects of this drug that W.V. must be taught to monitor? **[P/k/PI/ct]**
   - It inhibits rejection of transplanted tissues by inhibiting normal immune responses; the exact mechanism, however, is not known. It is thought to inhibit T-helper and T-suppressor cells and the production of T cell growth factor.
   - The most important side effects are tremors, HTN, nephrotoxicity, hirsutism, and gingival hyperplasia.

6. Because of the side effects of cyclosporine, how will W.V. know if he is experiencing organ rejection? **[A/ap/PI/ct,ni,tc]**
   - W.V.'s kidney will begin to fail if he experiences rejection; he should be taught to monitor his I&O, weight, and BP and immediately notify his physician of significant changes.
   - W.V. should be taught the signs/symptoms of hypersensitivity to cyclosporins: wheezing, dyspnea, flushed skin, hypotension, or hypertension.
   - Nephrotoxicity will be monitored through periodic serum BUN, creatinine, and Mg levels.
   - Hepatotoxicity is monitored through serum AST, ALT, alkaline phosphatase, amylase, and bilirubin levels.
   - Serum cyclosporine levels will be periodically evaluated and the dose adjusted accordingly.

7. If W.V. begins to reject his kidney, how would the rejection be classified, and what signs and symptoms would most likely be present? **[PD/k/PI/ct]**
   - Because he is 3 months posttransplant, the rejection would be classified as a chronic rejection.
   - W.V. would experience signs/symptoms of renal failure, such as weight gain, increased blood pressure, increasing BUN and serum creatinine, electrolyte imbalance, nausea, fatigue, and possibly abdominal tenderness or swelling of kidney.

8. Identify at least 4 ways that W.V. might experience difficulty adjusting to his organ transplant. **[PD/an/PI,PSI/ct]**
   - Financial difficulties r/t cost of immunosuppressive therapy.
   - Fear and anxiety over the possibility of organ rejection.
   - Dependency on medication for the remainder of his life.
   - Fear of infection r/t continual immunosuppression.
   - Adjustments in lifestyle patterns.
   - Guilt r/t receiving his kidney as the result of the death of another human being.

9. How can you best support W.V. and his family? **[P,I/an/PI,PSI/ct,ni,tc]**
   - Establish and maintain open communication; encourage W.V. and his family to ask questions; give straightforward, easily understood answers to all questions.
   - Offer support and assistance; make sure they have all important information in writing.
   - Teach W.V. and his family how to contact his physician or the transplant nurse if problems occur.
   - Provide education as needed.

10. Why is it necessary for W.V. to be concerned about infection? **[PD/c/PI/ct]**
    - W.V. is significantly immunosuppressed because of the cyclosporine and prednisone; persons who are immunosuppressed to prevent organ rejection are at increased risk for the development of a variety of infections, including tumors and opportunistic infections.

Case Study 6: Acquired Immune Deficiency Syndrome

Difficulty: *** *Setting:* Hospital

Index Words: Acquired immune deficiency syndrome

D.C. is a 32-year-old white clerical worker who lives with his 76-year-old grandmother, his primary caregiver. He was diagnosed as being HIV positive 3 months ago and has been under close outpatient medical supervision for the past 3 weeks because of persistent fever, pulmonary infiltrates, and nonspecific flu like symptoms. He is admitted to your nursing unit for fever, chills, sweats, myalgias, malaise, chest pain, dry nonproductive cough, axillary adenopathy, nausea, vomiting, and severe diarrhea. Admission VS are 108/84, 104, 30, 103.5°F. Following aggressive diagnostic workup, D.C. was diagnosed with AIDS complicated by *Pneumocystis carinii* pneumonia, cryptosporidiosis, oral candidiasis, and cytomegalovirus (CMV) infection.

Today is D.C.'s third day postadmission to the hospital. He remains acutely ill; however, his hydration status has improved and he is experiencing fewer than 8 diarrhea stools per day. He is not yet able to keep food or fluids down; therefore, TPN is being considered. D.C. complains of headache, nausea, continued fatigue, and muscle soreness. He is able to ambulate to the bathroom with assistance.

1. Why was D.C. diagnosed as having AIDS rather than complicated HIV infection? **[PD/c/PI/ct]**
   - When HIV infected individuals develop signs and symptoms of immune deficiency they are placed in the "AIDS" category.

2. Considering D.C.'s AIDS status, what findings are likely to be present when you receive the results of his lymphocyte studies? **[PD/c/PI/ct]**
   - Decreased total lymphocyte count: decreased absolute T cell and B cell counts and an inverse T-helper cell/T-suppressor cell ratio.

3. Provide a possible explanation for D.C.'s rapid conversion from HIV positive to AIDS. **[PD/an/PI/ct]**
   - The virus did not enter a dormant phase, which would have allowed D.C. to remain asymptomatic for a longer period of time.

     OR
   - An infection accelerated his development of AIDS.

4. As D.C.'s nurse, list at least 2 observations you would monitor in relation to each of the following infections: cryptosporidiosis, candidiasis, and CMV. **[P,I/an/PI/ct,ni]**
   - Cryptosporidiosis is an enteric parasite that causes severe diarrhea: you would observe and record the number, amount, and consistency of each stool; monitor for fluid and electrolyte imbalance; carefully inspect the skin around anus and buttocks for breakdown; assess weakness and fatigue levels because of the chronic inability to tolerate PO food or fluids, severe diarrhea, and electrolyte imbalance.
   - Candidiasis is type of fungal infection; oral mucous membranes should be visually inspected for erosions and plaques on the gingiva, palate, and hypopharynx; inspect around anus for signs of *Candida albicans* infection; administer nystatin (Mycostatin) oral suspension swish and swallow or troches as directed.
   - CMV is a member of the herpes virus family; note diarrhea, weight loss, and persistent fever; observe for blood in the stool.

5. Given the above possible problems that D.C. could encounter, which of the following nursing orders would be appropriate? Label each with "A" for appropriate or "I" for inappropriate and correct the inappropriate orders. **[E/an/S,PI/ct,ni]**

   ___ Monitor VS every 12 hours.
   ___ Assist with ADL as needed.
   ___ Keep perineal area clean and dry; use protective skin cream.
   ___ Regular diet.
   ___ Monitor lungs, skin, abdomen, and urine output once per shift.
   ___ Maintain complete bed rest.
   ___ Use toothettes or soft-bristled brush for oral hygiene.
   ___ Exclude diarrhea stool from I&O measurements.
   ___ Monitor IV site for signs of inflammation; change site if red or swollen.

   Answers:

   _I_ Monitor VS every 12 hours (q2-4h).
   _A_ Assist with ADL as needed.
   _A_ Keep perineal area clean and dry; use protective skin cream.
   _I_ Regular diet (once D.C. can tolerate PO, he should receive a mechanical soft diet).
   _I_ Monitor lungs, skin, abdomen, and urine output q shift (q2-4h).
   _I_ Maintain complete bed rest (activities as tolerated to maintain mobility).
   _A_ Use toothettes or soft bristled brush for oral hygiene.
   _I_ Exclude diarrhea stool from I&O measurements (included because diarrhea stools are an important part of D.C.'s fluid loss).
   _A_ Monitor IV site for signs of inflammation; change site if red or swollen.

6. D.C. is restless at times because of his muscle soreness. Upon entering his room you note that he has pulled out his peripheral IV and is bleeding. How should you respond? **[P,I/ap/S,PI/ct]**
   - First glove then apply pressure to the IV site to stop the bleeding; restart the IV in another area.

7. Cite at least 5 findings that would indicate D.C.'s condition is stabilizing or improving. **[PD/an/PI/ct]**
   - Clear lung sounds; soft, nontender abdomen with normal bowel sounds; return of normal stools; ability to tolerate PO food and fluids; return of oral mucous membranes to normal color and appearance; ability to perform his own ADL.

8. What assessment findings would the physician take into consideration when making the decision to place D.C. on TPN? **[E/an/PI/ct]**
   - Weight loss; presence of fluid and electrolyte imbalances; continued inability to tolerate PO foods and fluids; persistent diarrhea.

9. Given that D.C.'s grandmother is his primary caregiver, discuss the implications of D.C.'s diagnosis of AIDS. **[P,I/an/PI,PSI/ct,ni,tc]**
   - D.C.'s grandmother may not be financially, physically, or psychologically able to care for D.C. when his condition worsens. A social services consultation needs to be initiated to offer both D.C. and his grandmother assistance as his condition deteriorates.

10. Would D.C. require additional teaching regarding his ability to transmit HIV now that he has AIDS? **[PD/c/PI/ct]**
    - No, provided D.C. has already been taught about transmissibility of HIV; you should assess and reinforce his understanding of his disease.

11. D.C. begins to slowly respond to treatment, and discharge plans are begun. Cite at least 3 ways that D.C.'s post-AIDS care will differ from his pre-AIDS care. **[P,I/an/S,PI/ct,ni,tc]**
    - He is likely to develop infections more readily; he must avoid people with infections; he should be taught good handwashing techniques; must be taught how to quickly recognize sign/symptoms of infection and when to contact his physician.
    - He will be placed on a combination of antiretrovirus drugs, such as zidovudine (Retrovir) or cyanothymidine (CNT), and zalcitibine (DDC) or dideoxyinosine (DDI) to control the progression of the disease.
    - He may be a candidate for central line placement.
    - He will require closer follow-up monitoring.

12. How does AZT work to control progression of HIV? Can you confirm or refute this explanation? **[PD/c/PI/ct]**
    - AZT enters the virally-infected cells and is incorporated into the DNA of HIV. Replication is halted because AZT is a false building block that cannot replicate.

Case Study 7: Systemic Lupus Erythematosus

Difficulty: ***	*Setting:* Home, hospital
Index Words: Systemic lupus erythematosus	

D.W. is a 23-year-old married woman with 3 children under the age of 5. She presented to her physician 2 years ago with vague complaints of intermittent fatigue, joint pain, and low-grade fever. Her physician noted small patchy areas of vitiligo and a scaly rash across her nose, cheeks, back, and chest at that time. Laboratory studies revealed that D.W. had a positive antinuclear antibody titer, positive LE (lupus erythematosus) cell prep, elevated C-reactive protein and ESR (erythrocytesedimentation rate), and decreased C3 and C4 serum complement. Joint x-rays demonstrated joint swelling without joint erosion. D.W. was subsequently diagnosed with systemic lupus erythematosus. She was initially treated with sulindac (Clinopri) 200 mg PO bid and prednisone (Deltasone) 20 mg PO qd, bed rest, ice packs, and aspirin to control discomfort. She was counseled regarding her condition, advised to balance rest and activity, eat a well-balanced diet, use strategies to reduce stress, and avoid direct sunlight. D.W. responded well to treatment and was eventually told she could report for follow-up every 6 months unless her symptoms became acute. D.W. resumed her job in environmental services at a large geriatric facility.

1. What is the significance of each of D.W.'s laboratory findings? **[PD/ap/PI/ct]**
   - Positive antinuclear antibody titer: she has produced antibodies against the DNA of her own cells.
   - Positive LE cell prep: she has produced a particular cell indicative of lupus erythematosus.
   - Elevated C-reactive protein: she has an active inflammatory process taking place.
   - Elevated ESR: she is producing a large number of lymphocytes associated with an active inflammatory process.
   - Decreased C2 and C3 serum complement: serum levels are low, indicating the presence of an active immune response, in which complement has been summoned from the plasma to the area of immune response.

2. How does cutaneous lupus erythematosus differ from systemic lupus? **[PD/k/PI/ct]**
   - Cutaneous lupus is a milder form of the disease that generally affects only the skin; systemic lupus is a severe form of the disease that can affect all organs and cause severe damage.

3. What priority problems need to be addressed with D.W.? **[P,I/an/PI,PSI/ct,ni,tc]**
   - Impaired skin integrity.
   - Knowledge deficit regarding lupus, treatment, complications, and follow up care.

Eighteen months after diagnosis, D.W. sought out her physician because of puffy hands and feet and increased fatigue. D.W. reported that she had been working longer hours because of the absence of 2 of her fellow workers. Diagnostic evaluation revealed that her BUN and serum creatinine were slightly elevated, and that she had 2+ protein and 1+ RBC in her urine.

4. Of what significance are these findings, and what is the relationship of such findings to D.W.'s diagnosis of lupus erythematosus? **[PD/c/Pl/ct]**
   - She is likely developing glomerulonephritis secondary to her lupus; immune complexes are formed against connective tissues that are eliminated through the kidneys; the immune complexes are too large to be filtered and, thus, collect within the glomerulus, eventually destroying the basement membrane; as the process continues, D.W. is at risk for the development of chronic renal failure.

5. How will D.W.'s treatment and nursing plan likely change? **[PD/an/Pl/ct]**
   - Her dosage of prednisone will be increased, and her renal function will be closely monitored. If she does not respond, further immunosuppression may be necessary to prevent permanent renal damage. Nursing care will include measures to prevent and detect renal failure (monitoring urine output, blood pressure, electrolytes, BUN, serum creatinine, and other signs and symptoms of renal failure), as well as teaching D.W. about use of steroids and other immunosuppressive agents.

D.W. was seen in the immunology clinic twice monthly during the next 3 months. Although her condition did not worsen, her BUN and serum creatinine remained elevated. While at work one afternoon, D.W. began to feel dizzy and developed a severe headache. She reported to her supervisor who had her lie down. When D.W. started to become disoriented, her supervisor called 911 and had D.W. taken to the hospital. D.W. was admitted for probable lupus cerebritis related to acute exacerbation of her disease.

6. What preventive measures should be instituted to protect D.W. at this time? **[P/ap/S/ct,ni]**
   - Because D.W. is experiencing CNS involvement, seizure precautions and measures to protect her safety should be implemented.

7. What additional problems indicative of CNS involvement related to systemic lupus should D.W. be assessed for? **[PD/an/Pl/ct]**
   - Visual disturbances, vertigo, nystagmus, aphasia, insomnia, confusion, hallucinations, or further disorientation.

D.W. is again placed on IV methylprednisolone and started on plasmapheresis.

8. What major complications associated with immunosuppression therapy will D.W. have to be monitored for? **[PD/ap/Pl/ct]**
   - Infections, secondary malignancies, bone marrow suppression, and liver toxicity.

9. What does plasmapheresis do, and why might it reduce the signs and symptoms associated with systemic lupus? **[PD/c/PI/ct]**
   - Plasmapheresis involves filtering immune complexes from the blood. By removing immune complexes, there will be fewer complexes available to damage tissues or organs, thus, possibly reducing the signs and symptoms associated with systemic lupus.

10. What data would support the assumption that D.W.'s condition is stabilizing? **[PD/ap/PI/ct]**
    - An increase in her serum complement; a decrease in her BUN, creatinine, sedimentation rate, and anti-DNA antibody titer coupled with improvement in her symptoms.

11. Identify at least 4 topics that D.W. must be taught before she is discharged that may help her lead as normal a life as possible. **[P/an/PI,PSI/ct,ni,tc]**
    - Systemic lupus may progress in spite of all her efforts to avoid exacerbations.
    - Indications of exacerbating disease.
    - Indications of complications, such as lung infections.
    - The need for close follow-up care.
    - Medications and their potential side effects.
    - Methods for dealing with stress.
    - Support groups available in her area.

12. You note that D.W.'s husband is visiting her this afternoon. You enter the room to ask if they have any questions. D.W.'s husband states, "I have tried to tell her that she cannot go back to work. Sure we need the money but the kids and I need her more. I'm afraid that this lupus has weakened her whole body and it will kill her if she goes back to work. Is that right?" How would you respond to his concerns? **[PD/an/PI,PSI/ct,ni,tc]**
    - Lupus is a progressive disease that eventually involves the entire body. It is not wise for D.W. to work outside the home. Suggest that the social worker meet with them to discuss community services available to them.

CHAPTER 9. ONCOLOGIC/HEMATOLOGIC DISORDERS

Case Study 1: Infiltrating Ductal Carcinoma—Breast

Difficulty: *	*Setting:* Outpatient clinic, support group
Index Words: Breast cancer	

B.B., a 53-year-old divorced professional woman, was diagnosed with stage T1 N0 infiltrating ductal breast cancer based on a lumpectomy and axillary lymph node dissection over a year ago. After her radiation therapy (daily treatments for 6 weeks) was completed, she was placed on tamoxifen for an indefinite period. She has been coming to the clinic every 3 months for her checkup. In addition to working at the clinic, you are a volunteer consultant to the Encore-YWCA support group for women who have had breast cancer that B.B. attends regularly. The group invited you to present "Breast Cancer: Prevention, Screening, and Detection Guidelines" at their next meeting.

1. Describe estrogen replacement therapy (ERT) and the relationship to breast cancer. **[P/k/Pl/ct]**
   - Breast cancer tumors are thought to depend on hormones to stimulate their growth. Estrogen replacement therapy may contribute to an occurrence or recurrence of breast cancer. Many postmenopausal women receive ERT because it may help them feel better; in addition ERT may decrease their risk of coronary artery disease and osteoporosis. Current guidelines recommend that an individual discussion in which benefits and risks are evaluated should be conducted between the physician and the woman before initiating or continuing ERT.

2. What is tamoxifen? Why are women placed on long-term tamoxifen therapy as a treatment for breast cancer? **[P,I/c/Pl/ct]**
   - Tamoxifen is an antiestrogen drug. Most commonly, it is used to treat postmenopausal women with breast cancer whose tumor cells are positive for estrogen receptors.

3. What is an axillary lymph node dissection? Why did B.B. have an axillary lymph node dissection with her lumpectomy? **[PD/c/Pl/ct]**
   - When a woman has surgery for breast cancer, whether lumpectomy or mastectomy, the surgeon takes out a set of lymph nodes in the axillary area on the same side of the body. The cancer cells are examined by a pathologist who makes the diagnosis. The lymph nodes are examined to see if there is cancer in any of them; if so, the number of lymph nodes with cancer compared to the total number of lymph nodes removed are used to stage the person's breast cancer.

4. B.B. was diagnosed with stage T1 NO breast cancer. What does that mean? **[PD/c/PI,PSI/ct]**
   - This means that her breast lump was $\leq$2 cm and none of the lymph nodes was malignant. Tumor size and number of lymph nodes are the most important predictors for survival.

5. What risk factors for breast cancer will you include in your group presentation? **[A,P/k/PI,PSI/ct,tc]**
   - Risk factors include:
     - Gender (female > male).
     - Age (increases with age; e.g., most persons are diagnosed at 40 years of age or older).
     - Personal history of cancer (previous diagnosis of breast, ovarian, or endometrial cancer places one at greater risk).
     - Family history of cancer (first degree relative—mother/sister/daughter).
     - Early menarche and late menopause.
     - Reproductive history (women having no children or the first full-term pregnancy after age 30 has increased risk).
     - Obesity, especially with a male-pattern fat distribution (high waist-hip ratio).
     - Diet high in fat.
     - Radiation exposure.
     - Exogenous hormones (oral contraceptives and/or estrogen replacement therapy).

6. What will you teach them about early detection of breast cancer? **[A,PD/c/PI,HP/ct,ni,tc]**
   - *Monthly* breast self exam (BSE) should be performed by all women age 20 years and older; 90% of all palpable breast lumps are found through BSE.
   - A *thorough* clinical breast exam by a professional should be performed at scheduled health care visits.
   - Mammography is the only proven means of detecting breast cancer before it can be detected by BSE or physical exam; the size of the average lump found by BSE is >1 cm, the average size lump detected by mammogram is <0.5 cm. Mammography should begin at age 40; routine screening mammography every 1 to 2 years at ages 40 to 49, and every year past age 50. *A woman with known risk factors should discuss with her physician the frequency and specificity of mammography and clinical breast exams.*

7. What educational equipment can help women learn how to correctly perform BSE and how to detect lumps? **[A/k/PI,HP/ct]**
   - Breast molds are usually available from the local chapter of the American Cancer Society; in addition, the educational division of hospitals often use breast molds for demonstration and practice purposes. Have women describe and demonstrate BSE with return demonstration from all participants. Some women may have a spouse or significant other learn how to perform the breast exam on them.

<u>*Instructor Note:*</u> Many women who have had breast cancer report they found their lump in the shower when the skin over their breast was wet and slippery.

8. Describe the technique for performing BSE correctly. **[A,P/k/Pl/ct]**
   - Palpation is performed with the pads of the fingers; move your fingers in small circles, about the size of a dime; varying levels of pressure should be applied to each quadrant of the breast and the tail of spence; cover the entire breast in a clockwise motion (self-palpation is usually done lying down with the opposite arm under the head); inspect your breasts in a standing position with hands on hips, leaning forward, and hands behind your back; note any dimpling of tissue, erythema, presence of nevi, and/or skin retraction.
   - Perform BSE on a regular schedule (5 days postmenses in premenopausal women, the first day of the month for postmenopausal women).
   - Provide an American Cancer Society BSE brochure or written literature of similar quality to reinforce your teaching.

9. One of the women in the group shows you how the arm on the side with the breast cancer is more swollen than the other arm. She said she is having a lot of trouble with this. What do you think is happening? How will you explain this to her? What will you advise her? **[A,PD/an/Pl,PSI/ct,tc]**
   - This woman probably has developed lymphedema. Anyone who has surgery for breast cancer also has an axillary lymph node dissection for disease staging. The removal of lymph nodes can contribute to a back-up of lymph fluid in the affected arm. This can be serious as well as painful. She should ask her physician for a referral to a lymphedema specialist—usually a physical therapist—for treatment immediately. The more lymphedema is neglected, the worse it gets.

10. B.B. raises her hand and tells you she heard she should never have her blood pressure taken in her affected arm (the arm on the side of the breast cancer). You remember you told her this in the office but realize she was probably too anxious or tired to remember what you said. What will you advise her and the other women present? **[PD,P/c/Pl/ct,tc]**
    - Lymphedema is a serious complication of breast cancer. Some women have trouble with it almost immediately, whereas others never have a problem. In some cases, the person is fine for years, then has a sudden episode of lymphedema develop. Emphasize they must protect themselves from overzealous or ignorant health care workers. *Under no circumstances should they ever permit* someone to take a blood pressure in that arm, permit needle sticks or an IV, or allow that arm to be used for immunizations or similar procedures.

11. What are some other things breast cancer survivors can do to manage or prevent lymphedema (list 4)? **[PD,P/ap/S,CI,PSI/ct]**
    - Watch for any sign of infection or swelling in the affected arm.
    - Wear a glove on that hand when working in the garden or areas where they may injure themselves.
    - At the first sign of infection or injury, immediately seek professional attention.
    - Keep the affected arm elevated on a pillow during rest and long periods in a sitting position (such as a trip in a car).
    - Avoid adding extra salt in the diet.
    - Don't overexert with that arm (consult a physical therapist about specific guidelines).
    - Follow prescribed treatment regimens.
    - Avoid trauma to the affected arm.
    - Avoid wearing clothing with constricting bands.
    - Avoid carrying heavy object, or hanging a purse on the affected arm.

Case Study 2: Sickle Cell Disease

Difficulty: *	*Setting:* Hospital
Index Words: Sickle cell disease, pulmonary edema	

V.M. is a 39-year-old black man who has sickle cell disease (SCD) marked by frequent episodes of severe pain. His anemia has been managed with multiple transfusions, and he shows signs of chronic renal failure. He is a nonsmoker, nondrinker, and is on Social Security disability. His regular medications are pentoxifylline (Trental), oxycodone/acetaminophen (Roxicet), and folic acid (Folvite). In hematology clinic this AM, V.M.'s Hgb measured 6.7 g/dl. He received 2 units PRC (packed red cells) over 3 hours and then went home. V.M. developed dyspnea and shortness of breath approximately 1 to 1½ hours later, and his wife called 911. The EMS (emergency medical system) crew initiated oxygen and transported V.M. to the ED.

1. What is sickle cell disease, and how is it related to race? **[PD/c/PI/ct]**
   - Hemoglobin S (HgS) is genetically inherited. Separation of oxygen from the HgS distorts the RBC (red blood cell) into a sickle shape; repeated deoxygenation results in permanent sickling of the RBC.
   - There is a high prevalence in people of black African descent; however, SCD is not limited to people of black descent.

2. The stiff, sickled RBC tends to cause vascular occlusions with subsequent local infarction. As a rule, the spleen suffers so many vasoocclusive/infarction episodes that it is greatly reduced in size and is rendered nonfunctional by the time the individual is 6 years of age. What are the implications of having a nonfunctioning spleen? **[PD/c/PI/ct]**
   - The individual will be more susceptible to infections throughout his/her lifetime.

3. Identify 2 mechanisms that contribute to anemia in patients with SCD. **[PD/c/PI/ct]**
   - RBCs are friable and rupture more easily than normal RBCs, causing the Hct and Hgb values to decline.
   - Vascular occlusions occurring in the kidneys lead to renal failure and result in decreased erythropoietin production; because erythropoietin is not stimulating the bone marrow, RBCs are not replaced, and the Hct and Hgb decline even more.

4. On arrival to the ED, the physician asks V.M. if he is in pain and if he needs Demerol. V.M. answers "No" to both questions. Why did the physician ask these 2 questions? **[PD/c/PI/ct]**
   - The physician is trying to determine if V.M. is in sickle cell crisis (SCC). The pain of SCC is often severe and frequently includes bone pain. Episodes can last from a few days to several weeks. If the pain does not subside after 2 to 6 hours of IM or IV narcotic therapy in the ED, then admission for pain management is required; patients in crisis are typically hospitalized for 1 week.

5. V.M.'s ABGs on 9 L O_2/simple face mask are pH 7.34, PaO_2 74 mm Hg, $PaCO_2$ 33 mm Hg, HCO_3 18 mEq/L, BE -6. Is V.M. being adequately oxygenated, why or why not? **[PD/ap/PI/ct]**
   - No, he is not being adequately oxygenated: with an oxygen flow rate of 7 to 10 L/min, a simple face mask would deliver approximately 60% oxygen; V.M.'s PaO_2 of 74 mm Hg is very low for someone receiving 60% O_2.

6. V.M. complains of being short of breath. Do you believe his low Hgb level is responsible for his complaints? **[PD/ap/PI/ct]**
   - Not likely; although patients with SCD have marked anemia, it is usually well tolerated. This AM, V.M.'s Hgb was 6.7 g/dl before receiving 2 units PRCs; the transfusion should have increased his Hct by 3% per unit and his Hgb by 1 g/unit; his Hgb should be approximately 8.7 g/dl at this time.
   - He did not begin to experience SOB until 1 to 1½ hours after the transfusion.

You perform a quick assessment and note a systolic murmur and crackles in V.M.'s bases bilaterally. VS are 176/102, 94, 28, 97°F (oral). As you start an IV, you draw blood for CBC, Chem 7, calcium, and phosphorous and send it for analysis.

7. Your assessment findings are consistent with fluid overload. What 4 findings led you to that conclusion? **[PD/c/PI/ct]**
   - V.M.'s VS are elevated.
   - 2 units of PRC were transfused over 3 hours.
   - He began to experience SOB within 1½ hours of the transfusion.
   - You auscultated crackles in the bases of both lung fields, indicating fluid accumulation.

8. What action would you expect the physician to take next and why? **[PD/ap/PI/ct]**
   - The ED physician will prescribe Lasix for V.M. to stimulate diuresis.

The lab values return: Na 137 mEq/L, K 4.9 mEq/L, Cl 110 mEq/L, CO_2 16 mEq/L, BUN 27 mg/dl, creatinine 2.7 mg/dl, calcium 8.2 mg/dl, PO_4 4.7 mg/dl, WBC 4.3 mm^3, Hgb 7.8 g/dl, Hct 20.9%, platelets 208 mm^3.

9. What is the significance of the lab results and why? **[PD/an/PI/ct]**
   - The creatinine is elevated and the K is on the high side of normal; these results are consistent with CRF (chronic renal insufficiency).
   - The WBC is not elevated and he is not febrile; therefore, it is not likely that V.M.'s fluid overload was caused by a pulmonary infection; an inflammatory response would release vasoactive substances that alter the vascular permeability and allow fluid to leak out into the tissues.

The physician prescribes furosemide (Lasix) 20 mg IVP now, methylprednisolone (Solu-Medrol) 125 mg IVP, and ceftriaxone (Rocephin) 1 g IVPB after the Lasix.

10. Explain the significance of using each of these drugs. **[PD/c/PI/ct]**
    - The Lasix will promote diuresis and pull fluid out of the lungs.
    - The Solu-Medrol will inhibit any inflammatory response.
    - Because of his SCD, V.M. is very susceptible to pulmonary infections; the Rocephin is being used prophylactically to kill any invading organisms.

11. Why is it difficult to cross-match blood to transfuse V.M.? **[PD/k/PI/ct]**
    - Repeated transfusions of RBC over time result in alloimmunization: the sensitization to red blood cell antigens. The American Red Cross will need to match blood from their rare donor file; expect only 5 of every 1000 donors to match V.M.

As V.M.'s SOB is relieved, he shakes the physician's hand and thanks him for asking about the presence of pain and the need for pain medication. V.M. states, "One of my biggest fears is that I'll come here in crisis and the doctor won't treat my pain aggressively enough. I don't want to be labeled as a drug seeker or an emergency room abuser."

12. Why would V.M. be concerned about obtaining adequate pain control in the ED? **[PD/c/PSI/ct]**
    - It is easy for a patient like V.M. to become labeled as a drug seeker because there are no objective clinical signs by which to gauge if a patient is experiencing sickle cell pain crisis. Medical personnel must rely on the patient to indicate when pain relief is achieved. This uncertainty is uncomfortable for inexperienced physicians.
    - As a black man, V.M. belongs to a group that is highly stigmatized by health care professionals as substance abusers.

V.M. voids 1900 ml within 2 hours of the Lasix administration. On repeat assessment, the systolic murmur is audible, but all lung fields are clear. Repeat VS are 160/94, 82, 20, 98 °F (oral). V.M. is discharged to home on his previous medications.

13. What issues would you address with V.M. before he is discharged? **[P,I/an/S,PI/ct,ni,tc}**
    - Teach him that fluid overload may be prevented by administering each unit of blood over 3 to 4 hours; instruct him to inform the physician/nurse to infuse his blood over a longer period of time.
    - Discuss the need for him to plan his clinic visits to accommodate the expanded hours of RBC administration.
    - Allow V.M. to describe his symptoms related to transfusion overload, and reinforce that he seek medical attention at the first sign of fluid overload.

Case Study 3: Infiltrating Ductal Carcinoma—Breast

Difficulty: *	*Setting:* Outpatient clinic
Index Words: Cancer, breast cancer	

D.M. is a married, 36-year-old woman with 4 children who works part-time as a clerk. She is 68 in tall and weighs 135 lb. She has insurance through her husband's employer. She has never smoked and has an occasional social drink. She has PMH of plastic surgery for breast implants in August of last year. When she returned for her breast implant check-up 10 months later, a lump was discovered in her R breast. When a biopsy indicated the lump was malignant, she elected to have a lumpectomy and axillary lymph node dissection. Her CT scan and bone scans were negative. She was referred to the group oncology clinic where you are a staff nurse to receive chemotherapy. After she completes chemotherapy, she is scheduled to receive radiation therapy. Admitting diagnosis: infiltrating ductal carcinoma, stage T2 N1 MO, premenopausal, estrogen receptor-positive.

1. Explain the TNM method of staging malignancies. **[PD/k/PI/ct]**
   - T = the size, extent, and depth of the primary tumor. N = extent and location of involved regional lymph nodes. M = absence or presence of distant spread of disease.

2. D.M. wants you to explain exactly what stage T2 N1 MO means. What will you tell her? **[A,PD,P/c/PI,PSI/ct,ni,tc]**
   - First, assess how knowledgeable she is about cancer and what depth of knowledge she is capable of understanding.
   - Recognize that tumor size and number of involved lymph nodes are the two most predictive factors of survival chances in breast cancer.
   - T2 means the tumor is between 2 to 5 cm in diameter; N1 means there is metastasis to moveable ipsilateral axillary lymph nodes; MO means no distant metastases were discovered on her CT and bone scans.

3. She asks you to explain what her chances of survival are. How will you explain this to her? **[A,PD/c/PI,PSI/ct,ni,tc]**
   - The single most important predictor of disease recurrence and survival is the axillary lymph node status; survival is influenced by the number of lymph nodes involved.
   - Premenopausal estrogen receptor-positive infiltrating ductal breast carcinoma (stage T2; N1) usually requires more than one type of therapy to treat the disease. By combining surgery, combination chemotherapy, and radiation therapy, D.M. can have her best odds.

4. D.M. will be receiving 6 cycles of combination chemotherapy, consisting of doxirubicin (Adriamycin), cyclophosphamide (Cytoxan), and 5-fluorouracil (5-FU). What are the major side effects you want to prepare her for? **[PD/c/PI,PSI/ct]**
   - Major side effects are nausea and vomiting, hair loss, myelosuppression, and thrombocytopenia. You might suggest she think about getting a wig; reassure her the hair usually grows back in. Nausea and vomiting can frequently be controlled by medication. Her blood cell counts will drop: decreased WBCs result in immunosuppression; decreased platelet count contributes to greater risk of bleeding; and decreased red blood cells contributes to fatigue, dyspnea, and anemia.

5. What is a major complication in patients receiving a high amount of Adriamycin? **[PD/c/PI/ct]**
   - Patients receiving too much Adriamycin can develop heart damage; pulse and heart sounds should be monitored on a regular basis. Patients are only given a specific amount of Adriamycin to reduce the risk of damage.

6. Explain to D.M. in lay terms what she needs to know about immunosuppression. **[P,I/c/S,PI/ct,ni,tc]**
   - The drugs will affect her body so she won't be able to fight off infections and "germs" as well; this can be very serious because ordinary germs can make her sicker than usual. Sometimes this will be worse than other times in her cycle. There are things she can do to protect herself.
   - Stay away from people who are or think they are getting sick; children in daycare or school are especially likely to carry germs. Avoid crowded public places during her "low" times (when her WBC or AGC-absolute granulocyte count are down). Use her own, separate towel at home to dry her hands; use a dishwasher with the setting hotter than usual to wash dishes. Avoid raw fruits and vegetables during her "low" time. Use good mouth care with a recommended rinse to avoid infections. Avoid airline travel (some airplanes are poorly ventilated, and germs can spread through the air system).
   - Ask her to call you if she "catches" something; tell her not to wait until it gets too bad. Ask if she has a thermometer at home, and ask her to check herself for fever if she starts to feel ill. She should call you if she notices any of the following: (1) sore throat, cough, sniffy or stuffy nose; (2) burning or pain with urination or a bowel movement; (3) shaking chills; (4) pain, swelling, redness, and heat at skin injuries; or (5) drainage from eyes or ears. Although some clinics tell people to call with a temperature above 100.5°F (oral), this is highly individual. *Put these instructions in writing and give them to her.* Be sure to include the clinic's emergency telephone number with this information.

<u>*Instructor Note*</u>*:* Find out what the person's normal temperature is and adjust "fever" temperature accordingly. Some patients become extremely ill and never develop a fever. Recent research indicates that the "average" body temperature is closer to 97.6°F or lower rather than 98.6°F, especially in the AM.

D.M. completes her chemotherapy. She lost most of her hair and has been wearing a scarf but now her hair is beginning to grow back. She is being transferred to the radiation therapy department for treatment and is scheduled to begin radiation therapy.

7. What is hair loss called? Which drug was primarily responsible for the hair loss? **[A,PD/k/PI/ct]**
   - Hair loss is called alopecia; Doxirubicin is primarily responsible, but Cytoxan also contributes to alopecia.

You perform an admission assessment. Findings are: Wt. 148 lb. VS 104/70, 80, 20, 98.0°F (oral). Cardiovascular: S1 S2 without murmurs or rubs. Respiratory: clear to auscultation throughout. Neuromuscular/skeletal: negative, patient c/o of fatigue, no c/o bone pain. GI: without hepatosplenomegaly or masses. GU: negative. Integumentary/oral: hair growth ¼" over entire head, oral mucosa reddened and patient c/o soreness. Lymph node: no palpable adenopathy in the cervical, supraclavicular, axillary, or inguinal nodes.

8. What areas of the above assessment concern you? Explain. **[A/c/PI/ct]**
   - D.M. has gained 13 pounds during chemotherapy; this is a common experience during chemotherapy for breast cancer. Although the specific cause is unknown, it is probably related to changes in food preferences and decreased activity.
   - Fatigue is a common experience during and immediately following chemotherapy. She will also experience fatigue in response to radiation therapy; fatigue can seriously affect functioning and quality of life.
   - Her hair is starting to grow back. Sometimes, after doxirubicin, the hair grows back with a different color and texture.
   - Her mouth is still tender from the chemotherapy, but there is no evidence of white spots in her mouth to indicate infection.

D.M. received 6 weeks of daily (weekdays) radiation therapy treatments with a total dose of 6400 cGy. She had a terrible time with fatigue, and at one time, told you, "When I lie down, I can't be enough of the bed!" You helped her develop an activity-rest plan and supported her in obtaining outside help with housework. At her last visit, she tells you, "Now I hope I can see my kids grow up." She is scheduled to return to the oncologist every 3 months for follow-up care and monitoring.

9. D.M. comes to her scheduled follow-up appointment. She appears very anxious. When questioned she tells you, "I've been worried about my daughters. What if they get breast cancer? What can I do to help them?" What is your response? **[P/c/PI,PSI,HP/ct,ni,tc]**
   - Suggest community resources such as the American Cancer Society's I Can Cope, Reach for Recovery, and Y-ME as groups that may provide emotional support from others with similar experiences.
   - Explain breast cancer prevention guidelines for her daughters: BSE, frequency and onset of mammography, clinical breast exam (first-degree relatives have an increased risk for breast cancer occurrence).

10. You ask her if she has other questions. She tells you she is worried about the breast cancer coming back and wants to know if she would have to go through the chemotherapy and radiation therapy all over again. What can you do, and what will you tell her? **[A,PD,P/c/PI,PSI/ct,ni,tc]**
    - Assess her state of anxiety to see how much detail she can tolerate. If you think her anxiety is unusually high and/or if it is affecting her sleep or performance, ask the physician about prescribing something to help her obtain some relief. Many individuals find the posttreatment period to be very frightening and may benefit from pharmacologic, group, or counseling interventions.
    - Tell her that her worries are commonly experienced by other cancer survivors.
    - Be honest with her; yes, the cancer may come back. That is why she is being monitored. If her cancer comes back, there are a number of options depending on where it comes back. She may receive more radiation and/or chemotherapy, or she may be a candidate for bone marrow transplant.
    - Encourage her to continue performing BSE and come to her follow-up appointments so you can function as her "team" in helping look after her. Reassure her that she can call you between visits if she is concerned about symptoms she may be experiencing.

D.M. seemed to do fine for a while. On her 9-month follow-up visit, she tells you she has been having headaches for the past few weeks. Her MRI indicates she has metastases to the brain. She underwent a bone marrow transplant; unfortunately, it failed to stop her cancer. She died at the age of 38, leaving behind 4 children aged 4 through 14.

Case Study 4: Squamous Cell Carcinoma Anterior Tongue

Difficulty: **	*Setting:* Outpatient clinic
Index Words: Cancer, squamous cell carcinoma of the tongue	

A.V. is a 37-year-old, married housewife, with a 35 pack/year history of smoking. She says she "just can't quit." She denies ETOH use. Ht 67" Wt 115 lb. Her PMH includes C-sections for all 3 children ages 6, 14, and 18. She does not have insurance. She noticed a "canker sore" on the anterior lateral aspect of her L tongue several months ago. Over time, she developed a sore throat and ear pain. The family nurse practitioner at the low-income clinic sent her to a specialist who performed a biopsy of her anterior tongue. The diagnosis was squamous cell carcinoma—poorly differentiated—T2 N0. Before her surgery she had complete Panorex views of her mandible; fluoride trays were made followed by a partial glossectomy and excision of the floor of her mouth. Three weeks after surgery, multiple teeth are scheduled to be extracted. Afterward, she will be scheduled for 8 weeks of radiation therapy in your outpatient clinic.

1. Describe the rationale for this prophylactic treatment: teeth extraction, Panorex views, fluoride trays. **[P/c/PI/ct]**
   - Dental assessment is important before and during all head and neck surgery for prevention of oral complications during therapy. Data obtained from the patient assessment may include frequency of dental care; condition of teeth/dentures; bad breath odor; sore swollen gums; demonstrated gingival recession, hypertrophy, or decayed teeth should be treated before initiation of surgery/radiation therapy. A Panorex (full mouth x-ray) identifies the presence of teeth in edentulate patients and disease invasion into the mandible when radiation to this area is planned. Instruction on fluoride application and oral hygiene is initiated. Daily fluoride application should be encouraged as a part of preventive dental/oral care regimen. Fluoride is an anticaries agent with antibacterial properties that promotes remineralization of the enamel.

2. Identify and describe preop nursing care for partial glossectomy. **[P,I/c/PI,PSI/ct,ni,tc]**
   - Inform the patient about the purpose and rationale for the surgical procedure.
   - NPO status 8 hours before OR/anesthesia to minimize risk of aspiration.
   - Teach about and administer preop medications and their side effects.
   - Briefly describe the OR environment and what will happen.
   - Describe recovery room nursing interventions (airway and VS management) so she doesn't think something has gone wrong when she wakes up.
   - Instruct her that, upon awakening, there will be a feeling of discomfort in her mouth.
   - Tell her there will probably be sutures in her tongue, and it will feel very strange.
   - Tell her she will have an IV and will receive fluids through the IV.
   - Warn her about changes to expect when coughing, sneezing, or swallowing.
   - Tell her the nurse will frequently monitor her breathing, how her mouth looks, and her ability to swallow.

3. Identify and describe potential postop care for partial glossectomy. **[P,I/c/PI,PSI/ct,ni,tc]**
   - On a scheduled frequency:
     - Monitor signs and symptoms of respiratory distress: restlessness, agitation, confusion, air hunger, diminished or absent air exchange, inability to breathe, and dyspnea.
     - Monitor signs and symptoms of hemorrhage: continuous oozing of blood/bleeding around the surgical site, presence of unusual edema/drainage around the surgical site.
     - Monitor for signs and symptoms of hematoma formation: observe for clot/increased edema at the surgical site, note color/integrity of tongue tissue.
     - Monitor signs and symptoms of infection: change in VS, drainage/odor from tongue, intake and output.
     - Monitor signs and symptoms of nerve injury: if the hypoglossal nerve is severed, unilateral tongue paralysis will result causing impairment of speech and mastication.
   - Place the patient in a semi-Fowler's position; facilitate and monitor eating and drinking functions; provide privacy; know the location and use of emergent equipment and supplies (a functional suction set-up must be in place at the bedside).
   - Instruct the patient about postop complications and management.
   - Place the call light within reach, and instruct her to call for assistance when needed.

4. Identify and describe potential postop complications resulting from a partial glossectomy. Plan appropriate nursing interventions and patient teaching strategies to manage these complications. **[P,I/ap/PI,PSI/ct,ni,tc]**
   - The head and neck structures are responsible for the mechanics of respiration, speech, and swallowing. The tongue is located in the middle anatomical section of the head and neck area; partial removal of the tongue, flaps, and/or grafts to the tongue results in potential complications involving all 3 primary functions.
     - Respiration: surgical/radiation therapy treatment may alter the normal air-conditioning function of the upper air passageways, causing a cooling and drying effect on the trachea; postop obstruction of the airway passage may occur from a hematoma and/or hemorrhage at or near the suture site; infection may occur at the suture/graft site; an edematous tongue may result in airway obstruction.
     - Speech: the tongue serves a major function in speech formation, sounds, and clarity of verbal communication; edematous tissue and/or a hematoma at the suture site interferes with speech formation and enunciation.
     - Swallowing: the tongue is used to move food and fluids from the mouth to the esophagus as it enters the digestive tract; surgery and radiation therapy may interfere with normal healing of the tissue, resulting in limitation in ability to swallow; there is an increased potential for choking/aspiration of food; radiation therapy to this area will cause decreased salivary production (xerostomia).

5. When she returns for her first postop visit to your clinic, she appears to be quite distressed to hear about the radiation therapy. Although she still has considerable trouble speaking, she explains she really didn't think much about it before surgery. She seems quite embarrassed as she tells you her family has no insurance, and they were barely making it earlier. Now she says she is getting "nasty letters" from the hospital demanding payment. What can you do? **[A,P/an/PSI/ct,ni,tc]**
   - Reassure her this is nothing to be ashamed about. Many Americans today do not have insurance and live on the edge of financial disaster if they were to encounter an accident or illness; even those with insurance may lose it in the face of a disaster.
   - Ask if she has a copy of one of her bills with a specific name and number to notify (this will save time).
   - Advise her to keep a log of everyone she talks to, when, and about what in case she encounters "unresponsive" personnel or promises are not kept.
   - Call the hospital and ask to speak to a social worker or one of the billing advisors. Give A.V. the name of a contact person who can work with the family in arranging finances. Give her the name and number of the person in the clinic who handles the finances so her radiation treatments can be arranged.
   - Give her names and numbers of community resources that may help her and her family with some of their needs.

6. As she sits by you, she keeps her hand over her mouth and jaw. She is wearing her hair so if hangs down over her face. Her jaw and neck still are swollen from the surgery and tooth extraction. She avoids eye contact with you. How will you respond? **[A,PD,P/an/PSI/ct,ni,tc]**
   - Recognize that she probably is very self-conscious about her appearance; head and neck surgery for cancer is not a pretty thing, and patients are very conscious of the effect of their disfigurement on others. A.V. needs to know that she will look better when the swelling goes down, and after the radiation therapy is finished. (The sad thing is she probably lacks resources for good reconstructive surgery.)
   - Gently remind her that you work with people who have gone through surgery like hers every day, and you hope she can learn to feel as comfortable with you as you can be with her.
   - Explore self-esteem issues; also, evaluate for depression and suicidal ideation.

Case Study 5: Hodgkin's Disease

Difficulty: **	*Setting:* Outpatient clinic
Index Words: Hodgkin's disease, cancer	

A.T. is a 21-year-old college student. He works part-time as a manual laborer, uses a half can/week of smokeless tobacco, and drinks a 6 pack of beer/week. A year ago in September, he discovered a small, painless lump in his lower L neck. Over the quarter, he experienced increasing fatigue and a 10-lb weight loss that he attributed to "working and studying too hard." In the spring, he saw a nurse practitioner at the student health center who immediately referred him to an oncologist. A lymph node biopsy revealed Hodgkin's disease. The CT scan of the chest, abdomen, and pelvis; gallium scan; and bone scan all came back negative. A staging laparotomy was conducted a month later to confirm the diagnosis. His diagnosis was Hodgkin's disease stage IA mixed cellularity. You are a staff nurse in the outpatient oncology services when A.T. comes in.

1. A.T. wants to know what Hodgkin's disease is and how he "caught" it. What will you tell him? **[PD/k/PI,PSI/ct,tc]**
   - Hodgkin's disease is a kind of cancer of the lymphatic system; it is the most common cancer in his age group. It is not known how people "get it," and there are no identifiable ways of preventing someone from getting it.

2. A.T. wants to know what "stage IA" means; he also wants to know the significance of the test results. What are you going to tell him? **[PD/c/PI,PSI/ct,ni,tc]**
   - Keep in mind that the real question in A.T.'s mind probably is will he *live*. When people receive a diagnosis of cancer, they often think of dying. As you explain the staging and test results to him, watch his reaction to see how much information he wants and can handle. Commonly, it is necessary to explain things to patients several times because of the threatening nature of the information.
   - Stage IA Hodgkin's disease means his cancer was caught early; this is the earliest stage. The fact that his CT scans, the gallium scan, and bone scan all were negative is good news; it means his cancer probably has not spread.

A few days later, you see A.T. in the oncologist's office during his appointment to discuss the treatment regimen for radiation therapy. His prescribed radiation treatment regimen (outpatient) includes Monday through Friday with treatments scheduled for approximately 6 to 10 weeks. Admission assessment findings on his first visit to the outpatient oncology clinic at the end of January are Wt 183 lb, Ht 78 in. VS 124/66, 60, 16, 98.0°F (oral). Cardiovascular: heart rate regular. Respiratory: clear to auscultation. Neuromuscular/skeletal, GI, and GU: negative. Integumentary/oral: incision from staging laparotomy well-approximated without erythema, edema, pain, or drainage. Incision from lymph node dissection healing well, oral mucosa pink and moist, no palpable adenopathy.

3. What abnormal assessment findings do you find in the above information? **[A/c/PI/ct]**
   - None. The assessment findings are all within normal parameters.

4. A.T. jokes with you that he's going to get nuked and "glow." What information would you include in your teaching for someone like A.T. to prepare her/him for radiation treatments? **[P,I/c/PI,PSI/ct,ni,tc]**
   - Explain that the kind of radiation treatment he is getting is from high-energy, x-ray beams that attack cancer cells in a limited area of his body. Hodgkin's disease is very sensitive to radiation treatment.
   - He is going to have markings on his skin so the same area receives radiation every time; tell him not to try to wash these markings off.
   - A simulator is going to be used the first time to help the technician mark the correct area.
   - A custom shield will be used to protect healthy tissue from being harmed.
   - Side effects may include profound fatigue, skin "burns" or reactions, and loss of appetite; these side effects can seriously jeopardize quality of life. Patients should be encouraged to talk about how they are feeling throughout treatment.
   - Skin care should include checking the radiated area every day for changes, washing with cool water and a soft cloth; don't use soap; don't wear tight and/or synthetic materials; protect the treatment area from exposure to heat, cold, and sunburn.

   Instructor Note: Never count on people's memory, particularly when they are in health-threatening circumstances. Always be sure you have written/printed materials to give them that are appropriate to their educational level and interests.

5. You have developed a good relationship with A.T. during the multiple visits required for his radiation therapy. He shares some futuristic goals and says, "What are the chances that I will beat this cancer?" Respond to A.T.'s request. **[A,PD,P/c/S,PI,PSI/ct,ni,tc]**
   - Keep in mind that questions like this have fear of becoming impaired or dying behind them. They are serious questions that deserve thoughtful answers.
   - Survivorship begins with diagnosis and proceeds along a continuum through and beyond treatment to remission, recurrence, cure, and/or the final stages of life. This helps people recognize that cancer has long-term implications for living.
   - Multiple factors determine the occurrence, frequency, and severity of actual or potential effects; type and location of cancer; size and extent of primary disease; type and aggressiveness of therapy; age of the individual; general health; and, possibly, quantity and quality of psychosocial support available.
   - For statistical purposes, people are often considered "cured" if they are cancer-free 5 years after a cancer diagnosis or remain free of the disease after completion of therapy. How this is defined depends on the type of cancer; in addition, some types of cancer tend to recur faster than others.
   - There may be some long-term effects of treatment, including coronary artery disease where he had radiation treatment, fatigue, and loss of social functioning.

Other kinds of cancer may occur many years later as a result of the toxic effects of earlier treatment. This is one reason why cancer specialists are reluctant to use the word "cured."

6. What other issues of survivorship may affect patients like A.T. (e.g., insurance, employability)? **[PD,P/c/PSI/ct]**
   - Employment- or insurance-related problems may include avoidance by coworkers, being locked into a job for fear of losing benefits, and being denied insurance coverage.
   - Legal protection is provided through the Federal Rehabilitation Act of 1973, which prohibits discrimination; additional protection is provided by the Federal Rehabilitation Act under the Americans with Disabilities Act 1990. Federal and state laws specifically prohibit cancer-related employment discrimination.
   - Insurance can be a significant problem because it is usually linked to employment. Legal protection includes the Consolidated Omnibus Budget Reconciliation Act (COBRA) of 1986.
   - Research has shown that cancer consequences, such as lingering fatigue, can affect social and marital relationships long after the disease is in remission or "cured."

7. How and what are you going to counsel and teach A.J. about potential sterility/infertility side effects of treatment? **[P,I/ap/PI,PSI/ct,ni,tc]**
   - Promote open communication about sexual issues by bringing up the subject.
   - Assess for fear, anxiety, and diminished self-concept.
   - Discuss possible side effects of disease and treatment regimen on libido and sexual functioning; age and sex, stage of development, type/dose/duration of therapy are all integral factors in relation to reproductive tissue damage.
   - Provide privacy and a confidential environment when discussing sexual issues.

8. Six weeks into therapy, A.T. drags himself into the clinic one Friday, drops into a chair, and wearily states, "I'm quitting. If this is what life is like, it's not worth living." How would you respond to him? **[PD,P/an/PI,PSI/ct,ni,tc]**
   - Understand that this experience of fatigue is very common and can be very discouraging.
   - Remind him that there are only a few weeks to go, and this is an investment in a lifetime plan. Also, remind him how the fatigue gets better over the weekend, and Friday is his lowest day. Ask if he can wait until Monday and see if he still feels the same about quitting.
   - Assess his everyday activities and his fatigue patterns to identify possible nursing interventions to help him.
   - Help him evaluate his resources for help at school and home.
   - Check to be sure he is eating enough calories and drinking sufficient fluids (fatigued people rarely have an adequate calorie and fluid intake).

9. When A.T. checked in this week, he weighed 177 lb. When you express concern, he tells you he just doesn't have any appetite. How are you going to respond? List at least 4 interventions. **[P,I/ap/PI,PSI/ct,ni,tc]**
   - Fatigue often plays a role in weight loss with radiation; see if someone can prepare ready-made meals for A.T. so he can have 6 or more smaller, energy-rich snacks per day.
   - He should eat on a scheduled basis, even when he's not hungry.
   - Find out what flavors and foods are tolerable to him; even "unhealthy" salty or sweet foods are preferable to nothing at all!
   - Taking a nap before meals may provide some fatigue relief and enhance caloric intake.
   - Use commercial liquid preparations with regular (*not* low-fat) milk or cream to boost calories inexpensively, and use pasteurized egg substitute to enhance protein content.
   - If the odor or taste of foods is repulsive, try chilling them before eating so the taste/odor are weaker.
   - Unless there is an aversion to eating breakfast, try to get at least a third of the daily protein and calorie requirement at breakfast.

10. At his final appointment, A.T.'s laboratory values are WBC 3.3 mm^3, Hgb 14 g/dl, Hct 41%, and platelets 369 mm^3. His VS are 120/76, 84, 20, 98.0°F(oral). Wt 175 lb. Do any of these values concern you? Explain. **[A,PD/c/PI/ct]**
    - His WBC is decreased, but it should recover in the next few weeks. In addition he has lost nearly 20 pounds since the onset of his illness; he needs be especially careful to eat a well-balanced diet in the coming months to facilitate recovery of his immune system, and to replace much of the muscle-weight that is lost during treatment. It will take him a minimum of several weeks to recover his appetite.

A.T. was discharged from radiation and scheduled to see an oncologist every 3 months for follow-up care.

Case Study 6: Adenocarcinoma of Lung; Metastatic to Lymph Nodes, Liver, and Brain

Difficulty: **	*Setting:* Hospital
Index Words: Cancer, lung cancer	

C.W. is a 42-year-old, divorced woman with adenocarcinoma (cancer) of the lung with metastasis (spread) to the brain and liver. She is the single parent of a 17-year-old son, has experienced episodic health care, is currently unemployed because of poor health, and has no health insurance. She has smoked 1 to 2 packs/day for 20 years. PMH includes cholecystectomy, hysterectomy, and breast augmentation. In May of last year, she developed scapular and arm pain in her right side, was diagnosed with adenocarcinoma of the lung, and underwent a wedge resection of the upper right lobe of the lung. Because she had no insurance, she did not receive follow-up care (e.g., radiation therapy and/or chemotherapy).

C.W. developed pain in her right temple 48 hours ago and was seen in the ED, where she was given cephradine (Velosef). C.W. had a seizure 24 hours later, was transported to the ED, and was diagnosed as having an allergic reaction to the Velosef. She was instructed to call her family doctor. C.W.'s doctor was unavailable for 48 hours. After suffering a tonic-clonic (grand mal) seizure at home, she was admitted to a rural hospital. A CT scan revealed a large mass in the right frontal area of her brain. Dexamethasone (Decadron) was given IV, and an oncologist in the metropolitan area was consulted. C.W. was transferred to your oncology unit postseizure with slight slurred speech and intermittent bone pain. She has lost 22 lb. in the past year. She is receiving acetaminophen/hydrocodone (Lortab) 1-2 5 mg tabs every 3 to 4 hours, as needed. C.W.'s record lists codeine and milk allergies.

1. Identify the usual location, growth rate, and likelihood of metastasis of adenocarcinoma of the lung. **[A/k/Pl/ct]**
   - Adenocarcinoma usually presents as a slow-growing, peripheral mass and is associated with early metastasis; it tends to spread to the brain and liver.

2. Is the presence of bone pain and weight loss significant? **[PD/c/Pl/ct]**
   - Yes, bone pain and weight loss are associated with metastasis and worsen the prognosis.

3. What tests are likely to be performed to determine if C.W.'s adenocarcinoma has metastasized? **[A/c/Pl/ct]**
   - A CT scan of the head, chest, and abdomen will be done to look for metastasis to the brain, thorax, liver, and kidneys.
   - Liver enzymes and AFP (alpha fetal protein) tumor marker.

4. The tests are performed, and C.W. is diagnosed with adenocarcinoma of the lung with metastasis to lymph nodes, liver, and brain. She is scheduled to receive 10 radiation therapy treatments to the whole brain (3 as an inpatient, 7 as an outpatient). Identify 5 needs that you will address with C.W. and her son. **[P/an/S,PI,PSI/ct,ni,tc]**
   - Safety r/t seizures: administer IV corticosteroids as prescribed to decrease cerebral edema, initiate seizure precautions (pad siderails, keep airway and suction supplies at bedside, maintain quiet environment, monitor frequently for seizure activity).
   - Educate C.W. and her son about the side effects of radiation therapy: confusion, unsteady gait, blurred vision, headaches, N/V, and profound fatigue.
   - Obtain a social services consultation: C.W.'s son will need assistance to care for his mother; explore options for community agency resource availability and services provided; relatives and neighbors may arrange to come to stay at intervals in the home to assist with care needs, and need for scheduled home care agency assistance, such as hospice, church.
   - Nutrition: C.W. is unemployed, has lost 22 lb over the last year, and is about to begin radiation therapy to the head; all these factors place her at risk for malnutrition.
   - Pain: provide pain medication as prescribed; if the prescribed medication is inadequate, notify the physician and obtain an order for additional or alternative medications.
   - Emotional distress: talk to C.W. to determine if there is any family member, ex-husband, or close friend she can trust who can take her son when she dies. Discuss advanced directives with her; see if she has a will or would like to make one out.
   - Financial stress: has she applied for Social Security benefits for her son?

After her third radiation treatment, C.W. is discharged on the following medications: dexamethasone (Decadron) 4 mg PO q8h; propoxyphene/acetaminophen (Darvocet-N) 100 mg PO q4h PRN; prochloperazine maleate (Compazine Spansule) 15 mg PO q12h PRN; temazepam (Restoril) 30 mg PO q hs PRN.

5. What is the rationale for C.W. receiving each medication? **[P/c/PI,PSI/ct]**
   - Decadron is a long-acting corticosteroid that decreases the inflammatory response.
   - Darvocet-N is a nonopioid analgesic for mild to moderate pain.
   - Compazine is an antiemetic.
   - Restoril is a sedative/hypnotic (benzodiazepine).

Two months posthospital discharge and follow-up therapy, C.W. continues to have increasing symptoms of pain, anorexia, weight loss, edema in extremities, and insomnia. Her son accompanied her to the physician's office. While his mother is having her blood drawn, he asks the nurse what is going to happen to his mother.

6. How would you respond to him? **[A,P,I/an/S,PSI/ct,ni,tc]**
   - First, carefully assess his level of understanding and emotional status as you respond. Sit down with him and ask him to explain what he understands; ask him how the situation makes him feel. Discuss his mother's prognosis.
   - Establish what kind of support system he has. Perhaps a social worker may be able to assist with counseling.

7. He asks what he can do to help his mother. What information could you give him? **[A,P,I/an/S,PI,PSI/ct,ni,tc]**
   - Things he can do to help are:
     - Note the *severity* and/or *frequency* of his mom's symptoms, and report the information to the nurse/physician.
     - Provide a safe environment, simple step-by step instructions for tasks, positive reinforcement for accomplished tasks; encourage her to take frequent rest/naps, and reduce mental/physical activity late in the day; say "thank you for coming and goodbye" to visitors after a brief visit so she doesn't become exhausted by their presence.

   Instructor Note: It is important that C.W. have someone to talk to and confide in besides her son. He has his own stressors and needs someone to talk to, too. It is not appropriate or healthy for him to be her sole confidant.

8. As C.W.'s disease progresses, what signs and symptoms can be anticipated, and what kind of relief can be provided? **[A,P/c/S,PI,PSI/ct,ni]**
   - Brain metastasis changes may include headaches, seizures, aphasia, apraxia (inability to execute purposeful movements), inability to concentrate, memory loss, and disturbance in balance or gait; she will need increasing assistance with daily activities, ambulation, and self-care.
   - Liver metastasis changes may include abdominal distention/discomfort, diarrhea/constipation, nausea and vomiting, changes in skin/eye color (orange), diminished appetite and dyspepsia. Supportive comfort measures include diet of choice, small/frequent servings of food, and offer/provide pain medications and antiemetics on a scheduled frequency.
   - Pulmonary cancer will contribute to increased shortness of breath and decreased functioning; she should be positioned for optimal comfort, most likely in Fowler's position; palliative oxygen may provide some relief from the dyspnea.

9. C.W.'s son says he's never been around someone who is dying before. He expresses fear he won't know what to do. How can you help him? **[A,PD,P/ap/PSI/ct,ni,tc]**
   - Explore his thoughts and feelings about the meaning of death.
   - Discuss end-stage disease complications with him.
   - Provide social support and caretaker relief for him.
   - Tell him that the social worker and hospice nurse can help him through the dying process and will stay in contact with him after the death of his mother.
   - Discuss with him what things could be healing experiences.

Case Study 7: Acute Lymphoblastic Leukemia

Difficulty: ***	*Setting:* Hospital, outpatient clinic
Index Words: Acute lymphoblastic leukemia	

D.L., a 21-year-old, single, plumber's assistant developed low back pain "from a work injury" 2 weeks ago. He had no PMH and is a nonsmoker, nondrinker. He was instructed to take diclofenac (Cataflam) 50 mg PO tid for 6 doses and cyclobenzaprine (Flexeril) 10 mg PO tid for 6 doses. Within 2 to 3 days, he developed a fever (101.6°F, oral), and a rash developed over his entire body. He showed dramatic bruising; he also developed a decreased appetite and a sore mouth. He was taken to the ER at a rural hospital when he started vomiting blood. His labs were WBC 31.7 mm^3, Hgb 10.1 g/dl, Hct 29%, and platelets 16 mm^3. Arrangements were made to transfer him to the regional medical center, where you work on the heme/onc unit, to see an oncologist for a workup and to be admitted to the hospital for therapy. A bone marrow biopsy confirmed the diagnosis of acute lymphoblastic leukemia.

1. What is acute lymphoblastic leukemia (ALL), and what are other names for this same condition? **[PD/k/PI/ct]**
    - ALL is an unusually rapidly progressing form of leukemia, characterized by replacement of normal bone marrow by blast cells arising from a malignant, transformed hematopoietic stem cell. Correct classification of this type of leukemia is critical in planning treatment and establishing a prognosis. It is also called acute lymphocytic leukemia and is usually characterized by a sudden onset of symptoms that require intense therapy over a period of several weeks to months.

2. You are the leukemia support and education group leader for your hospital. Patients attending your sessions have acute/chronic lymphocytic leukemia, acute/chronic myelogenous leukemia, myelodysplastic syndrome, and multiple myeloma. Your topic for discussion today is the etiology of the hematologic diseases for the previously stated diseases. D.L.'s older brother, T.L., is a nursing student and he wants to know how many kinds of leukemia there are, and if they are caused by the same thing. List the related diseases in the leukemia family and what is thought to cause each. **[PD/k/PI/ct]**
    - Acute lymphocytic leukemia (ALL): etiology is unknown; exposure to radiation, chemicals, drugs, viruses, as well as genetic abnormalities have been implicated.
    - Acute myelogenous leukemia (AML): specific risk factors have been identified; people with certain genetic disorders, such as Down's syndrome, Bloom's syndrome, Klinefelter's syndrome, and Fanconi's anemia, are at an increased risk to develop AML; exposure to benzene (present in cleaning solvents and unleaded gas) and radiation are thought to be involved.
    - Chronic lymphocytic leukemia (CLL): appears to be related to autoimmune disorders such as lupus and hemolytic anemia.
    - Chronic myelogenous leukemia (CML): the incidence of CML increases with exposure to radiation, benzene, and alkylating drugs used in the treatment of cancer.
    - Myelodysplastic syndrome: associated with exposure to benzene products, radiation, and alkylating chemotherapy agents (e.g., busulfan, carboplatin, chlorambucil, cisplatin, cyclophosphamide, ifosfamide, nitrogen mustard, and thiotepa).
    - Multiple myeloma: chromosome abnormalities, host genetic factors, chronic antigenic stimulation, and viruses are thought to contribute to the development of plasma cell dyscrasias.

3. D.L. asks you what the chances are for someone, like himself, with ALL. What can you tell him? **[PD/c/PI,PSI/ct,tc]**
    - Keep in mind that D.L. is very frightened, very fatigable, and probably will not remember much detail. He is seeking reassurance, not just data. Watch his response to what you are saying throughout your discussion for clues as to how he is dealing with this.
    - The average survival is about 4 months after diagnosis without treatment.
    - There are several factors involved but his age is in his favor ($>$20 years old); however, the type of cells he has and a WBC $>$25 mm^3 are not as favorable.
    - Regardless of risk factors, the chance of initial remission is $\geq$90% in patients with ALL; the first goal of treatment is complete remission.

D.L. is scheduled to receive the initial *induction* combination chemotherapy by IV and IT (intrathecal) routes. He will be receiving doxorubicin (Adriamycin), vincristine and cyclophosphamide (Cytoxan) IVP, methotrexate IT, and prednisone PO. He will be hospitalized about 3 weeks. He will be scheduled for intense *consolidation* courses, and then *maintenance* therapy for 1 year. The induction and consolidation courses are intense drug therapies, requiring multiple blood product infusions and antibiotic therapy to aid recovery. Because of his recent employment and projected required course of therapy, he will be unable to work and will probably lose his insurance.

D.L.'s admission assessments are: VS 140/74, 90, 24, 103.3°F (oral); Wt 150 lb; cardiovascular: normal sinus rhythm, no S_3, S_4 rubs, or murmurs, all peripheral pulses present; respiratory: clear to auscultation; neuromuscular/skeletal: grossly intact; motor and sensory exam normal; GI: spleen about 5 fingerbreadths below the right costal margin-tender, liver is not enlarged, no ascites or intraabdominal mass or CVA tenderness; GU: rectal not done; integumentary/oral: HEENT, nomocephalic, pupils level, round, reactive to light in accommodation, no sclera icterus, conjunctivas very pale, fundoscopic exam is benign; oropharynx has some gingival lesions, mucous membranes are moist and pale; tympanic membranes are normal; neck: supple, trachea midline, thyroid normal, no murmurs or JVD distention. To facilitate D.L.'s chemotherapy and blood product infusion, a triple-lumen subclavian catheter is inserted.

4. Describe potential effects the acute leukemia, treatment, and rehabilitation have on the socioeconomic status and family relationships of people like D.L. **[A,PD/c,an/PI,PSI/ct]**
   - Developmental tasks in this age group include starting a career/family, finding a social group, and selecting a mate; diagnosis of an acute disease with intense (and expensive) therapy puts these tasks "on hold." Acknowledgment of the diagnosis and compliance with the intense therapy is the major goal. Support systems such as family/community groups provide psychologic support through listening, sharing of duties, consultation for financial management, and health care demands. Acute illnesses in early adulthood sometimes require young adults to return to their parents' home. Relationships within the family structure change with the added tasks of self-care management of the disease/side effects of therapy, inability to perform work duties/loss of income, unable to maintain separate living arrangements, inability to pay debts. Patient/family counseling may be necessary to identify strengths and weaknesses, explore coping strategies, deal with financial loss, and to meet the demands of the patient/family. Open communication, use of available community resources, and evaluation of patient and family needs are critical.

5. During the next 14 days, D.L. receives irradiated platelets and leukoreduced, irradiated RBCs. What is the rationale for using irradiated, leukoreduced blood products? Describe the nursing administration/monitoring procedure for these products. **[PD,P/c/Pl/ct,ni]**
   - Irradiated blood products are red blood cells and platelets that have been exposed to a measured amount of radiation; this renders the donor lymphocytes incapable of replication. This is done to prevent posttransfusion-related graft-versus-host disease in blood product recipients. Indications for these products are acute and aplastic leukemia, bone marrow transplantation, congenital immunodeficiency disorders, Hodgkin's or non-Hodgkin's lymphoma, intrauterine transfusions, low birth weight neonates, and first-degree family member blood donations.
   - Leukoreduced blood products are red blood cells that have filtration techniques, such as leukocyte depletion filters and/or blood bank processing, through centrifuge to remove 99.9% of the white blood cells; these cells are called NS-washed cells. Leukocyte depletion filters *are distinct separate products and are not interchangeable*. Leukocyte depletion techniques are utilized (1) to prevent recurrence of febrile, nonhemolytic transfusion reactions caused by donor white blood cell antigens reacting with recipient white blood cell antibodies, and (2) to reduce the incidence of urticarial and anaphylactic reactions.
   - Follow American Red Cross, American Association Blood Bank, and agency protocols to obtain blood products.
   - Initiate IV access; obtain appropriate transfusion supplies; verify critical elements; check name/product/ABO group/Rh type/ID number of the patient/blood product; verify consistency and compatibility, and record this data; 2 qualified individuals (another nurse or physician) must verify patient information and blood product information.
   - Obtain and record baseline VS; assess for pretransfusion symptoms (fever, rash).
   - Premedicate patient with prophylactic medications (antihistamines/ acetaminophen) as prescribed.
   - Initiate blood product infusion (2-5 ml/min) for initial 15 minutes; *observe for transfusion reaction.*
   - Repeat VS signs at 15 minutes, then 30 minutes after blood product is initiated, then hourly, then 1 hour posttransfusion.
   - Document blood product type, volume, ID numbers, date/time/duration and completion of product infusion.
   - Usual infusion time: RBCs 1 to 1½ hours with a 4 hour maximum; use leukocyte RC 100 filter with each red cell product infusion; platelets 150-200 ml/h with maximum transfusion time 4 hours; use leukofilter PL 100 with each product infusion.
   - Immediately document and report any acute transfusion reactions, such as acute hemolytic reaction, anaphylaxis, circulatory overload, febrile nonhemolytic reaction, and sepsis.

6. D.L. will continue to receive intense combination chemotherapy for several more weeks. Because of limited finances, his hospitalization stay will be cut short. What are the major self-care management issues for home care that need to be reinforced? **[A,P,I/an/PI,PSI/ct,ni,tc]**
   - D.L. must learn to care for his central venous access catheter because it will remain in place for his entire scheduled therapy.
   - Signs and symptoms to report immediately are:
     - Anemia: headache, shortness of breath, and dizziness.
     - Thrombocytopenia: bruising, petechiae, and/or bleeding from any body orifice.
     - Leukopenia: fever, chills, or myalgia.
   - Nutrition management; there is the potential for significant weight loss; teach D.L. how to maintain and increase calorie intake through milkshakes, puddings, food supplements, cheese, peanut butter, and cooked eggs.
   - Drug side effect management, such as nausea and vomiting, diarrhea, neuropathy, and excess fluid retention.

7. D.L. is going to be staying with his parents. T.L. has promised to help with D.L.'s care. In addition, a home care nurse will visit him twice weekly. You are going to teach D.L. and his brother, T.L., to care for and use his triple-lumen subclavian catheter. What will you tell them? **[P,I,E/an/PI/ct,ni,tc]**
   - A triple lumen subclavian catheter is inserted and anchored with sutures to the skin; the usual dwell time of a catheter is 6 to 12 weeks. The catheter requires a sterile environment at the catheter site for the duration of the catheter insertion; a sterile gauze dressing with occlusive tape is changed every 24 hours. To maintain catheter patency, each lumen of the catheter is flushed with heparinized saline solution (heparin 10-100 U/ml) 2 ml at least once a day.
   - Signs and symptoms to report immediately include air embolus, characterized by chest pain, dyspnea, increased pulse/respiration, and decreased BP. Catheter dislodgement is characterized by medication or fluid leaking from the catheter. Watch for infection, indicated by a fever $>101\,^{\circ}F$; an edematous, reddened, and/or painful catheter exit site.
   - Have them demonstrate with return demonstration correct sterile dressing change and catheter heparinization. Have the D.L. and T.L. verbalize who, where, and when to report symptoms and catheter-related problems. Include a printout with signs and symptoms to report and self-care management techniques for catheter site care.

Before he leaves, T.L. says, "You know, I've been studying about some of this stuff in my med/surg class, but I had no idea how bad it feels to go through this. I hope this makes me a better, more sensitive nurse."

Case Study 8: Small Cell (Oat Cell) Lung Cancer

Difficulty: ***	*Setting:* Outpatient clinic, hospital
Index Words: Lung cancer	

C.P. is a 61-year-old married farmer, with a PMH of hernia surgery in 1955 and prostate surgery in 1969 for BPH (benign prostatic hypertrophy). C.P. does not drink but he has smoked for 40 years; the past 3 years he has smoked 2 to 3 packs/day. He has no known allergies. Six months ago, C.P. visited the local rural health clinic with c/o progressive cough and chest congestion. Despite a week of antibiotic therapy, C.P. continued to worsen; he experienced progressive dyspnea, productive cough, and began to have night sweats. C.P. refused to be admitted to the hospital ("There's no one to look after the cows") but agreed to go for a CXR. The radiologist read C.P.'s CXR as left hilar lung mass—probable lung cancer. C.P. was scheduled for a diagnostic fiberoptic bronchoscopy with endobronchial lung biopsy as an outpatient to confirm the diagnosis.

1. What is fiberoptic bronchoscopy? What information will a fiberoptic bronchoscopy with endobronchial lung biopsy provide? **[PD/c/PI/ct]**
    - A fiberoptic bronchoscope is a flexible bronchoscope that is passed through the trachea and allows visual inspection of the tracheobronchial airways. The physician uses the scope to examine strictures, visualize inflammation, detect the site of bleeding, and/or locate foreign bodies in the bronchi. Bronchial washings and biopsies can be collected through the tube and sent to the lab for pathologic analysis; biopsy allows a definitive diagnosis. C.P.'s lung tissue will be examined for the presence of abnormal cells, particularly malignant cells, by a pathologist.

2. As the nurse who works with the pulmonologist, it is your responsibility to prepare C.P. for the fiberoptic bronchoscopy procedure. What would you include in your teaching plan? **[P/an/S,PI,PSI/ct,ni,tc]**
    - C.P. should take nothing by mouth for 6 to 8 hours before the test.
    - C.P. will be given IV medication (atropine) to dry-up his mouth and throat, and medication (midazolam [Versed]) to make him drowsy before the procedure.
    - C.P. will be sedated for the procedure; he should be accompanied by an adult because he will be unable to drive a car or operate equipment for 3 to 4 hours after the procedure.
    - Explain the procedure in language he can understand. A long tube will be passed through his nose or mouth and into his lungs; the physician will look at his breathing tubes; if he sees anything that doesn't look right, he will take out a little piece (biopsy) to be tested.

3. What will be your responsibility during and immediately after the bronchoscopy? **[P,I/an/S,PI/ct,ni]**
    - Monitor VS at regular intervals.
    - Continuously monitor SaO_2; if C.P. desaturates, immediately notify the physician.
    - Observe/monitor for pain, dyspnea, restlessness, bleeding, or desaturation, and immediately notify the physician of changes.
    - After the bronchoscopy, C.P. will remain NPO until his gag reflex returns.

4. C.P. tolerates the procedure well. He returns to the office in 4 days to learn the results of his test. The pulmonologist tells C.P. and his wife that he has oat cell lung cancer and explains that it is a very fast-growing cancer that has no cure. This kind of lung cancer is directly related to C.P.'s history of smoking. What is your role at this time? **[A,P,I/an/S,PSI/ct,ni,tc]**
   - Be present when the physician informs C.P. and his family of the results of the diagnostic procedure; realize that they are going to hear little or nothing beyond the diagnosis.
   - They are going to be in shock; provide privacy, tissues, and fluids.
   - Be supportive and listen to whatever they need to say.
   - Ask them what they understood and reexplain the disease/treatment information.
   - Put important points in writing for them to refer to later.

C.P. is scheduled to begin combination chemotherapy with cisplatin (Platinol) and etoposide (VePesid). He plans to continue to work the farm as long as possible; his brother-in-law has promised to help him.

5. How would you explain combination chemotherapy and how it works to C.P. and his wife? **[P,I/c/PI/ct,ni,tc]**
   - Chemotherapy works by stopping cancer cells from multiplying and making more of themselves; cells go through several steps when they multiply. Each chemotherapy drug "hits" the cancer cell at a different step; we know that using more than one drug can be more effective.

6. C.P.'s wife tells you she's heard that chemotherapy makes you really sick. How would you explain chemotherapy side effects? **[P,I/c/PI,PSI/ct,ni,tc]**
   - Chemotherapy attacks any cell that multiplies fast; cancer cells multiply really fast, so the chemotherapy attacks them. There are a lot of other cells in your body that multiply fast, such as the cells that make your hair grow, your red blood cells that carry oxygen around to all the cells in your body, white blood cells that fight infection, cells that make your blood clot, and cells in your bowels that help you digest and absorb the food you eat. The reason people get sick is because the chemotherapy is also attacking all those other cells. Different kinds of chemotherapy affect you in different ways; some people don't get very sick and others do.
   - Tell her there are measures that can be taken to make C.P. feel more comfortable.

7. What are the most common side effects of cisplatin and VePesid? **[PD/k/PI/ct]**
   - CisPlatin: neurotoxicity, nephrotoxicity, ototoxicity, and nausea/vomiting.
   - VePesid: hypotension, leukopenia, alopecia, and nausea/vomiting.
   - Profound fatigue, contributing to decreased functional status, is experienced by people taking either one or both of these drugs.

8. Based on your knowledge of the most common side effects, what interventions should be incorporated into his plan of care? **[P,I/ap/S,PI,PSI/ct,ni,tc]**
   - Explain to C.P. and his wife about what to expect and specific measures they can take so he experiences some relief.
   - Neurotoxicity: observe/report numbness or tingling in extremities; gait or balance disturbance; decreasing sensitivity to hot or cold; pain; presence or increase in confusion, disorientation, visual disturbance.
   - Nephrotoxicity: observe/report changes in amount/frequency/odor of urinary output; dysuria; flank pain; lethargy; changes in mental status. *Drink plenty of fluids!*
   - Alopecia: gradual and complete scalp/body hair loss; hair will return 2 to 3 months after completing chemotherapy; wear a hat or scarf to protect the head from heat/cold when outdoors. Use mild shampoos for head hygiene.
   - Nausea/vomiting: take prescribed antiemetics before and after chemotherapy infusion; eat cold foods and salty foods in small, frequent feedings; if nausea/vomiting continues for longer than 24 hours, notify physician/nurse so that s/he can assess C.P.'s hydration status.
   - Ototoxicity: observe/report change in hearing, such as diminished sounds or ringing in his ears.
   - Leukopenia: observe/report fever $>101°$ F, chills, pain, and/or erythema. Encourage prudent hygiene practices; avoid crowds/people with infectious diseases during immunosuppression (WBC <3.5 mm^3 or absolute granulocyte count <2.5 mm^3) episodes. Place the patent on reverse isolation.
   - Hypotension: observe/report episodes of dizziness and syncope; maintain hydration; use slow motion to change position from lying to sitting to standing.
   - Provide written/verbal information regarding the above side effects and interventions.

9. C.P. needs to have a working understanding of how to balance his treatments with his work. You sit down with C.P. to plan a daily work/activity/rest schedule to accommodate his treatments and side effects. What concepts would you emphasize? **[P,I/ap/S,PI,PSI/ct,ni,tc]**
   - Several disease- and treatment-related factors must be considered; profound fatigue, anemia, possible dehydration, difficulty concentrating and need for frequent breaks must be considered in the plans.
   - The above drugs require infusion time and recovery time before activities requiring concentration or complex physical activity may be resumed (e.g., operate machinery).
   - Describe sedative components related to antiemetic therapy and limitations on driving/operating machinery.
   - Farming encompasses many activities that have injury/infection potential for the patient with cancer receiving chemotherapy. Considerations for work/activity/rest will need planning and facilitation by him and his family members.
   - Explore social and community resources for help with C.P. and his wife; he will not be able to maintain his farm by himself.

10. C.P. receives cisplatin 60 mg in 100 ml NS IV over 1 to 2 hours daily, the first 3 days of each month for 6 months, and VePesid 200 mg in 250 ml NS IV over 1 to 2 hours daily, the first 3 days of each month for 6 months. What is the nadir for each drug and what implications does the nadir have for C.P.? **[PD/ap/PI/ct]**
    - The nadir is the lowest point reached in the peripheral blood cell count after chemotherapy is administered.
    - Cisplatin's nadir is 2 to 3 weeks with recovery in 4 to 5 weeks.
    - VePesid's nadir is 7 to 14 days with recovery in 20 to 22 days.
    - C.P. is receiving a dose of each drug the first 3 days of each month, and his blood counts will never return to optimal levels between doses. VePesid peaks in 1 to 2 weeks, and cisplatin peaks in 2 to 3 weeks; this means that C.P. will be maximally immunosuppressed for 2 weeks out of every month; he is most likely to acquire an infection during that time, and he is likely to be most fatigued during that time.

A month later, when C.P. returns for his second round of chemotherapy, he c/o SOB, chest tightness, and palpitations. He looks exhausted. ECG and CXR reveal atrial fibrillation and LLL pneumonia with L pleural effusion. C.P. is admitted to the hospital with the following laboratory values: WBC 2.5 mm^3, RBC 5.6 mm^3, Hgb 17.7 g/dl, Hct 51.7%, platelets 252.0 mm^3, PT 12.1 sec, PTT 29.7 sec, Na 131 mEq/L, K 4.2 mEq/L, Cl 90 mEq/L, CO_2 25 mEq/L, BUN 13 mg/dl, creatinine 0.8 mg/dl, glucose 175 mg/dl.

11. What do these lab values indicate? **[PD/c/PI/ct]**
    - The WBC is low: one of the side effects of VePesid is leukopenia. He is at increased risk for infection. You should review handwashing techniques with him, caution him against exposure to infections, and suggest he wear a mask when doing chores around the farm.
    - The Na and Cl values are low: cisplatin is salt-wasting. C.P. needs to increase the salt content in his diet, and may need to take supplemental electrolytes.
    - The creatinine level is not elevated; however, cisplatin is nephrotoxic so C.P. should be cautioned to drink at least 1 gallon of water each day.

    Instructor Note: Neutropenia can occur when the total WBC count is within a normal range (4,000-10,000 mm^3). It is necessary to calculate an absolute neutrophil count (ANC) to accurately assess a patient's risk of infection: ANC = WBC x (neutrophils in % + bands in %).

12. The pulmonologist performs a thoracentesis and prescribes cefotaximine (Claforan) 1 g IV and q8h erythromycin (Erythrocin) 500 mg IV q6h. What factor in C.P.'s background will complicate his diagnosis of pneumonia? **[PD/ap/PI/ct]**
    - C.P. has some degree of COPD (he smoked for 40 years), and he has been diagnosed with a smoking-related lung cancer.

13. C.P.'s condition continues to deteriorate. He tells you he doesn't want to live like this, but the doctor wants to continue with aggressive therapy. Discuss the pros and cons of continued therapy. **[PD/an/S,PI,PSI/ct,ni,tc]**
    - C.P. may be depressed; if the depression were treated, C.P. may want continued supportive therapy.
    - Oat cell cancer is not a surgically treatable disease, is associated with early and widespread metastasis, and the median survival rate is 1 year following aggressive treatment. The quality of life may be decreased by administration of chemotherapeutic drugs. Have C.P. and his wife been given all the information they need to make an informed choice?
    - C.P. and his wife stated their wishes early in his course of treatment; his wishes should be honored. If the physician can not accept this, C.P. should get another physician who will accommodate his wishes.
    - Does C.P. have advanced directives? If not, he and his wife should work this out ASAP.
    - C.P. has the right not to suffer; he should be given the option of receiving hospice care at home.

C.P. was given the second round of chemotherapy and was discharged to home. He never returned to the hospital for further treatment. He died 2 weeks later.

Case Study 9: Colon Cancer

Difficulty: ***	*Setting:* Hospital
Index Words: Colon cancer	

You are caring for J.B., a 56-year-old woman with colon cancer. PMH includes colon resection followed by combined chemotherapy approximately 18 months ago; recently diagnosed with recurrence of colon cancer and chemotherapy was administered for 5 of the 8 scheduled cycles; previous significant weight loss (current Ht 67", Wt 105 lb); 50 pack/year (2 PPD x 25 yrs) smoking history. J.B. was admitted for acute nausea, vomiting, and dehydration. She is nutritionally depleted. Her physician determines that diagnostic evaluation requires exploratory laparotomy. VS 150/90, 124, 26, 100°F.

1. What are the major risks and potential complications for J.B.? **[PD/an/Pl/ct]**
   - Potential for bowel obstruction.
   - Potential for electrolyte imbalance and third spacing fluid postoperatively.
   - Potential for infection; she will undergo abdominal surgery and already has a compromised immune system r/t chemotherapy treatments.
   - Nutritional compromise: she has lost a significant amount of weight, has suffered from acute N/V to the point of dehydration, may have a bowel obstruction, the side effects of chemotherapy would promote nutritional depletion, and the surgical procedure will render her unable to take PO nutrients.
   - Potential for respiratory infection: she has a 50 pack/year smoking history, she is at risk for third spacing fluid postoperatively, and she will be given general anesthesia for surgery.
   - Hypothermia: her body temperature will be decreased during surgery, and she will receive cool IV fluids during surgery.

2. The physician performs an exploratory laparotomy for lysis of adhesions, small bowel resection, colectomy, and colostomy with Hartman's pouch. After surgery, J.B. is admitted to the SICU with a large abdominal dressing. You roll J.B. side-to-side to remove the soiled surgical linen, and the dressing becomes saturated with a large amount of serosanguinous drainage. Would the drainage be expected after abdominal surgery? **[PD/c/Pl/ct]**
   - Yes: a patient undergoing abdominal surgery would have the abdominal cavity flushed with several liters of NS, and a Penrose drain placed through the abdominal wall before the surgeon would close the abdominal cavity.

3. Traditionally, the physician performs the first dressing change. Why is this done? **[PD/c/Pl/ct]**
   - The physician should observe the suture line, surrounding tissue, and drainage on the original surgical dressing. After the physician is satisfied that all is well, the nurses are requested to perform subsequent dressing changes.

4. The physician removes the surgical dressing. The wound edges are well approximated, the suture line is edematous, the staples are intact, the transverse colostomy rosebud looks pink in the middle and dark around the edges, and there is a Penrose drain in the RMQ. Do any of these findings concern you and why? **[PD/ap/PI/ct]**
   - The rosebud should be pink throughout; dark edges may mean that the tissue is not viable.

The physician prescribes the following TPN orders: amino acids 10% - 100 ml; dextrose 70% 1000 ml; water for injection 1000 ml; sodium acetate 20 mEq; sodium phosphate 20 mEq; potassium acetate 20 mEq; KCl 90 mEq; calcium gluconate 20 mEq; magnesium sulfate 10 mEq; regular insulin 10 units; multivitamins 1 amp; heparin 1200 units. Infuse 3000 ml volume over 24h daily.

5. What nursing management activities should you provide to minimize the potential side effects for J.B.? **[P,I/an/PI/ct.ni]**
   - Observe and monitor the infusion rate per infusion device.
   - Ensure sterile technique when connecting/disconnecting the TPN tubing to the central venous catheter.
   - Monitor and report critical laboratory values: glucose, serum albumin, sodium, potassium, and chloride.
   - Administer sliding scale insulin as prescribed.
   - Provide sterile CVC dressing changes per hospital protocol schedule.
   - Monitor and report changes in mental status, VS, respiratory distress, and I&O.

6. The TPN infusion is complete, the alarm is sounding, and the pharmacy has not delivered the next bottle of TPN. What action should you take and why? **[P,I/an/PI/ct,ni,tc]**
   - Hang a bag of $D_{10}W$, call the pharmacy and tell them she needs the TPN right away, and monitor for changes in glucose level. If the high glucose solution is abruptly stopped, J.B. may experience a profound hypoglycemic episode.

7. You explain to J.B. that she needs to dangle at the side of the bed for a few minutes, then get out of bed and sit in the chair. As J.B. attempts to stand at the bedside, the oxygen tubing pulls her head backward. You remove the oxygen while assisting J.B. to be seated in the chair, then replace the nasal cannula. What are the implications of your action? **[PD/ap/S,PI/ct]**
   - J.B. is being denied oxygen during activity—when she needs it the most.

8. Within minutes of sitting in the chair, you note that J.B. is becoming increasingly pale and diaphoretic. Her pulse is rapid and irregular and she c/o being nauseated and dizzy. What actions should you take next? **[P,I/an/S,PI,PSI/ct,ni,tc]**
    - Turn on the nurse's light and call for help.
    - Get J.B. back to bed and raise all side rails while reassuring her that you are going to stay with her until she is stable.
    - Obtain a full set of VS, check pulses, and obtain a STAT glucose level.
    - Obtain oximeter reading and increase oxygen flow rate as needed to maintain $SaO_2 > 90\%$.
    - Observe the abdomen and ask J.B. about abdominal discomfort.
    - Determine if the wall suction unit is functioning, the tubing is connected securely, and the NGT is patent.
    - Notify the physician and document the incident.

9. J.B. looks at you and tells you that she knows she is never going to leave the hospital alive. She says she has a lot of regrets. She confides that she used to drink a lot and wasn't a good mother to her 3 children; her son hasn't spoken to her in 15 years. How should you respond? **[P,I/an/PSI/ct,ni,tc]**
    - Do not try to deny J.B.'s feelings; listen to her.
    - Talk to her; tell her that most people do things that they are not proud of. She is still alive, and as long as she can draw a breath, she has the opportunity to make things right.
    - Ask her if she wants you to call her children and have them come to visit.
    - Ask her if she would like to talk to a clergy person.
    - Encourage her to make peace with her "Higher Power," if that is part of her belief system, then try to make peace with her family.
    - Remind her that anytime can be a time for healing.

CHAPTER 10. MULTIPLE SYSTEM DISORDERS

Case Study 1: Burns

Difficulty: *	*Setting:* Hospital
Index Words: Burns	

You are working the day shift on the medical-surgical unit in a small, rural community hospital. Your assignment includes an 18-year-old woman, A.N., admitted at night. She was burned in a house fire. She sustained 30% body surface and partial-thickness burns on her legs and back.

1. A.N. is undergoing burn fluid resuscitation using the standard Baxter (Parkland) formula. She was burned at 0200 and admitted at 0400. She weighs 110 pounds. Calculate her fluid requirements, and specify how much will be given and what time intervals will be used. **[P/c/PI/ct,ni]**
   - Crystalloids are the fluids of choice during the first 24 hours. Ringer's lactate is the fluid used in the Baxter (Parkland) formula. The calculation for fluid needs during the first 24 hours = 4 ml x weight in Kg x % of body surface area burned. In this case it would be: 4 x 50 x 30 = 6000 ml of Ringer's lactate. The first half will be given during the first 8 hours since the time of the burn. So, 3000 ml will be given by 1000. In the next 8-hour period, ¼ of the total fluid will be given. The same amount will be given during the last 8-hour period. So, she will receive 1500 ml of Ringer's lactate from 1000 to 1800, and 1500 ml from 1800 to 0200. Crystalloids and colloids will be used in the next 24-hour period.

2. A.N. was sleeping when the fire started and managed to make her way out of the house through thick smoke. You are concerned about possible smoke inhalation. What assessment findings would corroborate this concern? **[A/k/PI/ct,ni]**
   - You will assess A.N. for burns to the face and neck, singed nasal hair or facial hair, dry cough, hoarseness, copious sputum with or without evidence of charcoal or soot, whether she was burned in a closed space, smoke odor, and signs of respiratory distress.

3. A.N. is very concerned about visible scars. What will you tell her to allay her fears? **[I/k/PI/ct,ni]**
   - Based on her admitting diagnosis, her burns are partial thickness and no scarring should occur. However, the burns may be deeper than they initially appeared, so it will take a few days to know for sure.

4. A.N. is in severe pain. What is the drug of choice for pain relief following burn injury, and how should it be given? **[I/k/PI/ct,ni]**
   - The drug of choice for pain management is morphine sulfate. It should be given intravenously in small increments. Intramuscular and subcutaneous injections should be avoided. Many burn units initially administer morphine sulfate or midazolam (Versed) by PCA pump.

5. A.N.'s burns are to be treated by the open-method with topical application of silver sufadiazine (Silvadene). What is the major drawback to this method of treatment? **[P/c/PI/ct,ni]**
   - Chilling. The patient loses more heat through the burned areas because of injury to the vascular bed that normally regulates heat loss. Heat lamps, increased room temperature, avoidance of drafts, and humidification of the room air will help prevent or treat this.

6. A special burn diet is ordered for A.N.. She has always gained weight easily and is concerned about the size of the portions. What diet-related teaching will you provide? **[I/c/PI,PSI/ct,ni,tc]**
   - The patient who has been burned needs extra protein and calories to promote wound healing. The registered dietitian will calculate the number of calories needed for wound healing. During recovery, she needs to eat approximately twice as much as she did before the burn. In addition to her meals she should also eat between-meal snacks. The extra calories will be used by her body to heal, so she should not gain weight.

7. Tissues under and around A.N.'s burns are severely swollen. She looks at you with tears in her eyes and asks, "Will they stay this way?" What is your answer? **[A,I/c/PI/ct,ni]**
   - No, following a burn, capillary damage occurs, causing capillary leak. There is a rapid fluid shift from the vasculature to the interstitial spaces, resulting in massive swelling. This usually lasts 2 to 3 days. Once the capillaries have repaired themselves, the fluid is reabsorbed and then excreted.

8. Following significant burn injury, the patient is at high risk for infection. What nursing measures will you institute to prevent this? **[P/c/PI/ct,ni]**
   - The patient should be placed in a private room. Protective isolation procedures should be initiated. Aseptic technique with sterile gloves should be used during dressing changes. All supplies necessary to care for the patient should remain in the patient's room. No one with an actual or potential infection should care for or visit the patient.

9. A.N. has one area of circumferential burns on her right lower leg. What complication is she in danger of developing and how will you monitor for it? **[I/c/PI/ct,ni]**
   - She is in danger of developing circulatory compromise distal to the circumferential area. You need to closely monitor the foot for signs of decreased circulation or sensation. Compare the two feet for quality of pulses, warmth, color, capillary refill, level of sensation, swelling, and pain. Report signs of decreased circulation or sensation immediately.

Case Study 2: Multiple Trauma

Difficulty: *	*Setting:* Hospital
Index Words: Multiple trauma, fracture	

You are working evenings on an orthopedic floor. One of your patients, J.O., is a 25-year-old man who was a new admission on day shift. He was involved in a motor vehicle accident (MVA) during a high-speed police chase. His admitting diagnosis is status post (s/p) open reduction and internal fixation of the R femur, which was performed under general anesthesia, multiple rib fractures, sternal bruise, and multiple abrasions. He speaks some English but is more comfortable with his "home" language. He is under arrest for narcotics trafficking, so one wrist is shackled to the bed and he has a guard with him continuously. Another drug dealer has told him "he's coming to get him." Hospital security is aware of the situation.

Your initial assessment reveals stable VS of 116/78, 84, 16, 98.6°F. His only complaint is pain, for which he has a PCA pump. He has crackles in lung bases bilaterally. His abdomen is soft and nontender. He has an indwelling Foley catheter and an nasogastric tube connected to low wall suction. His IV of D_5 LR is infusing in the proximal port of a L subclavian triple lumen catheter, the remaining two ports are heparin locked. His R femur is connected to skeletal traction. The dressing is dry and intact over the incision site.

1. J.O. wants to smoke a cigarette. He usually smokes a pack a day and has had none since the accident. He is irate because the day nurse would not let him smoke. What is your major concern about J.O.'s smoking? **[PD/an/S,PI/ct]**
   - It may be illegal or against hospital policy (depending on your state) and it would constitute a hazard to safety.
   - The evidence of chest trauma, crackles in both bases, general anesthesia, history of smoking, and the traction-enforced bed rest put J.O. at high risk of pulmonary complications, especially ARDS or atelectasis. He is also at high risk for pulmonary embolism resulting from a thomboembolus from prolonged bed rest or a fat embolus from his fractured femur. Cigarette smoking decreases oxygen absorption, constricts arteries and arterioles (compromises his circulation), and may further complicate his condition.

2. J.O.'s right leg is connected to 10 pounds of skeletal traction. As you troubleshoot the system, you note that the ropes are knotted at connection sites, the pulleys have rope running along the center tracts, the leg is slightly flexed at the knee, the leg is 6 inches above the mattress, and the 10-pound weight is resting on the floor. Are any of these findings of concern to you? If so, how would you fix it? **[A/ap/PI/ni]**
   - The weight should not be resting on the floor.
   - Call a second person to maintain traction on the rope while you untie the knot around the weight. Reposition the weight so that it no longer rests on the floor, and retie the knot. Have the second person slowly release manual traction once the weight is repositioned.

The nurse in the emergency room phones to tell you that J.O.'s immunization status could not be determined when he arrived so no tetanus immunization was given. When you ask J.O. the date of his last tetanus shot, he looks puzzled and asks you what a tetanus shot is. When asking about his childhood, you find that he was born and raised in Colombia. He immigrated to the United States 5 years ago. He does not know if he has ever had a tetanus shot. You inform the physician and he orders diphtheria/tetanus toxoid 0.5 ml IM and Hypertet (tetanus immune globulin) 250 U deep IM.

3. Why is J.O. getting two injections? **[P,I/k/HP/ct,ni]**
   - The diphtheria/tetanus toxoid is given to J.O. as the first dose in his general immunization against tetanus. A second dose will be given in 1 to 2 months, and the third dose in 6 to 12 months. Thus, he will not be fully immunized against tetanus for 6 to 12 months. Hypertet supplies passive immunity to tetanus following injury for those people who have not had a complete set of tetanus immunizations. It is given to prevent tetanus from occurring as a result of this injury.

4. J.O. has a Foley catheter inserted to drain his urine. What should the nurse assess for in relation to the Foley catheter? **[A/c/PI/ct]**
   - Quantity of urine output is important for J.O., as it is in any victim of multiple trauma. The nurse should expect a minimum of 30 to 60 ml per hour of urine output.
   - Color is also an important parameter in this case because J.O. was involved in a high-speed accident that can result in acceleration/deceleration injuries. The kidneys are often damaged. The urine should be observed for frank blood and tested for microscopic blood and rhabdomyolysis following such severe bruising and muscle injury.

5. While assessing distal to the fractured femur, the nurse notes that his toes are cold to the touch. What other assessment findings should be gathered? **[A/c/PI/ni]**
   - The nurse should check temperature of the toes on the unfractured leg, capillary refill in both feet, quality of peripheral pulses in both feet, quality of sensation in both feet, color of both feet, presence of pain in the foot of the fractured leg, and presence of swelling in the foot of the fractured leg.

6. J.O. has an antiembolism stockings ordered for his L leg. What is the rationale for putting stockings on only one leg? **[I/ap/PI/ct,ni]**
   - The right leg is immobilized in skeletal traction, so the hose cannot be applied to this leg. However immobilization will necessitate a prolonged period of bed rest. Prevention of thromboembolism in the unaffected leg is important to prevent complications. Application of an antiembolism stocking to the unaffected leg is one way to prevent thromboembolism.

7. At 1800 J.O.'s guard summons you to his room. J.O. is cold and clammy, groaning, pale, agitated, and slightly confused. VS are 70/palp, 140, 28, 98.0°F. His pulse is weak and thready. His abdomen is painful and appears to be increased in size. You summon the physician. What else can you do? **[P,I/an/PI/ct,ni]**
   - Elevate the patient's unaffected leg and remove the pillow under his head. This will place the patient in modified Trendelenburg and assist venous return to the heart. Increase the rate on the IV to increase intravascular volume and, hopefully, blood pressure. Repeat VS every 5 minutes.

8. The physician arrives and wishes to perform a peritoneal lavage. Explain why peritoneal lavage is being done, and describe the procedure. **[A/k,c/Pl/ct,ni]**
   - This is a diagnostic procedure used to detect blood in the peritoneal cavity.
   - A single puncture (using a trochar) is made through the abdominal wall into the peritoneal cavity, a peritoneal lavage catheter is inserted and a standard 1 L bag of Ringer's lactate (never a solution with dextrose) is hung and infused through regular IV tubing. When it is fully infused, the IV bag is then lowered below the height of the abdomen so the fluid can drain back out. A sample of the bag contents is sent to the laboratory immediately for analysis for blood, bacteria, or food contents/contaminants. Significant blood loss usually is obvious from the color of the solution.

9. What are the nursing responsibilities in preparation for this procedure (in order)? **[P/ap/Pl/ct,ni]**
   - Explain the procedure to the patient, assess VS, insert a Foley catheter to decompress the bladder (J.O. already has one in place), and a nasogastric tube to decompress the stomach (if not already in place). Obtain a peritoneal lavage tube, prepare 1 L LR to be used as lavage fluid, and assemble additional supplies as needed.

10. The physician begins the diagnostic peritoneal lavage procedure. Upon insertion of the trochar into the abdomen, bright red blood under pressure returns. What happens next? **[E/an/Pl/ct]**
   - The test is over, as this is a grossly positive result. The trochar is removed. J.O. will be taken to the OR for an exploratory laparotomy ASAP. Depending on the extent of injury, he may return to the orthopedic unit or an intensive care unit following surgery.

11. In view of the threat made on J.O.'s life and his vulnerable situation, what precautions should the nursing unit take to protect him? **[P/ap/S/ct,ni]**
   - Check the hospital's policy and procedures regarding prisoners and security risks. Keep security apprised of the situation. Request shift and responsibility details from the guard (e.g., who will be working what hours). Ask that the guards check in at the nurses' station and show picture identification; *anyone* can rent a uniform. Require that they never leave J.O. alone (not even for a cigarette or for a break). Do *not* place J.O.'s real name on his door. Guard his chart carefully; do not place his name or room number anywhere it can be seen. Do *not* use "John Doe" as an identifier, it's too obvious. Some hospitals assign a false name; this can be dangerous because it can result in medication errors or making entries on the wrong chart. Calmly ask any individuals you do not know who are in the charting or nurses' station area for identification; *anyone* can wear scrubs or a lab coat. Obtain a list and description of approved visitors, and require identification. Do not give out information over the telephone unless it is to an identified next-of-kin. Report strangers who appear to be wandering around to security immediately. Keep his door closed and your eyes open. Threats on a patient's life jeopardize every other individual on the unit, patients, visitors, and staff included.

J.O. recovered for several weeks in the hospital before being sent to jail to await trial. Shortly before his trial date, he was found stabbed to death in his cell. Although there was an investigation, the murder weapon was never found, and no one was ever charged in his death.

Case Study 3: Pulmonary Edema

Difficulty: ** *Setting:* Hospital

Index Words: Pulmonary edema, chronic obstructive pulmonary disease, myocardial infarction

You are working on the cardiac unit. One of your patients, J.H., is 52 years old and has had an acute anterior wall myocardial infarction (MI). He is a police detective who is overweight, smokes 2 packs per day, drinks daily, sporadically takes his antihypertensive medication, and is angry that he is in the hospital. He suffered his MI during a heated argument with his wife. He initially blamed her for all of his current problems and refused to cooperate, but he has now consented to participate in the cardiac rehabilitation program. From his barrel chest and history, you also assume he has COPD, although that has not specifically been diagnosed.

Upon arrival at his bedside you note that he is extremely short of breath. He is having difficulty talking and has gurgling respirations and a moist cough. You are surprised to see his IV is empty. He tells you that the nurse told him he could go have a cigarette after his IV antibiotic was finished, so he "opened the valve to make-it run faster."

1. You suspect he has pulmonary edema. What other assessment findings would confirm your suspicion? **[A/c/PI/ct]**
   - Anxiety, restlessness, blood-tinged frothy sputum, use of accessory muscles for breathing, central and peripheral cyanosis, nasal flaring, ashen color, cold and clammy skin, peripheral edema, crackles on auscultation, wheezing, elevated blood pressure, tachycardia, and S_3 gallop rhythm.

2. What position will J.H. find most comfortable during this episode? **[I/ap/PI/ct]**
   - Fluid overload is the reason for his pulmonary edema. Positions that pool blood in the extremities result in less blood return to the heart. High-Fowler's with legs in the dependent position will most effectively decrease venous return to the heart.

J.H. has the following medications ordered: furosemide (Lasix) 40 mg IV q6h, potassium (K-Dur) 20 mEq PO bid, digoxin (Lanoxin) 0.25 mg PO qd, lisinopril (Prinovil) 10 mg qd, morphine 2-4 mg IVP prn, 2 L O_2/nc HS and prn. He has not had any medications yet this morning.

3. What medications might you give him before the arrival of the physician? State your rationale. **[P/an/PI/ct,ni]**
   - All but the K-Dur would be effective in pulmonary edema. However, the patient's ability to drink fluids and take oral medication is compromised and aspiration may occur. The onset of action of oral medications is also not rapid enough for this situation. Give:
     - Lasix 40 mg IV: a loop diuretic that is rapid-acting and will decrease the fluid overload.
     - Morphine sulfate 4 mg IV: drug of choice in acute pulmonary edema. Decreases anxiety and causes vasodilation to decrease venous return to the heart.
     - Oxygen: 2 L O_2/nc will increase the concentration of available oxygen inhaled into the lungs, thus increasing blood levels.

4. You summon the physician STAT. An additional intravenous dose of Lasix 40 mg is ordered. How fast can Lasix be administered IVP? What is the onset of action? **[P,I/c/PI/ct,ni]**
   - Give over 2 minutes because you can give up to 20 mg per minute. The onset of action can be as rapid as 5 minutes. Have a urinal or bedpan handy or insert a Foley catheter quickly.

5. J.H. diureses effectively and begins breathing more comfortably. He does not understand how such a small amount of fluid from his antibiotic could cause such big problems. He asks you to explain it. **[I/k/PI/ct,ni,tc]**
   - His heart has been damaged from his recent heart attack and is not capable of handling rapid increases in the amount of fluid effectively. Rapid infusion of even small amounts of intravenous fluid can result in the problems he experienced.

6. In view of his recent diuresis, what 2 lab values would you especially need to monitor? **[PD/ap/S,PI/ct,ni]**
   - Potassium and magnesium are both lost in diuresis and are essential for effective myocardial functioning.

7. Once J.H. has recovered from his episode of pulmonary edema, you decide to take advantage of the "teachable moment" to reinforce the concept of fluid overload. List 3 other ways J.H. can cause an overload of fluid in his body. **[I/ap/PI/ct,ni,tc]**
   - Increased fluid intake, particularly sodium-rich fluids.
   - Increased use of table salt.
   - Eating sodium-rich foods (e.g., peanuts, chips, pizza).
   - Avoiding foods rich in potassium, calcium, and magnesium (they help the body to balance sodium).
   - Failure to take his prescribed diuretic.

8. J.H. tells you that his favorite things to eat and drink are ham sandwiches, peanuts, coffee, beer, iced tea, apple juice, colas, and milk. Which ones can he continue to eat or drink on a low-sodium cardiac prevention diet? **[PD/c/PI/ct]**
   - He can continue to drink apple juice. He may modify the milk to skim milk and continue drinking it. He can drink decaffeinated coffee or tea. Peanuts, ham, colas, and beer are high in sodium and should be avoided.

9. J.H. becomes short of breath while he is walking with you. He panics and is absolutely certain he is going into pulmonary edema again. You believe he is suffering from dyspnea on exertion. Explain the difference between dyspnea on exertion and pulmonary edema. **[E/ap/PI/ct]**
   - Both conditions cause respiratory distress. Dyspnea on exertion following MI is usually a result of deconditioning and mild dehydration; muscle deconditioning from the inactivity of hospitalization results in increased fatigue, and bed rest contributes to gravitational dehydration (resulting from extended time in the horizontal position). It is important to rest when fatigue occurs, but slowly increasing activity will recondition muscles and decrease fatigue. His episode of acute pulmonary edema was a result of a sudden overload of fluid.

10. Pulmonary function tests are performed while J.H. is in the hospital, and COPD is confirmed. From J.H.'s history, what factor probably contributed to both his cardiac and pulmonary disease? **[A/an/Pl/ct]**
    - His heavy smoking was likely the biggest contributor to both his cardiac and pulmonary disease.

J.H.'s wife has had enough. She goes home, throws out all the ashtrays, and comes into his room announcing he will either quit smoking or she is going to throw him out. J.H. tries to get sympathy from you. "Sorry, Marlboro Man," you tell him, "She's right this time, and you're on your own." He glares at you both for a few minutes, then shrugs and pulls out his "secret stash" of cigarettes and his lighter, hands them to you, and tells you it's OK to trash them. "Guess what?" you cheerfully inform him, "We've got a smoking cessation class starting this afternoon and it's going to be full of a bunch of tough guys like you!"

Case Study 4: Abdominal Aortic Aneurysm

Difficulty: **	*Setting:* Hospital
Index Words: Abdominal aortic aneurysm, paralysis, dehiscence	

You are working on a telemetry unit and have just received a transfer from the intensive care unit. The 50-year-old male patient, T.A., had a repair of an abdominal aortic aneurysm (AAA) measuring 8 cm in diameter. This is his second day postop. He is an attorney with a very active practice. He considered himself to be healthy before diagnosis of the aneurysm, although he took medication for gastric hyperacidity. He has had progressive weakness of his lower extremities and decreasing urine output since surgery. T.A. also has a 10-year history of type II diabetes mellitus; he has been requiring animal-based insulin the last 6 months to keep his glucose levels under control.

1. T.A. is very concerned about the leg weakness since his surgery. He states, "If I had knowm this was going to happen, I never would have agreed to the surgery. I was fine before. I'd still be fine now if I hadn't been operated on, wouldn't I?" Your response based on the knowledge of aortic aneurysm should be: **[I/c/PI/ct,ni,tc]**
   - No. Because of the size of his aneurysm, he was at great risk for rupture. Aneurysms less than 4 cm in diameter can be managed medically. Those that are 4 to 6 cm are carefully managed medically. Those greater than 6 cm should be surgically repaired because the risk of rupture and subsequent mortality is extremely high. Aneurysms typically grow at 0.5 cm per year. So, T.A. was not fine before the surgery; he was at high risk for sudden death and didn't know it.

2. You are performing your initial assessment of T.A.'s legs. What findings should you record? **[A/ap/PI/ct,ni]**
   - Neurosensory findings in the legs are particularly important in the patient who has had repair of an abdominal aortic aneurysm. Sensation, movement, color, capillary refill, pulse quality, and symmetry of the legs should be recorded. Any abnormalities should be rapidly reported.

3. Four hours after admission to your floor you note that T.A. has had a urine output of 75 ml of dark amber urine. You examine the catheter and tubing for obstructions and there are none. What other assessment data should you gather to determine if a problem exists? **[PD/ap/PI/ct]**
   - The concern here is acute renal failure. Many patients have a lower than normal output in the first few days following surgery because of decreased intake. The first item to review in this case is patient intake. If possible, determine the amount of weight gain in the presence of an intake greater than an output. Next review lab results for increases in renal lab values (BUN, creatinine, urinalysis, and urine osmolality). If these tests have not been done, now is the time to suggest them. Next, scan the surgical notes to see if the aneurysm was above or below the renal arteries. Crossclamping the aorta to repair the aneurysm above the level of the renal arteries may have resulted in anoxic renal damage.

4. Laboratory tests reveal renal damage. T.A. is placed on a fluid restriction and a renal diet. T.A. asks what he is going to be able to eat on his diet. You reply: **[P,I/c/PI/ct,ni]**
   - Renal diets restrict those products that increase nitrogenous wastes and increase serum potassium levels; thus, they are high in carbohydrates and fats but low in protein and potassium. Acute renal failure also results in nausea, which makes adequate dietary intake problematic.

5. T.A. has a dialysis catheter inserted into his left subclavian vein. You are preparing to administer an intravenous antibiotic and find that his only other intravenous access, a peripheral line, is obstructed. What should you do? **[P/ap/PI/ct,ni]**
   - You should insert another peripheral IV. The dialysis catheter is dedicated for dialysis access and should not be routinely used for scheduled intravenous medications. Administration of medications through the catheter is usually restricted to those medications given during hemodialysis.

6. Upon return from his first dialysis, T.A. complains of headache and nausea, is slightly confused, restless, and has an elevated blood pressure. You suspect disequilibrium phenomenon. You notify the physician. What nursing measures can you institute at this point? **[P,I/ap/PI/ct,ni]**
   - Keep him quiet, reduce environmental stimuli, closely supervise him to prevent injury, and give a mild analgesic for the headache if he has one ordered. Following stabilization, notify the dialysis unit of the event, so that they can monitor for problems in subsequent dialysis sessions.

7. T.A. has an episode of severe vomiting. His abdominal wound dehisces, and a loop of his intestines eviscerates. Another staff member has summoned the doctor. What care should you render before the physician's arrival? **[I/ap/PI/ct,ni,tc]**
   - First, cover the intestines with sterile gauze moistened with warm, sterile normal saline, and elevate the head of the bed or knees to decrease pressure within the abdominal cavity. Next, assess VS frequently because shock may occur. Third, reassure the patient. Fourth, notify the nursing supervisor/OR of the evisceration.

8. You are concerned that the weakness in Mr. Andrew's legs may result in muscle atrophy. What nursing interventions can you take to prevent this? **[P,I/ap/PI/ct,ni]**
   - Recognize the significance of this problem and request a physical therapy referral for specialized and focused intervention.
   - Passive range of motion is crucial to the maintenance of joint mobility and should be performed twice daily at a minimum. Foot drop and knee flexion must also be prevented by careful positioning. Encouraging T.A. to move his legs to the extent possible for him will also help prevent muscle atrophy.

A sliding scale human recombinant insulin plan has been instituted, but T.A.'s glucose levels have been ranging from 62 to 387 mg/dl. "That's funny," he tells, you. "You're giving about the same amount about the same times as I gave it to myself at home. I don't understand why it's not working!" You explain to him that the dialysis and the surgery both profoundly affect his insulin needs. In addition, although it may look similar in the syringe, he is getting a different dose of insulin than he has been getting at home.

9. Based on recent findings contrasting the metabolism of human insulin versus animal insulin sources, explain why T.A. may be having trouble regulating his glucose levels. **[P,I,E/ap/PI/ct]**
   - Recent research has indicated human insulin has faster-acting metabolic action than the animal-based insulins, with a more rapid time/action profile (onset, peak, and duration). In addition, there is increasing recognition of the profound interindividual differences in response to insulin that must be respected to achieve glucose control.

10. T.A.'s wound is not healing. You call the enterostomal therapy (ET) RN to evaluate what can be done. After looking at T.A.'s wound, he looks at T.A.'s chart, sighs, and points to the glucose levels. "Here's your problem," he says. "The way this is going, he'll never heal." Based on recent findings in diabetes management, explain what he means. What other health care professionals may help you with T.A.'s glucose regulation? **[A,PD,I,E/an/PI/ct,ni]**
    - Recent research indicates that unless glucose is kept near 140 mg/dl or lower, wounds won't heal. A registered dietician or registered nurse Certified Diabetes Educator (CDE) may help you understand how to adjust meals, insulin, and activity so T.A. maintains a therapeutic glucose level and has an optimal healing environment. It may take days to weeks for T.A.'s glucose to come under control as recommended for wound healing to occur.

Case Study 5: Deep Vein Thrombosis

Difficulty: *** *Setting:* Hospital

Index Words: Deep vein thrombosis, cerebrovascular accident, chronic obstructive pulmonary disease, congestive heart failure

T.M., a long-haul trucker, has arrived as an emergency department admission. He has a history of chronic bronchitis that has been controlled on an outpatient basis for the last 10 years. After a 10-day road trip, he noted that his left leg was swollen and painful. A scan revealed a deep vein thrombosis (DVT) of the left leg (a 24-cm clot in the left femoral vein). His admission VS are 190/110, 76, 24, 100°F. His admission assessment shows barrel chest; male pattern obesity ("beer belly"); heart sounds that are distant secondary to lung sounds; rhonchi and wheezes intermittently in all lung fields; enlarged palpable liver; and a left lower leg that is red, edematous, warm, and significantly larger than the right. He has been told by his physician to quit smoking, drinking, lose weight, and increase exercise. He has decreased his drinking to weekends when he is not on the road and has switched to light beer. But, he still smokes 2 packs per day and remains overweight. He takes theophylline (Theodur) 300 mg PO q8h and uses an ipratropium (Atrovent) inhaler q4h prn to help keephis COPD under control.

1. Upon admission, T.M. states, "I just don't know how this happened....I've been taking my drugs and cut back on my beer. I've even lost 10 pounds. This healthy living stuff is overrated!" List and explain his risk factors for DVT versus the primary contributing factor to his DVT. **[PD/c/HP/ct]**
   - His risk factors for DVT are immobility (occupational hazard; he sits in one position during trips for long periods of time), disease processes (his smoking), and COPD (chronic bronchitis) contributes to polycythemia, which thickens his blood), pressure on the vessel (his obesity puts extra pressure on the vessels of his legs when he sits), and clotting dysfunction (the increased viscosity of his blood from polycythemia predisposes him to this).
   - Venous stasis in the legs is the primary contributing factor to DVT.

2. T.M. wants to know why his liver is enlarged when he has just about quit drinking. How are you going to explain this to him? **[PD/an/PI/ct,tc]**
   - Chronic bronchitis is a progressive disease that eventually causes failure of the right side of the heart because of the increased pumping pressure needed to pump blood through the lungs. One of the signs of right-sided heart failure is a back-up of blood into the liver, resulting in enlargement.
   - Alcoholic liver disease is also a progressive disease. Although he has decreased his drinking, he drank for years in excessive amounts. This also can result in liver enlargement.
   - His enlarged liver may be from his chronic bronchitis, from his previous high alcohol intake, or from a combination of both.

3. The physician ordered total bed rest. T.M. says he can't possibly stay in bed all the time, he has to go outside to smoke and he absolutely has to go to the bathroom. He tries to bargain with you not to get up to smoke if he can go to the bathroom. He thinks you are being unreasonable and asks why you won't at least let him get up to the bathroom. How are you going to respond? **[P,I/an/PI,PSI/ct,tc]**
   - There are several reasons why bed rest is essential. Foremost is to prevent the thrombus from becoming an embolus. Migration of the clot to the lungs or brain could result in death. The second reason is that elevation decreases swelling and increases venous return to the heart, preventing further clotting. The third is that immobilization decreases pain in the leg.

4. T.M. is placed on 2 L O_2/nc, a heparin drip, an IV antibiotic, and his usual COPD medications. Four days after admission, his wife calls you to the room "because he's acting weird." When you arrive, you observe he is very confused; he was lucid an hour ago. What should you do? **[P,I/an/PI/ct,ni]**
   - First, check the oxygen setting. Hypoxia is the most frequent cause of acute confusion.
   - Next STAT page the physician. While awaiting his arrival, get VS and perform an assessment. Pay particular attention to subtle changes in the neurologic exam and the pulmonary exam.
   - Check SaO_2 if a pulse oximeter is available.

You note decreased strength and movement in the L side of his body. He also has a mild facial droop on the L side of his face. The physician arrives and orders a STAT CT scan of the head with and without contrast.

5. According to his wife, T.M. has no drug allergies; he's only allergic to shrimp. What significance does this allergy have? **[A/c/S,PI/ct]**
   - Allergy to shellfish is a contraindication to receiving contrast material. He will not be able to receive the dye used for contrast during the CT scan. This information needs to be given to the physician immediately; also, make sure the radiologist knows it and that it's written on the front of the chart before the exam. Document what you have done.

6. An x-ray transporter arrives to take T.M. to x-ray. Additional floor personnel who could go to the x-ray include 3 certified nurses aides (CNAs), licensed practical nurse (LPN), 3 RNs, and the physician. Who should accompany T.M. to x-ray and why? **[P,E/an/PI/ct]**
   - His most likely diagnosis is cerebral thrombosis from a DVT embolus. His stroke is still evolving, so *he is extremely unstable at this point.* At the least, an RN should accompany him to assess for further changes. The physician also should accompany T.M. The chances for further embolus formation increase with movement to the transport stretcher and x-ray table. This is a high-risk situation that may evolve into a CODE.

7. CT scan reveals a right hemispheric cerebral thrombosis from an embolus. On return from the CT scan you observe his level of consciousness has decreased, and he no longer responds to questions. Although the doctor explained the findings to her, his wife keeps asking you when he is going to wake up. What should you do? **[I/an/PSI/ct,ni,tc]**
   - Ask her to tell you what the physician told her. She may not understand what she has been told. Reinforce the explanation. Answer her questions honestly. Suggest she give you the number of a family member or friend who can come be with her. Contact the social worker or chaplain, if she chooses.
   - Ask her if T.M. has advanced directives or health care power-of-attorney. See if you can elicit what her feelings are on his behalf.

8. If he survives this current crisis, which complication of CVA is T.M. at greatest risk of acquiring? **[PD,P/an/PI/ct]**
   - T.M. is at highest risk for developing pneumonia. He already has a compromised pulmonary system because of his COPD. The decreased mobility that will result from the stroke will decrease his ability to clear secretions. Aggressive pulmonary toilet and respiratory therapy need to be instituted to prevent this complication.

Case Study 6: Alzheimer's Disease

Difficulty: *** *Setting:* Hospital

Index Words: Alzheimer's disease, urosepsis, cerebrovascular accident, decubitus ulcers, malnutrition

You are working nights on an inpatient geriatric unit. An 82-year-old woman, M.B., is admitted from an extended care facility with urosepsis, Alzheimer's disease, and a history of hypertension and CVA. Her right side is flaccid. She does not communicate, moans when in pain, and hits, kicks, and claws with her left arm and leg when disturbed. Her initial assessment shows emaciation and multiple pressure ulcers. She has an indwelling Foley catheter and one peripheral IV of D_5 NS at 75 ml/h. Her initial VS are 86/50, 108, 24, 104.6°F. Her initial WBC is 34.2 mm^3.

1. Four hours after admission you note that M.B.'s Foley catheter has not drained any urine. You cannot begin her antibiotics until you collect a urine culture. What should you do? **[E,A/an/Pl/ct,ni]**
   - First check the age of the catheter. If the patient arrived with the catheter in place, it may be clogged with debris and need replacing. If the catheter is newly inserted, check placement. Elderly women often have atrophy of the genitalia with retraction of the urethral opening into the vagina. That, coupled with vaginal atrophy, often results in erroneous insertion into the vagina. If there is correct placement of a new catheter and there is no increase in urine output, the patient may be dehydrated. A request for an increase in the 75 ml/h rate of the IV might be warranted. If this does not work, the patient should be evaluated for acute renal failure.

2. M.B. has 2 intravenous antibiotics, gentamicin (Garamycin) and ticarcillin (Ticar), ordered for 1000. Her morning serum creatinine is 3.2 mg/dl. Her admission serum creatinine was 2.0. Which medication can you safely give? **[I/an/S,Pl/ct,ni]**
   - Both. Gentamicin is nephrotoxic but Gentamicin nephrotoxicity rarely occurs after the first dose; typically occurring after 7 days of therapy. The dose of Gentamicin must be administered in more conservative doses and serum levels must be monitored more closely. Ticarcillin, although not nephrotoxic, should be used cautiously in renal impairment. The physician should be notified of the serum creatinine values before the administration of either antibiotic, and adjustments should be made in the treatment regimen.

3. M.B.'s diet is "mechanical soft." The certified nursing assistant (CNA) tells you that M.B. often spits food during feeding. She also becomes agitated and tries to hit and kick the CNA during meals. Her total intake is less than 25% of the food she is supposed to receive. You believe she may be suffering from protein caloric malnutrition. What assessment findings would you gather to support this? **[A/an/Pl/ct,ni]**
   - Signs of protein caloric malnutrition include emaciation, poor skin turgor, evidence of infection, poor nutritional intake, nonhealing pressure sores, decreased serum albumin, and decreased serum total protein.

4. M.B. has a PEG tube inserted and is started on continuous tube feedings at 100 ml/h. During your morning assessment you note that her gastric residual is 175 ml. There are no specific orders regarding residual amount. What should you do? **[PD/ap/PI/ct,ni]**
   - Continue the feeding but monitor the residual closely. Residuals of greater than 2 times the hourly feeding infusion rate should be reported to the physician. A residual of 175 is close to the 2-hour total of 200.

5. M.B. is at high risk for pulmonary aspiration of her tube feedings. What nursing measures can decrease the chances for this complication? **[P,I/ap/S/ct,ni]**
   - Nursing measures to prevent pulmonary aspiration include tinting the formula with blue coloring, keeping the head of bed elevated at least 30 degrees, measuring gastric residual at least every 4 hours, and assessing for the presence of bowel sounds every 4 hours.

6. M.B. has a large, stage IV decubitus ulcer over her sacrum and stage II decubitus ulcers over both trochanters. You are initiating a turning schedule for M.B.. What would be the most effective positions and schedule? **[P/ap/PI/ct,ni]**
   - Because of the existing pressure sores over the bony prominences of the back, right, and left sides, the most effective schedule should not include these areas. Turning from left to right every 2 hours and positioning in the 30 degree position removes weight from all of these areas and allows for healing.

7. The enterostomal therapy nurse orders Elase ointment to the sacral decubitus followed by wet-to-moist dressing. What observations are important to note following dressing changes? **[A,E/an/PI/ct,ni]**
   - Elase ointment is an enzymatic debriding agent that is effective only in a moist environment. The wound should be evaluated for debridement of necrotic tissue and appearance of healthy tissue. Once all necrotic tissue is removed, the Elase ointment should be discontinued. The enterostomal therapy nurse will need to specify a different type of therapy at this point. Be aware that a moist environment facilitates the migration and proliferation of epithelial cells in the wound resurfacing process.

8. What could you do to improve M.B's quality of life? **[A,P/an/PSI/ct,ni]**
   - Contact the ECF she came from and find out if M.B. responds positively to anything (music, massage, foot rub, special foods, colors) that could be used to address her needs.
   - Evaluate M.B. for the possibility of pain, and see if anything can be done about it.
   - Check M.B.'s mouth and teeth to see if there is any reason she would have trouble eating. Can she swallow?

   Instructor Note: So often, basic comfort and pleasure needs of older adults are ignored by our health care system. It is difficult to imagine how miserable life can be when one cannot communicate basic needs and preferences. Unfortunately, students often work with nurses or ancillary personnel who do not have time or interest to investigate these issues.

One of the CNAs at the extended care facility said M.B. always "perked up" when their therapy dog, Cindy, came for a visit. Although hospital policy prohibited dogs (except for companion and helper dogs) visiting in patients' rooms, special permission was obtained for Cindy to visit M.B. "It was miraculous," the afternoon nurse told her colleague at report, "M.B. perked up and smiled for the first time since she came here. She petted that dog for the longest time and seemed more relaxed and cooperative afterward than you ever could imagine. Maybe all she needed was a little loving. Anyway, they left a picture of Cindy for her to keep on her bedside stand. It seems to have a calming effect on her."

Case Study 7: Immunosuppression

Difficulty: *** *Setting:* Hospital, ICU

Index Words: Immunosuppression, idiopathic cardiomyopathy, cardiac transplant

You are admitting a 30-year-old woman, J.L., to your telemetry unit with the diagnosis of status postcardiac transplantation and fever of unknown origin (FUO). She was healthy until the birth of her only child at age 27. She developed idiopathic cardiomyopathy following childbirth and underwent cardiac transplantation at age 29. There is a family history of early death from "heart problems."

1. Admitting has assigned J.L. to a semiprivate room. Her roommate is on day 4 of intravenous antibiotic treatment for pneumonia and now has a near normal WBC level. Is this assignment appropriate? What is your response? **[E,I/an/S/ct,ni]**
   - No. Although 4 days of antibiotic therapy may be sufficient to prevent infection in other patients, J.L. is immunosuppressed. She should be admitted to a private room, and every precaution should be taken to prevent nosocomial infections. Call admitting immediately and tell them she requires a room assignment change.

2. Fever is a sign of 2 major complications of organ transplantation. What are they? **[PD/k/PI/ct]**
   - Sepsis: immunosuppression medications necessary to prevent organ rejection predispose the patient to infection.
   - Rejection: fever may represent the body's attempt to reject the organ. Cardiac catheterization with myocardial biopsy will be needed to assess for rejection.

3. What other signs and symptoms of organ rejection should the nurse assess for in this patient? **[A/an/PI/ct,ni]**
   - Malaise, weight gain, extra heart sounds, edema, shortness of breath, and vague chest discomfort.

4. What other signs and symptoms of sepsis should the nurse assess for in J.L.? **[A/an/PI/ct,ni]**
   - Pain (general or specific), swelling, redness or warmth to the skin, productive cough, discolored nasal drainage or sputum, dysuria, cloudy urine, vaginal odor with discolored discharge, earache, and swollen lymph nodes. The patient should be pan-cultured, and those results in addition to WBC count with differential and urinalysis results should be reviewed.

5. While you are assessing J.L., she tells you that she always urinates frequently, because of her diuretics. However, she has experienced burning with urination for the last 2 days. You wish to collect a urine specimen for laboratory analysis. What do you suspect may be causing the burning, and what type of urine specimen should you obtain? **[PD,P/c,ap/PI/ct,ni]**
   - Clean-catch is probably the best option in this situation. In-and-out catheterization may cause additional trauma and will increase the risk for additional infection. Plain urinalysis is inappropriate because a culture will be needed.

6. The physician tells you that J.L. is to be started on antibiotics as quickly as possible. She has just had a PICC line inserted, and her first dose of intravenous antibiotics has just arrived from the pharmacy. Is there other information that you would like to know before you begin her antibiotics? **[A,I/ap/PI/ct,ni,tc]**
   - Yes, it is important to determine if all of the necessary cultures have been performed before initiating the antibiotic therapy. You would also need to know medication allergies.

7. J.L. says she has complained to her physician that she is constantly short of breath running after her 3-year-old. She says her physician told her that this is to be expected but did not tell her why. Why does she become dyspneic with exertion? **[I/an/PI/ct]**
   - There is no central nervous system control for J.L.'s heart rate since the heart transplant. Increased activity does not lead to a normally occurring increase in heart rate. Her shortness of breath results from increased tissue demands for oxygen following exertion that is not compensated for with an increased heart rate.

8. J.L. tells you that her husband's parents have given her child their cat because they play so well together. She jokingly says, "They gave him the play and me the work! My husband is going to have to help. I'm not up to looking after a cat, too." What job does her husband need to do? **[P,E/ap/PI/ct,ni,tc]**
   - Her husband should be responsible for emptying the litter box. Because she is immunosuppressed, she is at risk for toxoplasmosis. The organism causing it is frequently found in cat feces. Emptying the litter box increases her exposure and risk for infection.

9. You would like to teach J.L. some practical things she can do to protect herself from infection. List 5. (*Hint:* this would include many of the same things cancer patients on chemotherapy are taught.) **[P,I/c/S,PI,HP/ct,ni,tc]**
   - Use a separate towel to dry her hands at home and change it frequently.
   - Avoid food that cannot be washed or cooked when eating in public places.
   - Avoid contact with people who "are coming down with something" or "think they have a bug."
   - Go shopping or to the mall during less busy times.
   - Wash her hands in public like nurses do, and teach her to use the towel to open the restroom door (so she doesn't recontaminate herself).
   - Stay well hydrated, especially when traveling (it keeps mucosal membranes functional as barriers).

CHAPTER 11. EMERGENCY SITUATIONS

Case Study 1: Respiratory Arrest

Difficulty: *	*Setting:* Long-term care
Index Words: Respiratory arrest; airway obstruction	

The American Heart Association has two different classifications of certifications, one for lay people and one for all health care providers. As a nursing student you should use the health care provider guidelines to answer the following questions.

You are on duty in an extended care facility, when you enter a patient's room and find the patient unconscious and not breathing. The patient's meal tray is in front of her, and you notice part of an orange on it.

1. What is the first action you should take? **[A,I/k/PI/ct,ni]**
   - You should know the code status of each patient. If this patient has DNR (Do Not Resuscitate) orders then you do *not* resuscitate. If she is in full code, then establish unresponsiveness by shaking the patient gently and saying, "Are you okay?"

The patient does not respond.

2. What would you do next? **[A,I/k/PI/ct,ni]**
   - Open the airway and check for breathing.

3. How would you open the airway? **[I,E/k/PI/ct,ni]**
   - Jaw thrust, chin lift.

The patient is not breathing.

4. What is your next action? **[I,E/k/PI/ct,ni]**
   - Give two deep breaths.
   - Call a code or dial 911 of you are not equipped to handle an emergency.

After attempting rescue breathing, the patient's chest does not rise.

5. What should you do next? **[I,E/k/PI/ct,ni]**
   - Blind finger sweep to attempt to remove a possible obstruction. Do not do this if the patient is seizing.

You detect no obstruction.

6. What should you do next? **[I,E/k/PI/ct,ni]**
   - Proceed with Heimlich maneuver.

After repeated maneuvers, the situation remains unchanged.

7. What should your next action be? **[I,E/k/Pl/ct,ni]**
   - Attempt ventilations again, and repeat Heimlich maneuver until obstruction is dislodged.

The paramedics arrive and attempt to manually ventilate the patient with a bag-valve mask device. They are unable to ventilate the patient's lungs. They then attempt to intubate the patient. While visualizing with the laryngoscope, the paramedic notices dentures and a piece of orange in the patient's airway.

8. How could this obstruction have occurred? **[E/c/Pl/ct]**
   - The patient could have aspirated them herself.

The obstructions were removed, the patient was intubated, manually ventilated, and transported to the hospital. She suffered a cardiac arrest in the ambulance and all attempts to resuscitate were unsuccessful. The patient was pronounced dead on arrival at the hospital.

9. What 3 could have been taken in the above scenario that may have averted this outcome. List preventive measures first. **[P/an/S,HP/ct,ni]**
   - Don't give an elderly person large pieces of fruit. Serve fruit in small pieces.
   - Make sure patients receiving solid food are able to chew and swallow safely and that their dentures fit well.
   - Always check the throat for dentures in a nonbreathing victim if you cannot find them.
   - Always LOOK into the airway of an unconscious, nonbreathing victim.

Case Study 2: Status Epilepticus

Difficulty: *	*Setting:* Hospital
Index Words: Status epilepticus, substance abuse, seizure disorder	

You are the nurse on a medical unit taking care of a 40-year-old man, T.Z., who has been admitted with peptic ulcer disease (PUD) secondary to chronic alcoholism. You enter T.Z.'s room and find him having a grand mal (tonic-clonic) seizure.

1. List 5 things you would do. **[A,PD,P,I/k/S,PI/ct,ni]**
   - Protect the airway the best you can.
   - Administer oxygen.
   - Protect T.Z., especially his head, by making sure the environment is safe.
   - Do not leave the patient unattended.
   - Call for help.
   - Time the seizure.
   - Observe the progression of the seizure activity.

   Note: Placing any objects, including an airway into the patient's mouth at this point is contraindicated, due to the possibility of patient or caregiver harm.

T.Z.'s seizure activity does not appear to be subsiding and he is becoming cyanotic. The physician is notified and orders diazepam (Valium) 5 to 10 mg IV until seizure activity subsides.

2. What is the rationale for giving T.Z. diazepam? **[A/c/PI/ct]**
   - Diazepam decreases abnormal electrical impulse production associated with status epilepticus.

3. What is status epilepticus? **[A/k/PI/ct]**
   - A series of seizures lasting 30 minutes or more without recovery of the baseline neurologic status between the seizures.

4. What would you be particularly alert for when giving diazepam intravenously (list 3)? **[A/k/S,PI/ct]**
   - Respiratory depression.
   - Respiratory arrest.
   - Cardiac arrest.

By the time the physician arrives, T.Z.'s seizure activity has not subsided. The physician administers an additional 10 mg of diazepam, without effect. Fifteen minutes has elapsed since you found T.Z. having seizure activity.

5. What is the significance of this? **[A/c/PI/ct]**
   - Hypoxemia with subsequent CNS damage (people do not breathe during generalized seizure activity).

The physician decides to administer vecuronium (Norcuron) and intubate T.Z.

6. What is vecuronium and why is it being administered to T.Z.? **[A,P/k,c/S,Pl/ct]**
   - Intermediate acting, nondepolarizing skeletal muscle relaxant.
   - Vecuronium will paralyze T.Z. and he will not be able to breathe. Therefore, he must be intubated and mechanically ventilated until the Norcuron wears off.

T.Z. has been intubated; the physician orders 600 mg phenobarbital IV and transport to ICU.

7. What is the rationale behind giving phenobarbital? **[A/k/Pl/ct]**
   - A long-acting barbiturate that interferes with impulse transmission in the cerebral cortex. It is given for long-term management of seizure activity or status epilepticus.

8. List 2 nursing diagnoses for T.Z. **[PD/ap/S,Pl/ct]**
   - Ineffective airway clearance r/t strong clonic/tonic movements.
   - Risk for injury r/t seizure activity and uncontrollable movement.
   - Alteration in tissue perfusion r/t hypoxemia.

9. Given T.Z.'s above history, state at least 2 possible causes for his grand mal seizure. **[PD/c/Pl/ct]**
   - Seizure activity could result from alcohol withdrawal.
   - T.Z. may have been "smuggled" alcohol in his room.
   - Seizure may have been from street drugs smuggled in to him.
   - T.Z. may have an undiagnosed, underlying seizure disorder independent of or exacerbated by his substance abuse.

T.Z's seizure was successfully treated with diazepam and phenobarbital, and he has had no further seizure activity. As you are writing up his release papers, you overhear T.Z. telling his girlfriend to have his car brought to the hospital so he can drive home.

10. How should you respond to this situation? **[A,P/an/S,HP/ct,tc]**
    - In view of the fact that he has had a seizure, it is illegal for T.Z. to drive. You should instruct him to inform the state division of motor vehicles that he has had a seizure. Although laws vary from state to state, people who have had a seizure are prohibited from driving for a specified period of time (usually ranges from 1 to 2 years). If he remains seizure-free throughout that period, he may qualify to regain his license. His physician will be involved in this decision. Suggest to T.Z. that his girlfriend or another friend come take him home.

Case Study 3: Compartment Syndrome

Difficulty: **	*Setting:* Outpatient clinic, hospital
Index Words: Compartment syndrome, trauma	

It is 0800, and the outpatient clinic where you work as an RN has just opened. R.W., a 40-year-old man, hops into the clinic complaining of severe pain and swelling in his right lower leg. He tells you he was walking between two cars the night before, when one of the cars was backed up, catching his lower leg between the bumpers. He states he didn't think it was "hurt that bad" and went home to wash the abrasions. He woke up at approximately 0400, and states "My leg was killing me."

1. How would you transport R.W. to the examining room? **[P/c/S,Pl/ct,ni]**
   - Wheelchair. Anyone who is having severe lower limb pain should not be allowed to walk on the extremity, or hop. The person could fall while hopping and sustain further injury.

R.W. is placed in the examining room and asked to remove his trousers and put on a gown. R.W. is unable to lay his leg on the exam table without pain. You observe that his right lower leg is grossly edematous and pale.

2. What should your next priority be? **[A/k/Pl/ct]**
   - Assess the limb for presence of pedal and posterior tibial pulses, sensation, temperature, and motor function.

There are no pulses in the distal extremity, sensation is diminished, the extremity is cold to touch, and any movement is extremely painful.

3. What should your next action be? **[I/ap/Pl/ni]**
   - Contact the physician immediately!

The physician is with another patient, and asks you to wait a minute.

4. How should you respond? **[I/ap/S,Pl/tc]**
   - Explain to the physician that you think this situation is urgent, and the patient needs immediate attention.

After assessing the patient, the physician determines that R.W. should be transported to the nearest ED. The clinic physician notifies the ED physician that R.W. is coming in by ambulance with possible compartment syndrome of the right lower leg.

5. Explain the pathophysiology of compartment syndrome and clarify its significance. **[A/k,c/Pl/ct]**
   - Trauma to the soft tissue causing edema, which increases pressure within the fascia surrounding the muscles. The increased pressure restricts blood flow, causing ischemia of the muscles, resulting in excruciating pain. Compartment syndrome is a medical emergency.

6. How is compartment syndrome treated? **[A/k/Pl/ct]**
   - Fasciotomy. The surgeon makes an incision medially and laterally, relieving the pressure and facilitating the return of blood flow.

7. While waiting for the ambulance, R.W. starts to tell you "one-leg" jokes. How will you respond? **[P/ap/S,Pl,PSI,HP/ct,tc]**
   - It's important to recognize that there are many confusing and threatening things happening to R.W. Patients often try to use humor to cover their fear. Clearly, R.W. is afraid he is going to lose his leg. He may even fear he is going to die. This is a good opportunity to talk to R.W. about the nature of his injury and how it will be treated. It is common for patients to require several explanations before they begin to understand what is happening. Talking in general terms about recovery and rehabilitation is a good way to orient patients to the need for good follow-up care and helps instill hope. Remind R.W. of the need to follow instructions and take care of his leg after surgery.

8. How would you manage the fasciotomy once it has been performed? **[I/ap/S,Pl/ct,ni]**
   - The open surgical wounds would be covered with a topical antibiotic ointment such as silver sulfadiazine (Silvadene) ointment, and either left open to air or covered with a sterile dressing. The dressings will be removed, the wounds cleansed, an ointment applied, and sterile dressings applied. (Treatment protocols may vary according to institutional policy and procedures.)

Given that this is a crush injury, the physician orders a urine for myoglobin on R.W.

9. What is the rationale behind this order? **[PD/c/S,Pl/ct]**
   - Disintegration of striated muscle fibers from injury causes rhabdomyolysis, leading to excretion of myoglobin in the urine (myoglobinuria), which can damage the glomeruli in the kidneys and lead to renal failure.

10. How is rhabdomyolysis treated? **[A/k/S,Pl/ct]**
    - Large amounts of intravenous fluids to flush the kidneys.

After an uneventful 5-day stay on the surgical unit, R.W. is being discharged to home care services and has been referred for physical therapy.

11. As you question him about his living conditions, you discover that R.W. lives alone in a third story apartment; there are no elevators. What other information do you need from him in preparation for discharge? **[E/an/S,Pl,HP/ct,ni,tc]**
    - Is there anyone he would be able to stay with for several weeks (family, friends)? If so, get name, telephone number and address so the home health agency can make appropriate arrangements. If not, R.W. may need to go to an extended care facility. In either case, this necessitates an urgent social services consult to ensure follow-up and promote continuity of care.

Case Study 4: Insulin Shock

Difficulty: ** *Setting:* Outpatient clinic

Index Words: Insulin shock, type I diabetes mellitus, hypoglycemia

T.R. is a 22-year-old college senior who lives in the dormitory. His friend finds him wandering aimlessly about the campus appearing pale and sweaty. He engages T.R. in conversation and walks him to the campus medical clinic where you are on duty. It is 1050. He explains to you how he found T.R., and states that he knows T.R. is a diabetic and takes insulin. T.R. is not wearing a medical warning tag.

1. What do you think is going on with T.R.? **[PD/an/PI/ct]**
   - Given his limited history, T.R. probably is experiencing an insulin reaction characterized by hypoglycemia.

   Instructor Note: Individuals who have had IDDM for 5 to 10 years, or more, may not exhibit a typical adrenergic response to blood glucose as low as 30 mg/dl. Unconsciousness, seizures, or altered levels of consciousness may be the first warning signs of hypoglycemia in this population.

2. List 2 nursing diagnoses for T.R. **[PD/ap/S,PI,HP/ct]**
   - Risk for injury r/t, altered LOC, and possibility of seizure activity.
   - Knowledge deficit r/t dietary management.

3. What is the first action you would take? **[P,I/an/S,PI/ct,ni]**
   - Get a blood glucose on T.R. via glucometer and draw blood for a laboratory blood glucose level.
   - If a glucometer is not immediately available, assume he is hypoglycemic and treat accordingly.

4. Because the glucometer reading is 50 mg/dl, what would your next action be? **[I/an/S,PI/ct,ni]**
   - Give T.R. a cup of orange juice (glucose 50-80 mg/dl).

   Instructor Note: Although some protocols call for adding sugar to the juice, this tends to result in a rebound hyperglycemia. A safer practice is to use a cup of juice and recheck blood glucose levels 15 minutes later. Although much depends on what and when T.R. ate and the time and dose of his insulin, this usually is followed by a half-sandwich and additional milk or juice (blood glucose <60 mg/dl). Intervention practices and protocols vary widely. The 1994 American Diabetes Association nutrition recommendations and principles for people with diabetes mellitus and recent research findings have been used as guidelines in this workbook.

5. When you enter the room to administer the orange juice, T.R. is unresponsive. What should your next action be? **[E/an/S,PI/ct,ni]**
   - Check and maintain airway, breathing, and circulation. Always keep this in mind regardless of what else is happening. This is your first priority. Check vital signs.

6. T.R. is breathing at 16 breaths per minute, has a pulse of 85 and regular, but remains unresponsive. What should your next action be if (1) your clinic is well-equipped for emergencies, and (2) your clinic has no emergency supplies? **[I/ap/S,PI/ct,ni]**

   Since this is an outpatient setting, your resources may vary:

   - If glucagon is available, administer 0.5-1.0 mg IM or SC (some patients with IDDM carry glucagon syringes on their persons).

   and/or

   - Start IV of 0.9% NaCl; administer one ampule of 25 g of 50% dextrose IV push.

   and/or

   - If you have no emergency resources in the clinic, dial 911. In this case, use an IV solution of 5% or 10% dextrose (the highest concentration available) until the medics arrive.

A few minutes after dextrose is administered, T.R. begins to awaken. He becomes alert and asks where he is and what happened to him. You orient him, then explain what has transpired.

7. What questions would you ask to find out what precipitated these events? **[A/k/PI/tc]**
   - How much, what type, and when did he take his insulin?
   - What has T.R. had to eat today?
   - Has this ever happened to T.R. before?
   - What kind of a diet is T.R. on?

T.R. tells you he took 35 units human NPH and 12 units of regular human insulin at 0745. He says he was late to class so he just grabbed an apple on the way. He adds this has happened twice in the past, but he recognized it and treated it with candy and then ate a meal. He says he is on a 2000 calorie ADA diet (newer research is calling into question the older "ADA calorie diet" approach, but it still is commonly taught and used).

8. Based on your knowledge of different types of insulin, when would you expect T.R. to experience an insulin reaction? **[A/k/PI/ct]**
   - Because regular human insulin peaks at approximately 2 to 3 hours after administration, T.R. would be expected to experience a reaction midmorning or before lunch time.
   - Because NPH human insulin peaks between 4 and 10 hours after administration, T.R. could have a reaction in midafternoon.

   <u>Instructor Note</u>: Recent research is challenging traditional beliefs about insulin action. Human insulin tends to peak and act faster than animal insulin. This may explain why many diabetics have had difficulty regulating their glucose levels in the past. For instance, human NPH insulin commonly is given at bedtime rather than at supper to prevent 0300-0600 hypoglycemic episodes. Also, students should note the wide individual variability in response time for the insulins. Students can anticipate significant new approaches to the treatment of diabetes in the next few years.

9. In discussing your teaching plan with T.R., list at least 4 important points that you would stress. **[P/ap/S,PI,PSI,HP/ct,ni,tc]**
   - The importance of eating an appropriate breakfast after taking his morning insulin.
   - When to expect an insulin reaction (both morning, afternoon, and during night time sleep).
   - Carry glucose tablets with him at all times.
   - The importance of letting friends and significant others know that he is diabetic.
   - The importance of wearing a medical warning tag.
   - Check with his physician or nurse practitioner about a prescription for a glucagon kit for emergency use.

Case Study 5: Drug Abuse and Withdrawal

Difficulty: **	*Setting:* Hospital
Index Words: Substance abuse, overdose, nurse practice act	

You are on duty in the ED when a "Code Blue" is called overhead. As the code nurse, you grab the crash cart and run to the code, which is in the employee lounge of the operating room. On the couch you find a nurse unconscious, cyanotic, and barely breathing. Her scrub shirt has been cut off, and you attach ECG leads to her chest. Her pulse is 45; respirations are 8 and shallow. She is intubated, an intravenous line is started with 0.9% NaCl, and she is given an ampule of 50 ml D_5W, 0.4 mg naloxone (Narcan), and 0.5 mg atropine IVP. Her respirations improve slightly, and pulse increases to 56. She is transported to the ED.

1. What is the purpose of giving the 3 above-mentioned drugs in this case? **[A/c/S,Pl/ct]**
   - D_5W is given to an unconscious patient whose history is unknown. The patient may be a diabetic and having an insulin reaction; the D_5W would provide a source of glucose for the brain.
   - Naloxone is a narcotic antagonist, which helps reverse the effects of narcotic-induced sequelae.
   - Atropine is given to reverse the bradycardia.

After additional naloxone, the patient woke up and was extubated.

2. What additional information do you want to know? **[A,E/an/Pl/ct,tc]**
   - Is she diabetic?
   - What is her blood glucose level?
   - Is she abusing drugs?
   - Does she have heart problems?

In response to your questions, Z.H. tells you that she had taken fentanyl IM. She then asks you to call a friend to come stay with her.

3. What information would you give her friend over the phone? **[I/c,a/PSI/ct,ni,tc]**
   - Inform the friend that Z.H. is in the ED at your hospital.
   - Z.H. is ill and requests that she come to the hospital for support.

   <u>*Instructor Note:*</u> It is a breach of patient confidentiality to give out any information but that she is in the ED and is requesting her friend to come.

4. The friend asks you what is wrong. How do you respond? **[I/ap/PSI/ct,ni,tc]**
   - Z.H. is OK, you cannot give additional information over the phone; Z.H. will be able to tell her when she arrives.

5. Identify 5 nursing diagnoses that may apply in this situation. **[PD/ap/S,PS,PSI/ct,ni]**
   - Impaired gas exchange r/t hypoventilation.
   - Decreased cardiac output r/t hypoventilation and drug action.
   - Risk for self-harm r/t impaired judgment.
   - Risk for injury r/t impaired judgment.
   - Anxiety r/t loss of control.
   - Ineffective individual coping: anger, dependence, or denial r/t inability to constructively manage stressors without drugs/alcohol.
   - Self-esteem disturbance r/t guilt, mistrust, or ambivalence.

Z.H. is admitted to the ICU for 24-hour observation and then transferred to the chemical dependency unit.

6. What is chemical dependency? **[PD/k/S,PI,PSI/ct]**
   - It is the psychologic and/or physical dependence on mood-altering substances causing a compulsion to seek and obtain those substances.

One of Z.H.'s colleagues calls on the phone to ask how she is. She tells you that she thought something was wrong with Z.H. because her behavior was so erratic, but "I had no idea it was drugs. I didn't think Z.H. would ever do anything like that!" Keep in mind that patient confidentiality extends to health care professionals not directly involved in Z.H.'s care. You cannot give information on how Z.H. is doing.

7. What is the profile of an impaired nurse (list 5 characteristics). **[A/k/PSI/ct]**
   - Tend to start using chemicals for a physical condition rather than for recreation.
   - Tend to take chemicals in isolation.
   - Have a heightened sense of responsibility.
   - Hold very demanding jobs (ICU, ED, OR).
   - Highly respected for excellent work.
   - Very demanding of themselves.
   - Very ambitious and achievement oriented.
   - Usually doesn't use street drugs (obtain drugs through work or physician).
   - No history of delinquency.
   - Have a higher level of education than most other groups of substance abusers.

8. What 4 are problems associated with impaired nurses who are practicing? **[A/k/S,PSI/ct]**
   - Patient safety is compromised.
   - Trust among colleagues is jeopardized.
   - The nurse's safety is compromised.
   - The nurse's career is jeopardized.
   - Liability increases for the impaired nurse and her colleagues.

Z.H. asks her nurse what is going to happen to her career.

9. What are the regulatory issues r/t impaired nurses that will guide your response (list at least 5)? **[A/k/S/ct,tc]**
   - Many nurse practice acts require that impaired nurses be reported to the licensing body.
   - Nurses are usually required to appear before the designated board or committee regulating nursing practice.
   - They are subject to random urine drug screens.
   - They are required to report on rehabilitation progress to the designated board or committee regulating nursing practice.
   - They are required to have follow-up aftercare posttreatment.
   - They are denied access to controlled substances for a specified period of time.
   - They are required to attend support group meetings for chemically dependent nurses.
   - They are scheduled to attend regular meetings with the regulatory body for the duration of probation.
   - If the nurse complies with the terms of probation, the license may be fully restored. If it is violated in any way, further action is taken.

   Instructor Note: These stipulations vary according to individual state regulatory laws and nurse practice acts. Encourage students to become familiar with the policies of your state.

Z.H. successfully completed treatment and continues to practice as a nurse. She is now serving as a sponsor for another nurse undergoing treatment for chemical dependency.

Case Study 6: Acute Head Injury

Difficulty: **	*Setting:* Hospital, ED
Index Words: Head injury, trauma	

J.R. is a 28-year-old man who is doing home repairs. He falls from the top of a 6 foot step ladder, striking his head on a large rock. He experiences momentary loss of consciousness. By the time his neighbor gets to him, he is conscious but bleeding profusely from a laceration over the R temporal area. The neighbor drives him to the ED of your hospital. As the nurse, you immediately apply a cervical collar, lay him on a stretcher, and take J.R. to a treatment room.

Instructor Note: Stress importance of calling 911 and never trying to transport a head-injured individual. Also stress the importance of cervical immobilization until the C-spine is proved to be intact. All patients who sustain a blow to the head should be treated as having a possible neck injury until proven otherwise.

1. What steps should you take to assess J.R.? **[A/k/Pl/ct/ni]**
   - ABCs.
   - Neuro exam.

2. List at least 5 components of a neuro exam. **[A/k/Pl/ct]**
   - Glasgow coma scale (GCS) is composed of eye opening, best motor response, best verbal response.
   - Level of consciousness.
   - Pupil size, shape, and reaction to light.
   - Sensation.
   - Observation of bilateral symmetry.
   - Behavior status (e.g., combative, cooperative, calm).

You complete your neuro exam and find the following: GCS 15, PERRLA, and has full sensation. He complains of a headache; he is becoming increasingly lethargic.

3. As the radiology technician performs a portable cross table lateral c-spine x-ray, J.R. begins to speak incoherently and appears to drift off to sleep. What is the next action you would take? **[A/c/Pl/ct,ni]**
   - Immediately begin reassessing neurologic status.

You find J.R. has become unresponsive to verbal stimuli and responds to painful stimuli by abnormally flexing his extremities (decorticate movement). He has no verbal response. The right pupil is larger than the left, and does not respond to light.

4. What is J.R.'s Glasgow coma scale (GCS) score at this time? Indicate what this means. **[A/k/Pl/ct]**
   - GCS = 5. This is a medical emergency, and the physician must be summoned immediately.

5. Based on his GSC score, what are the next steps you should take? **[P/an/S,PI/ct,ni]**
The physician already has been summoned. You proceed to:
   - Apply oxygen per nonrebreather mask at 15 L/min.
   - Start an IV with a large-bore catheter.
   - Draw trauma labs: CBC with differential, Chem 20, UA, type and screen, PT/PTT, ABGs, blood alcohol level, toxicology screen.
   - Institute cardiac monitoring.
   - Initiate blood pressure monitoring with automated blood pressure device.
   - Insert a Foley catheter to straight ("down") drain.
   - Prepare for CT scan of the brain.

   Instructor Note: IV fluids should not be infused in large quantities, but infused at a keep-open rate in patients in whom head injury is the only problem. Automated blood pressure readings should be checked for accuracy against the standard cuff method.

6. What is the significance of the dilated and fixed pupil on the right? **[PD/c/PI/ct]**
   - Increased intracranial pressure causes pupil dilation on the side of the injury due to pressure on the oculomotor nerve.

The physician orders 500 ml of 25% mannitol solution IV.

7. What is mannitol, and why is it being used on J.R.? **[PD/c/PI/ct]**
   - Mannitol is an osmotic diuretic that draws fluid from the interstitial to the intravascular space, where it is eliminated by the kidneys. It is being administered in J.R.'s case to reduce cerebral edema and prevent transtentorial (uncal) herniation.

   Instructor Note: Mannitol should be administered using a micron filter needle to filter large molecules that could cause microemboli. Mannitol can cause a rebound increase in ICP approximately 12 hours after administration; therefore, it is usually followed up with dexamethasone (Decadron), which will be administered for several days until the patient is out of danger of further cerebral edema.

J.R. is transported to CT scan where he is found to have a large epidural hematoma on the right with a hemispheric shift to the left. He will be taken to the OR from CT scan for evacuation of a right epidural hematoma.

While en route from the CT scan to the OR, the physician instructs the respiratory therapist to initiate hyperventilation of the patient to "blow off more CO_2."

8. What is the rationale for this action? **[I/c/S,PI/ct]**
   - CO_2 acts to dilate blood vessels, which contributes to increased intracranial pressure. CO_2 levels are therapeutically decreased to protect the brain tissue from further damage. This intervention prevents edema and vasodilation, contributes to oxygenation of neural tissue, and minimizes further damage to brain tissue.

9. Explain at least 6 nursing interventions you would use to prevent increased ICP in the first 48 postoperative hours. **[I/c/S,PI/ct,ni]**
   - Elevate HOB 30 degrees to decrease cerebral edema.
   - Maintain oxygenation (monitor oxygen delivery and respirations).
   - Minimize level of environmental stimulation (e.g., lights, sounds, stressors, talking around the patient, movement).
   - Group care activities in brief intervals to allow for longer periods of rest and recovery.
   - Limit suctioning.
   - Carefully monitor I&O.
   - Do not flex the patient's neck.
   - Talk to the patient softly and explain what is happening, even if the person does not appear to be conscious.
   - If the patient is awake, caution him or her *not* to perform a Valsalva maneuver.

   Instructor Note: Hypercapnia and hypoxemia are powerful contributors to cerebral edema.

While he is in surgery, J.R.'s family arrives at the ED. They ask that their faith healer anoint J.R. and pray over him.

10. What should the nurse say? **[P/ap/PSI/ct,ni,tc]**
    - Take them to a private place where you can talk.
    - Explain you're very sorry they missed him, but they had to take him to surgery immediately. Everything possible is being done for him.
    - Offer to make them comfortable—is there anything they need?
    - Find out whether this is the family's faith healer, or J.R's faith healer (in other words, would J.R. want the faith healer involved in his care).
    - Call the OR and notify the physician that the family has arrived and where they will wait to talk to him/her postop.
    - Instruct the family where they can wait to talk to the doctor.

Case Study 7: Spinal Cord Compression

Difficulty: **	*Setting:* Hospital ED
Index Words: Spinal cord compression, rehabilitation, trauma	

B.J. is a 34-year-old woman who has been thrown from a galloping horse in a remote area. She was flown to the trauma center by helicopter from a rural hospital with spinal cord compression due to spinal fracture and disk fragments in her lumbar spine. Her cervical spine is free from injury. She arrives strapped to a rigid backboard and begins to vomit.

1. What would you do to keep B.J. from aspirating? **[I/c/S,PI/ct,ni]**
   - Keep B.J. strapped to the backboard.
   - Have suction readily available to aspirate vomitus from the mouth and oropharynx.
   - Place an NG tube and connect to low continuous suction.

2. What would you do to assess B.J.? **[A/k/PI/ct,ni]**
   - Complete the ABCs (airway, breathing, circulation).
   - Do a complete neuro check, including Glasgow coma scale.
   - Get a full set of vital signs.

You find that B.J. is hypotensive and bradycardic. She has an IV of 1000 ml LR with a large-bore catheter at 75 ml/h.

3. What is causing the hypotension and bradycardia? **[PD/c/PI/ct]**
   - Spinal cord edema with subsequent edema can block sympathetic outflow from the cord and cause a shock syndrome. Loss of sympathetic tone causes peripheral vasodilation and severe hypotension.

The neurosurgeon arrives in the ED and examines B.J. He finds her areflexic below the lumbar region of the spinal cord. There is absence of sweating in the region, and no sensation below the level of the lesion. He writes the following orders: CT scan of the spine; myelogram; prepare for surgery; admit to ICU; 10 mg dexamethasone (Decadron) IV now.

4. Why did the physician order both a CT scan and a myelogram? Differentiate between the diagnostic value of each. **[PD/c/PI/ct]**
   - A CT scan will visualize the bony structures and disks of the spine and indicate whether they are fractured and/or dislocated, causing pressure on the spinal cord.
   - The myelogram is done by doing a lumbar puncture, aspirating spinal fluid, and injecting radiographic contrast into the subarachnoid space. The patient is placed in various positions, and radiographic images are seen and recorded. It allows visualization of the nerve roots and surrounding structures.

5. What is dexamethasone, and why is it being used on B.J.? **[PD/c/PI/ct]**
   - Dexamethasone is a corticosteroid used in the treatment of inflammatory conditions. It is being used in B.J. to help reduce spinal cord swelling.

6. List 5 nursing diagnoses for B.J. **[PD/ap/S,PI,PSI/ct,ni]**
   - Ineffective airway clearance r/t immobilization and vomiting.
   - Decreased tissue perfusion r/t spinal cord shock.
   - Anxiety r/t uncertainty of future.
   - Self-care deficit r/t sensory motor deficit.
   - Pain r/t spinal cord compression.
   - Fear r/t loss of independence.
   - Fear r/t injury.
   - Fear r/t paralysis.
   - Impaired physical mobility r/t spinal cord compression.

7. What are complications and problems associated with spinal cord shock (minimum of 7)? **[A/k/PI/ct]**
   - Hypotension.
   - Bradycardia.
   - Hypotension may result in acute tubular necrosis.
   - Paralytic ileus may result from spinal cord shock.
   - Constipation.
   - Altered skin integrity.
   - Deep vein thrombosis.
   - Contractures.
   - Pain.

8. How would you detect complications from spinal cord shock (list 6)? **[A/k/S,PI,PSI/ct]**
   - Monitor blood pressure every 30 minutes and prn.
   - Observe heart activity continuously with cardiac monitor.
   - Monitor the urine output at least hourly. Adequate urine output (1 ml/kg/hour) implies adequate renal perfusion.
   - Increase in gastric secretions, abdominal pain, abdominal distention, and absence of bowel sounds.
   - Document bowel movements (quantity, caliber, and consistency of stool).
   - Assess skin when turning patient.
   - Assess for changes in pulses, swelling, color, temperature, and sensation.
   - Assess ease of range of motion.
   - Ask the patient to rate the pain on a scale of 0 to 10, 0 being no pain at all and 10 being as bad as it can get.

9. What are 8 interventions that could be initiated to prevent or treat complications from spinal cord shock? **[I/an/S,PI,PSI/ct,ni]**
   - Adequate hydration and vasopressors.
   - Administer atropine if symptomatic bradycardia is present.
   - If the urine output is inadequate, you could give a fluid challenge, give a diuretic, or start a intropin (Dopamine) drip to dilate the renal arteries.
   - Give metoclopramide (Reglan) to stimulate the bowel.
   - Stool softening agents, mild laxatives, oil retention enemas, digital stimulation, and diet high in dietary fiber.
   - Make sure the patient is turned and given good skin care.
   - Sequential compression devices, TED (thromboembolic deterrent) hose.
   - Physiotherapy for active and passive range of motion.
   - Pain relief measures such as positioning, guided imagery, or analgesics.

B.J. went to surgery directly from x-ray for decompression of her spinal cord, and was admitted to ICU on absolute bed rest. From ICU she was transferred to the surgical unit, fitted for a back brace, and began physiotherapy. After undergoing surgery for a bone graft and spinal fusion, she was transferred to a rehabilitation facility. After months of intense physiotherapy, B.J. regained the use of her legs and basic functioning and was discharged to home.

Case Study 8: Cardiac Tamponade

Difficulty: **	*Setting:* Hospital
Index Words: Cardiac tamponade, trauma	

You are working on the intermediate cardiac care unit in a large hospital. You are taking care of R.J. who was admitted for a chest contusion he sustained in an auto accident and fractured 4th and 5th ribs on the left side. About 2000, his wife runs up to you at the nurse's station and says "I think my husband just had a heart attack. Come quick!" She follows you into his room, where you find him face down on the floor. He is breathing, is cyanotic from the neck up, and his pulse is very weak.

1. What should your first action be? **[A,PD,P,I/an/PI/ct,ni,tc]**
   - Recognize this is an emergency condition. You need to call a code STAT.

2. Suddenly, you remember R.J.'s wife, who is anxiously hovering over you in the room. What are you going to do? **[I/an/S/ct,ni,tc]**
   - Calmly but quickly thank her for calling you. Ask her to wait for you down in the visitor's area, and explain you'll see her as soon as you can to explain what happened. It's important she not get caught in the code "stampede."
   - Some facilities are now allowing next-of-kin to stay during emergenices. If this is the case, assess her ability to deal safely with this situation.

The code team arrives. R.J.'s trauma surgeon is making rounds on your unit when the code is called, and he runs to the room. R.J. is intubated, and the NS lock is changed to an IV of LR. The trauma surgeon recognizes Beck's triad and calls for a cardiac needle and syringe. He inserts the needle below the xiphoid process and aspirates 50 ml of unclotted blood.

3. What is Beck's triad and what causes it? **[A/k/PI/ct]**
   - Beck's triad is a syndrome identified by distended neck veins (in the absence of shock), hypotension, and distant heart sounds. It is caused by pericardial tamponade.

4. Explain the rationale for the surgeon performing a pericardiocentesis. **[A/c/PI/ct]**
   - The surgeon approached the heart from beneath the diaphragm to lessen the risk of causing a pneumothorax or entering the great vessels of the thorax. He aspirated blood from the pericardial sac to allow expansion of the ventricle during diastole, thereby improving stroke volume and cardiac output.

R.J. is transferred to the thoracic intensive care unit for observation.

5. List 3 nursing diagnoses for R.J. **[PD/ap/PI,PSI/ct]**
   - Decreased cardiac output r/t pericardial tamponade.
   - Impaired gas exchange r/t decreased tissue perfusion.
   - Ineffective breathing pattern r/t tissue injury.
   - Pain r/t disrupted nerves and tissues.
   - Fear r/t invasive procedures and threatening environment.

6. As the team prepares R.J.'s transfer, you go to find R.J.'s wife to tell her what has happened. Briefly, and in everyday terms, how would you explain what happend to her husband? **[I/c/PI,PSI/ct,ni,tc]**
   - Reassure her that her husband is being well cared for. Relate this crisis to his accident so she understands this is not a "new" problem. You might use the image of a blood-filled balloon or a similar metaphor for the pericardial tamponade. Explain that the physician had to stick a needle through the balloon to remove the blood so his heart had room to work again. Tell her that he is being transferred to the intensive care unit for observation, and prepare her for the shock of this environment. If you can't accompany her yourself, give her good directions on how to get to the TICU, and then call the unit so they know she is coming.

7. As you both get up to leave, Mrs. J. suddenly turns pale and says she feels very dizzy. What are you going to do? **[I/an/S,PI,PSI/ct,ni,tc]**
   - Have her lie down and elevate her legs or sit on the floor with her head between her knees. Place a cold cloth on her forehead or neck and get some juice for her. While you are doing this, ask her questions: When did she eat last? Has anything like this ever happened before? Does she have any medical conditions? Is she taking any medications? Take her vital signs. Continue to observe her as you talk. Inform her that you would like to take her to the ED for a checkup. Use a wheelchair. Even if she refuses and wants to go to the TICU to see her husband, offer to take her in a wheelchair and inform the TICU nurses that she had a "near-syncopal" episode on your unit. If she becomes unconscious at any point, take her to the ED for treatment. Document your actions in an incident report.

Case Study 9: Anaphylaxis

Difficulty: **	*Setting:* Hospital ED
Index Words: Anaphylaxis	

You are working in the ED when a patient comes in having an allergic reaction to bee pollen she has eaten. She brought the jar of bee pollen with her. Your nurse colleague, curious as to how bee pollen tastes, ingests a small amount. A few minutes later your colleague begins to experience itching in her throat and ears, hives, and mild respiratory distress. The respiratory distress rapidly progresses to audible wheezing. You notice that your colleague appears to be in distress.

1. What do you think is wrong with your colleague? **[PD/c/S,PI/ct]**
   - Severe allergic reaction.
   - Anaphylaxis.

2. Given that your colleague is having a possible allergic reaction, what actions should you take (list 6)? **[A,P,I/ap/S,PI/ct,ni]**
   - Get her into a treatment room and start her on oxygen.
   - Notify the ED physician STAT and ask her about additional allergies.
   - Start an intravenous infusion of D_5W.
   - Give epinephrine (Adrenalin) subcutaneously as ordered.
   - Give diphenhydramine (Benadryl) IV as ordered.
   - Give IV methylprednisolone (Solumedrol) as ordered.
   - Make certain that airway and resuscitation equipment is readily available at the bedside.

3. What is the rationale behind giving the medications you identified in answer 2 above? Indicate their usual dosages. **[A/k/S/ct]**
   - Epinephrine is a sympathomimetic that acts to dilate the airways to promote breathing, and constrict vasculature to correct hypotension that accompanies anaphylactic reactions. The drug also acts as an antihistamine to block release of histamine during an allergic reaction.
     Dosage: 0.2 to 0.5 mg subcutaneously, repeated every 5 minutes as needed.
   - Diphenhydramine is an H1 blocking agent that prevents the release of histamine from mast cells during an allergic response. Histamine acts locally to produce vasodilation and vascular permeability, leading to loss of fluid and protein into the interstitial space.
     Dosage: 25 to 50 mg IV not to exceed 400 mg per day. May be followed up with oral therapy.
   - Methylprednisolone is a synthetic corticosteroid used in the treatment of inflammatory conditions and anaphylaxis. It stabilizes capillary walls to decrease fluid shifts out of the vasculature.
     Dosage: 100 mg to 1 g IV.

4. Identify 3 nursing diagnoses for B.J. **[PD/ap/S,PI/ct]**
    - Impaired gas exchange r/t bronchoconstriction.
    - Fluid volume deficit r/t histamine release.
    - Altered tissue perfusion r/t circulatory collapse.
    - Altered protection r/t antigen antibody reaction in anaphylaxis.
    - High risk for respiratory failure r/t airway swelling.

The nurse begins to improve. She states that the itching has subsided and the hives are fading. She reports that she no longer has acute shortness of breath. On auscultation of her lungs, you note that the wheezing has resolved. She wants to return to work.

Instructor Note: It is imperative that the patient's lungs be auscultated and the patient be carefully observed. The patient may report no acute distress and still have wheezing on auscultation. It is common to hear patients say they "feel fine" when the condition is only partially resolved.

5. Is it appropriate to allow her to return to duty? Why? **[E/c/S,PI/ct,ni,tc]**
    - No.
    - The nurse can have a delayed reaction from the bee pollen later.
    - The nurse is under the influence of medications that have the potential to alter her judgment. Diphenhydramine has a sedative effect and can cause drowsiness, especially when given IV.

A decision is made to discharge the nurse to her home.

6. What issues should you address in discharge teaching of this nurse (list 3)? **[PD/ap/S,PI,HP/ct,ni,tc]**
    - A friend should stay with her after she gets home, so she isn't alone if she should have another reaction.
    - She should be warned about operating a vehicle or working while taking antihistamines.
    - Caution her to avoid bees and bee products.
    - Encourage her to obtain and wear a medical warning ID tag.

7. Should you allow the nurse to drive herself home? Why? **[E/ap/S,PI.ct,ni]**
    - No, for the reasons stated above.

A friend was called to come and drive your colleague home, and she was discharged. She lived to nurse another day.

Case Study 10: Diabetic Ketoacidosis

Difficulty: ***	*Setting:* Outpatient clinic, hospital ED
Index Words: Diabetic ketoacidosis, type I diabetes mellitus	

You are working in an outpatient clinic when a mother brings in her 20-year-old-daughter, C.J., who has type I diabetes mellitus and has just returned from a trip to Mexico. She's had a 3-day FUO (fever of undetermined origin), and diarrhea with N&V. She has been unable to eat and has tolerated only sips of fluid. Because she has been unable to eat, she has not taken her insulin.

Because C.J. is unsteady, you bring her to the examining room in a wheelchair. While assisting her onto the examining table, you note that her skin is very warm and flushed. Her respirations are deep and rapid, and her breath is foul smelling. C.J. is drowsy and unable to answer your questions. Her mother states "she keeps telling me she's so thirsty, but she can't keep anything down."

1. What additional information do you need to elicit from C.J.'s mother (list 4)? **[A/an/Pl/ct]**
   - What have C.J.'s blood sugars been running?
   - How much fluid has C.J. been able to keep down over the past 3 days?
   - How often has C.J. been vomiting over the past 3 days.
   - How often has C.J. voided over the past 3 days?
   - How long has C.J. been drowsy?

   Possible answers:
   - "Blood glucose has been 'high' (glucometer does not read above 400)."
   - "Sips of ginger ale."
   - "About every other time she drinks."
   - "Well, when she first got home, she went a lot, but yesterday she hardly went at all, and I don't think she has gone today."
   - "She went to bed early last night, and I could hardly wake her up this morning, that's why I brought her in."

2. Describe the pathophysiology of diabetic ketoacidosis. **[A/k/Pl/ct]**
   - Diabetic ketoacidosis often follows an acute illness and occurs as the result of a relative lack of insulin leading to the body's increase in metabolism in a less efficient attempt to use other sources for energy. The result is burning of lipids from fat stores. Ketones are formed as a result of lipolysis, and metabolic acids are produced. Serum osmolality increases slightly, drawing fluid and sodium from cells, resulting in dehydration and increased urine output. Blood lactate levels rise, further complicating the acidosis.

3. Explain the patient's presenting signs and symptoms (list 6). **[A,PD/ap/PI/ct]**
    - Probable infection contracted in Mexico leading to diarrhea, nausea, and vomiting and elevated temp.
    - Decreased intake, increased output, and high glucose levels result in dehydration and thirst.
    - Lack of insulin resulting in elevated blood glucose.
    - Lipolysis for energy resulting in ketone formation leading to halitosis.
    - Dehydration, increased metabolism, and fever from probable infection leading to skin warmth and flushing.

4. Her current VS are 90/50, 124, 36 and deep; temperature is 101.3° F (tympanic temp). Are these vital signs appropriate for a woman of C.J.'s age? Why or why not? Discuss your rationale. **[PD/c/PI/ct]**
    - None of the VS is appropriate for a woman this age.
    - Blood pressure is low due to dehydration and hypovolemia secondary to limited intake, vomiting, diarrhea, and serum hyperosmolarity.
    - Pulse is elevated as a compensatory mechanism for reduced fluid volume and fever.
    - Respirations are rapid and deep in an attempt to compensate for metabolic acids produced during diabetic ketoacidosis by blowing off carbon dioxide.
    - The patient has a fever due to dehydration, increased metabolic activity, and the possibility of a parasitic or infectious process.

5. Write 3 nursing diagnoses for C.J. **[E/ap/PI,HP/ct]**
    - Decreased cardiac output r/t dehydration and hypovolemia.
    - Fluid volume deficit r/t hypovolemia, dehydration, and lack of insulin for cellular metabolism.
    - Increased thirst r/t dehydration from hyperosmolar diuresis.
    - Altered urinary elemination r/t dehydration.
    - Risk for injury r/t decreased level of consciousness.

A decision has been made to transport C.J. by ambulance to the local ED. After evaluating C.J., the ED physician writes the following orders.

6. Carefully review each order to determine if it is appropriate or inappropriate as written. Place an "A" in the space provided if appropriate; place an "I" in the space provided if inappropriate and underline the inappropriate part. Explain why it is inappropriate and correct the order. **[A/an/S,Pl/ct,ni]**

___ 1000 ml LR IV STAT.
___ Give 36 units lente and 20 units regular insulin SC (sub-Q) now.
___ CBC with differential; Chem 20 (electrolytes, glucose, enzymes); blood cultures x 2 sites; clean catch urine for UA and C&S; stool for ova and parasites, *C. difficile* toxin, and C&S; serum lactate, ketone, and osmolality; ABGs on room air.
___ 1800 calorie ADA diet.
___ Ambulate qid.
___ Tylenol 650 mg (10 gr) PO.
___ Lasix 60 mg IVP now.
___ Urine output every hour.
___ VS q shift.

Inappropriate orders:

- IV fluids. Initially, you would want to rapidly administer 0.9% NaCl. 0.9% NaCl is an isotonic solution and is needed to expand intravascular volume to bring blood pressure back in line with normal, and facilitate renal perfusion. After initial fluid resuscitation, hang D_5 ½ NS which promotes intracellular fluid replacement and provides needed glucose for metabolism while IV insulin is being administered.
- Insulin. The patient should receive an IV bolus of regular insulin, followed by a continuous sliding scale drip of regular insulin via an infusion pump.
- Laboratory tests. Clean catch urine cannot be obtained due to the patient's decreased LOC. A Foley catheter will need to be inserted, and urine for lab studies obtained at that time. The rest of the labs are appropriate.
- Diet. The patient is vomiting and cannot tolerate PO intake at this time.
- Activity. C.J. should be on bed rest until her condition stabilizes.
- Acetaminophen (Tylenol). Due to vomiting, C.J. should receive acetaminophen rectally per suppository.
- Furosemide (Lasix). Due to dehydration, this patient should not receive a diuretic.
- Vital signs. A full set of vital signs should be obtained at least every 2 hours.

Appropriate orders:

- Urine output every hour.

Omissions:

- Antibiotics. The patient would receive prophylactic broad-spectrum antibiotics after all cultures have been obtained.
- Blood glucose checks via glucometer have not been ordered. They should be performed every hour until glucose stabilizes within normal limits.
- Insulin drives potassium into the cell; therefore, the nurse should monitor serum potassium levels to prevent the occurrence of complications such as dysrhythmias, altered LOC, and seizure activity.

All orders have been corrected and initiated. C.J. has received fluid resuscitation and is on a sliding scale insulin drip via infusion pump. Her latest glucose was 347 mg/dl.

7. What is the rationale behind using an infusion pump for the insulin drip? **[P/ap/PI/ct]**
   - Large amounts of regular insulin are added to 0.9% NaCl to provide a continuous infusion (hospital policies on mixture vary). An infusion pump is critical to the safety of the patient to prevent a large bolus of regular insulin, which can lead to profound hypoglycemia and/or death.

C.J. is ready for transport to the medical ICU. C.J.'s mother is beginning to realize that C.J. is more acutely ill than she thought. She leaves the room and begins to cry.

8. How would you handle this situation? **[I/an/PSI/ct,ni,tc]**
   - Provide C.J.'s mother with tissues. Ask her if there is anything you may do to help. Ask her what her perception of C.J.'s condition is. Provide clarification as needed.
   - Type I diabetics typically can become ill very rapidly. If this is the first experience C.J.'s mother has had with DKA, explain that it can happen acutely and, when she sees this same pattern in the future, to seek care right away.

9. C.J.'s mother asks where she can get more information on how C.J. can control her diabetes. What are some resources she may find useful? **[I/k/S,PI,PSI/ct,ni/tc]**
   - Give her the number of the local chapter of the American Diabetes Association. In addition, your own hospital or clinic may have classes or support groups for diabetics. Libraries and bookstores also have excellent information to help consumers manage their diabetes.

C.J. was transported to the MICU in slightly improved condition. She continued to improve, and was discharged from the hospital 3 days later.

Case Study 11: Gastrointestinal Hemorrhage

Difficulty: ***	*Setting:* Hospital ED
Index Words: Gastrointestinal hemorrhage, hypovolemic shock	

You are the nurse on duty on the intermediate care unit and you are scheduled to take the next admission. The ED nurse calls to give you the following report, "This is Barb in the ED and we have a 42-year-old man with lower GI bleeding. He is a sandblaster with a 12-year history of silicosis. He is taking 40 mg of prednisone per day. During the night, he developed severe diarrhea. He was unable to get out of bed fast enough and had a large maroon-colored stool (hematochezia) in the bed. His wife 'freaked' and called the paramedics. He has been seen here and is coming to you. His VS are stable: 110/64, 110, 28, and he's a little agitated. His temperature is 36.8° C. He hasn't had any stools since admission but his rectal exam was guaiac positive and he is pale but not diaphoretic. We have him on 5 L O_2/nc. We started a 16-gauge IV with LR at 125/hour. He has an 18-gauge Salem sump to continuous low suction; the drainage is guaiac negative. We have done a CBC with differential, Chem 20, PT/PTT, and a T&C for 4 units PRCs and a UA. He's all ready for you."

1. How should you prepare for this patient's arrival? **[P/an/Pl/ct,ni]**
   - Pad the bed in preparation for significant bleeding.
   - Make sure there is an oxygen flow meter, oximeter, and IV pole, suction set up, 1 L of NaCl, and catheter-tip syringe at the bedside.

K.L. arrives on your unit. As you help him transfer from the ED stretcher to the bed, K.L. becomes very dyspneic and expels 800 ml of maroon stool.

2. What are the first 3 actions you should take? **[P/an/Pl/ct,ni]**
   - Take a set of vital signs.
   - Ask K.L. if he feels sick to his stomach, or is getting thirsty (signs of hypovolemia).
   - Call the physician.

   Instructor Note: Elderly individuals and those with chronic illnesses often lose their thirst response to hypoglycenia.

K.L. reports that he is getting nauseated, but not thirsty. VS are 106/68, 116, 32.

3. What additional interventions would you need to institute? **[I/an/S,Pl/ct,ni]**
   - Initiate pulse oximetry.
   - Connect him to a cardiac monitor.
   - Obtain ABGs.
   - Clean K.L. and change the bed linen.

The ABG results are as follows (these results reflect values at sea level): pH 7.45; $PaCO_2$ 33 mm Hg; PaO_2 65 mm Hg; HCO_3 23 mEq/L; BE +1.0 mEq/L; SaO_2 91%.

4. Interpret the preceding ABGs. What do they tell you? **[PD/c/PI/ct]**
   - Respiratory alkalosis with hypoxemia.

The gastroenterologist was notified by K.L.'s physician and arrives on the unit to perform a colonoscopy and endoscopy. You are going to be giving K.L. midazolam (Versed) and meperidine (Demerol) IV during the procedures.

5. Given the above history, what do you think significantly contributed to the GI bleed? **[PD/an/PI/ct]**
   - Chronic prednisone therapy.

6. What are midazolam and meperidine, and why are they being given to K.L.? **[PD/k/PI/ct]**
   - Midazolam is a short-acting benzodiazepine and is indicated for use in conscious sedation before endoscopic procedures. Midazolam also has an amnesic effect on the patient.
   - Meperidine is a Class II controlled substance (opiate) given for pain and sedation during diagnostic procedures.

During the colonoscopy, K.L. begins passing large amounts of bright red blood. He becomes more pale and diaphoretic, and begins to have an altered level of consciousness.

7. Identify 5 immediate interventions you should initiate. **[PD,I/an/PI/ct,ni]**
   - Switch oxygen to nonrebreather mask at flush flow rate (100% O_2).
   - Start another large-bore IV with 0.9% NaCl.
   - Call blood bank for 2 units of PRCs STAT, and order fresh frozen plasma (FFP)
   - Put K.L. in a modified Trendelenburg position.
   - Get a set of vital signs.
   - Reassure K.L. that you're with him and you won't abandon him—don't forget the person behind the crisis.

   Instructor Note: Fresh frozen plasma must be thawed in the blood bank (usual time to thaw is 20 minutes).

8. List 4 nursing diagnoses for K.L. **[PD/ap/S,PI/ct]**
   - Fluid volume deficit r/t GI hemorrhage.
   - Altered tissue perfusion r/t hypoxemia and hemorrhage.
   - Fear r/t critical illness.
   - Ineffective breathing pattern r/t blood loss and hypoxemia.
   - Altered protection r/t decreased LOC.

K.L. has been stabilized with fluids, blood, and FFP. There has been no further evidence of active bleeding. He received ranitidine (Zantac) 50 mg IV push, and is receiving an infusion of 8 mg/h via infusion pump.

9. Later, when he seems to be feeling better, K.L. tells you he's really embarrassed about the mess he made for you. How are you going to respond to him? **[A/an/PSI/ct,ni,tc]**
    - Many adults are embarrassed and humiliated by "messing in the bed" or similar problems. It is important we not minimize their feelings but to reassure them that, as professionals, this is something we are accustomed to. Focus the conversation back to K.L. and how he is doing now. If he is strong enough, this may be the time to gain some psychosocial history (occupational risks, history of substance abuse) in a nonjudgmental setting. This is a good opportunity for trust building.

It was concluded that the GI hemorrhage was prednisone-induced. The physician will discharge K.L. and attempt to decrease his maintenance dose of prednisone while monitoring his respiratory status (the prednisone is being used to suppress the progression of silicosis).

Case Study 12: Pulmonary Embolism

Difficulty: ***	*Setting:* Hospital
Index Words: Pulmonary embolism, trauma	

S.K., a 51-year-old roofer, was admitted to the hospital 3 days ago after falling 15 feet from a roof. He sustained bilateral fractured wrists, and an open fracture of the left tibia/fibula. He was taken to surgery for open reduction and internal fixation (ORIF) of all his fractures. He is recovering on your orthopedic unit. You have instructions to begin getting him out of bed and into the chair today. When you enter the room to get S.K. into the chair, you noticed that he is very agitated and dyspneic, and says to you, "My chest hurts real bad. I can't breathe."

1. Identify 5 possible reasons for S.K.'s symptoms. **[A/an/Pl/ct]**
   - Myocardial infarction.
   - Spontaneous pneumothorax.
   - Pleurisy.
   - Pneumonitis.
   - Lung contusion.
   - Onset of adult respiratory distress syndrome (ARDS).
   - Pulmonary embolism (PE).

You auscultate S.K.'s breath sounds. You find that they are diminished in the LLL. S.K. is diaphoretic, tachypneic, and has circumoral cyanosis. His apical pulse is irregular and 110 beats per minute.

2. List in order of priority 3 actions you should take next. **[P,I/an/Pl/ct,ni,tc]**
   - Initiate pulse oximetry if readily available.
   - Initiate oxygen therapy, or increase the flow rate if he already has oxygen.
   - Secure intravenous access.
   - Notify the physician of S.K.'s condition (STAT page).

The physician orders the following: arterial blood gases (ABGs), chest x-ray (CXR), ECG, and ventilation/perfusion (V/Q) lung scan. The blood gas results come back as follows (these results reflect values at sea level): pH 7.47, $PaCO_2$ 33.6 mm Hg, PaO_2 52 mm Hg, HCO_3 24.2 mEq/L, BE -3.4 mEq/L, SaO_2 83%, and A-a gradient 32 mm Hg.

3. What is your interpretation of the blood gases? Give your rationale. **[E/c/Pl/ct]**
   - The pH indicates the patient is alkalotic.
   - The $PaCO_2$ is low, indicating alkalosis.
   - The PaO_2 indicates hypoxemia.
   - HCO_3 is normal.
   - BE is low, indicating the patient is using up base.
   - Oxygen saturation is 83%, which indicates hypoxemia.
   - A-a gradient is twice as high as it should be, indicating shunting.
   - This is a picture of respiratory alkalosis with hypoxemia.

4. Based on the ABGs and your assessment findings, what do you think is wrong with S.K.? **[E/an/Pl/ct]**
   - S.K. is suffering from a pulmonary embolism.

5. List 3 nursing diagnoses for S.K. **[A/ap/S,Pl/ct]**
   - Ineffective breathing pattern r/t hypoxia.
   - Impaired gas exchange r/t hypoxemia.
   - Altered tissue perfusion r/t hypoxemia.
   - Pain r/t P.E.
   - Injury r/t pulmonary infarction.
   - Anxiety r/t fear of current problems.

The physician writes the following orders for S.K.:

__ Transfer to MICU.
✓ Heparin 20,000 units IVP now, and 20,000 units in 1000 ml/D_5W to run at 1000 units per hour.
__ PT and PTT every 4 hours. Call house officer with results.
✓ 3 L O_2/nc
✓ PCA pump with morphine sulfate: loading dose 10 mg; dose 2 mg.; lockout time 15 minutes; maximum 4-hour dose 30 mg.
__ Streptokinase, 250,000 IU IV over 30 minutes, then 100,000 IU per hour x 48 hours.
__ Solucortef 1 g IV now.
✓ Albuterol (Proventil) MDI (metered-dose inhaler), 2 puffs q6h.

6. Of the orders *listed above*, identify inappropriate orders by placing a check mark (✓) in the space provided. Give a rationale for your decision. **[A/ap/S,Pl/ct]**
   - Heparin loading dose is inappropriately high, maintenance dose is appropriate.
   - Oxygen per cannula is inappropriate. S.K. should be on 100% oxygen via nonrebreather mask at flush flow rate.
   - Loading dose of morphine is inappropriately high. Should be 2 to 4 mg.
   - Albuterol (Proventil) inhaler is inappropriate. A better mode of delivery would be a small-volume nebulizer (SVN) given by a respiratory therapist (the patient is unlikely to have the coordination to properly use an inhaler).

   Instructor Note: The IV heparin drip will be adjusted to maintain PTT between 1.5 and 2.5 times the normal baseline. Warfarin (Coumadin) will be given 2 to 3 days before discontinuation of the heparin drip. The daily dose will be based on PT results.

All orders have been corrected. S.K.'s V/Q scan indicated a pulmonary embolism in the LLL, and antithrombolytic therapy was initiated. Repeat ABGs show the following values (these results reflect values at sea level): pH 7.45, $PaCO_2$ 35 mm Hg, PaO_2 82 mm Hg, HCO_3 24 mEq/L, BE -2.4 mEq/L, SaO_2 90%, A-a gradient 28 mm Hg.

7. What do these gases generally indicate? **[E/c/Pl/ct]**
   - S.K.'s ABGs are improving.

The physician orders Lasix 20 mg IV now.

8. Why do you think the physician ordered furosemide (Lasix) for S.K.? **[A/c/PI/ct]**
   - To prevent the onset of pulmonary edema, which is often a sequela of pulmonary embolism.

S.K. was watched very closely for the next several days for the onset of pulmonary edema. Thrombolytic therapy, oxygen, pulse oximetry, daily chest x-rays and blood gas analysis, and pain management were continued. When he was stable, S.K. was transferred back to your orthopedic unit.

9. The next day, S.K. suddenly exploded and threw the physical therapist out of his room. He yelled, "I'm sick and tired of having everyone tell me what to do." How are you going to deal with this situation? **[I/an/S,PI,PSI/ct,ni,tc]**
   - It is not uncommon for patients to become discouraged during a hospitalization and feel profound loss of control. This is often reflected in such emotions as helplessness, anger or depression. Behavioral manifestations of these emotional problems often include belligerence, withdrawal, hostility, or regressive behaviors. S.K.'s dignity as a human being and right to some control in his life should be recognized. Giving him a chance to talk in a supportive, noncritical environment may help. In addition, he should be offered some meaningful choices in his care to help him regain a sense of control. It is important to remember that the neurobiochemical effects of bed rest and some of the medications contribute to emotional lability. As much as possible, involve S.K. in his continued care, and show respect for his feelings and wishes.

Case Study 13: Disseminated Intravascular Coagulation

Difficulty: ***	*Setting:* Home care
Index Words: Disseminated intravascular coagulation	

D., a 38-year-old woman diagnosed with ruptured appendix, was hospitalized for an appendectomy. She developed peritonitis and was discharged 9 days later with a left peripherally-inserted central catheter (PICC line) to home care for IV antibiotic therapy. You work for the home care department for the hospital. You have been assigned to D.'s case, and this is your first home visit to her. You are to do a full assessment on D. During the assessment, you notice a large ecchymotic area over the right upper arm. You question her about the bruise and she tells you, "the nurses took my blood pressure so many times it bruised."

1. Do you accept D.'s explanation? Why or why not? **[A/c/Pl/ct]**
    - No, a blood pressure cuff should not induce this type of trauma.

In examining D. further, you find a fine, nonraised, dark red rash over her trunk.

2. What questions would you ask D. to elicit additional information? **[A/k/Pl/ct]**
    - How long has the rash been present?
    - Does it itch?
    - Does it hurt?
    - Has she ever had something like this before?

D. hadn't noticed the rash before you pointed it out. The rash does not itch or cause pain. She has never had one like it before.

3. What other information would you want to gather? **[A/c/Pl/ct]**
    - Look for signs of the rash on other areas of the body.
    - Get a full set of vital signs.
    - Ask D. if she is having any other symptoms.
    - Ask D. about any allergies she may have to anything.
    - Check what antibiotics D. was receiving in the hospital.
    - Check the surgical wound for integrity, drainage, and color.
    - Palpate the abdomen for tenderness.
    - Check the IV site for evidence of infection or infiltration.

The wound is not discolored or draining; the abdomen is not tender to deep palpation. There is oozing of serosanguinous fluid around the PICC insertion site. The rash is confined to the trunk. You have made a decision to call the physician regarding your assessment findings.

4. What vital information would you relay to the physician? **[A/an/Pl/ni]**
    - Brief history of the patient.
    - Ecchymosis on the right upper arm.
    - Truncal rash (describe).
    - Oozing around the IV insertion site.

The physician orders blood to be drawn for coagulation studies and a CBC with differential. He says he would like to evaluate D. for disseminated intravascular coagulation (DIC).

5. What laboratory tests would you expect to see performed in coagulation studies? **[PD/c/PI/ct]**
   - PT, PTT.
   - Fibrin split products.
   - Platelet count.
   - Fibrinogen level.
   - Clot retraction time.

You give D. her antibiotic, draw her blood, and take it to the lab. You return 6 hours later to administer another dose of antibiotics. D. greets you at the door very upset and ushers you to the bathroom where you find blood in the toilet. She tells you that she has been urinating blood for the past 2 or 3 hours. She also shows you a tissue in which she has bloody-appearing sputum. She tells you she has been coughing up blood. You notify the physician who instructs you call 911 and get the patient to the ED immediately. You call the ED and give report to the triage nurse on duty.

6. What are you going to tell the triage nurse? **[P/an/PI/ct,ni]**
   - Identify yourself and give the patient's name, age, and doctor. The patient is a 38-year-old woman who was discharged from the hospital yesterday after a 9-day stay for a ruptured appendix with subsequent peritonitis. You saw her today in her home and noted ecchymosis on her right upper arm and a rash on her trunk. The rest of her assessment was unremarkable. You notified the doctor, who ordered a coagulation profile and CBC with differential. You drew the blood and took it to the lab. When you went back 6 hours later, the patient was very upset and had been having hemoptysis and hematuria for approximately 2 to 3 hours. Her physician is sending her in to be evaluated. She is being brought in by ambulance with paramedic assistance. You tell the triage nurse that the physician suggests the patient may be developing disseminated intravascular coagulation (DIC).

7. Are the patient's presenting signs and symptoms consistent with DIC? Explain. **[PD/c/PI/ct]**
   - Yes. DIC is a syndrome with an unknown cause marked by widespread intravascular clotting which depletes both platelets and clotting factors, leading to profound hemorrhage. Presenting signs and symptoms are organ specific. This patient has presented with ecchymosis, petechiae, hematuria, and hemoptysis.

The following labs were prolonged: PT, PTT, split fibrin products, and D dimer. The following labs were decreased: platelets, platelet aggregation time, clot retraction time, and fibrinogen level. CBC is all within normal range, with the exception of the WBC, which is 12.5 mm^3, and platelet count, which is 46 mm^3. D. is diagnosed with DIC.

8. List 4 nursing diagnoses associated with DIC. **[PD/ap/S,PI,PSI/ct,ni]**
   - Fluid volume deficit r/t hemorrhage.
   - Altered urinary elimination r/t microthrombi.
   - Altered tissue perfusion r/t microthrombi.
   - Impaired gas exchange r/t pulmonary hemorrhage.
   - Risk for injury r/t abnormalities in clotting factors.
   - Fear r/t disabling illness and hospitalization.
   - Anxiety r/t insufficient knowledge of causes and treatment.

9. List at least 3 priority needs for D. **[P/an/S,PI,PSI/ct,ni,tc]**
   - High-flow oxygen therapy with 100% oxygen with a nonrebreather mask.
   - Fluid volume replacement with volume expanders such as lactated Ringer's solution, hetastarch (Hespan) and blood products.
   - Anticoagulant therapy with sodium heparin.
   - Emotional support for D. and her significant others.

D. was stabilized with oxygen, fluids, and blood products, and medication therapy was initiated. She was transferred to the ICU in guarded condition.

Instructor Note: The prognosis for someone with DIC is very poor.

Case Study 14: Open Pneumothorax

Difficulty: ***	*Setting:* Hospital ED
Index Words: Pneumothorax, trauma, respiratory distress	

You are the trauma nurse working in a busy tertiary care facility. You receive a call from the paramedics that they are en route to your facility with the victim of multiple gunshot wounds to the chest and abdomen. The paramedics have started two large-bore IV lines with LR, O_2 by mask at 15 L/minute. The patient has a sucking chest wound on the left and a wound in the upper right quadrant of the abdomen. Vital signs are 80/36, 140, 42. The patient is diaphoretic, very pale, and confused. ETA (estimated time of arrival) is 4 minutes.

1. List at least 6 things you are going to do to prepare for this patient's arrival. **[P/c/PI,ct]**
   - Call a "trauma code." Calling a trauma code will get personnel from the OR, laboratory, x-ray, respiratory therapy, and social services to the ED immediately. The trauma surgeon on call will also be alerted. The trauma code also alerts the ICU staff of a possible admission to their unit.
   - Set up a thoracostomy tray and chest drainage system setup in the trauma room.
   - Prepare the blood warmers and patient warming lights.
   - Have intubation equipment readily available.
   - Prepare a Foley catheter with a temperature probe for insertion.
   - Make sure high-flow trauma IV tubing is available.
   - Set up for arterial line and CVC (central venous catheter) insertion.
   - Set up for NG tube insertion.

On arrival to the ED, your patient, B.W., is cyanotic and in severe respiratory distress. When he is transferred to the trauma stretcher, you notice that there is an occlusive dressing over the sucking chest wound. It is taped down on all sides.

2. Is taping the occlusive dressing on all sides appropriate? Explain. **[PD/k/S,PI/ct]**
   - No, the occlusive dressing should be taped only on three sides, with one side left open for the escape of air from the chest, thus preventing a tension pneumothorax.

3. Who usually responds to a trauma code and what are the functions of the people from the various departments? **[PD/c/S,PI/ct]**
   - OR (anesthesiologist, OR nurse) will assess the patient situation and alert other OR personnel of the possibility of surgery.
   - Laboratory phlebotomist will draw all trauma lab blood and take it to the lab; trauma labs include clotting profile, CBC with diff, Chem 20, toxicology screen, blood alcohol level, type and cross for 4h WB.
   - X-ray to take portable chest x-rays and CT scans.
   - Respiratory therapy to intubate and manage the airway and draw ABGs.
   - Social services to act as a "crisis team" for family and significant others.

4. Prioritize the actions of the physicians and nurses in the trauma situation. **[A,PD,P,I,E/an/S,PI,PSI/ct,ni,tc]**
   - ED MD performs initial assessment (airway, breathing, circulation), insert chest tube, establish central lines, and monitor overall patient condition.
   - Trauma nurse performs initial assessment (airway, breathing, circulation), make sure all ordered procedures are carried out, place Foley catheter and NG tube, hang IV fluids and blood, assist with chest tube insertion, accompany patient to CT scan, monitor vital signs continuously, administer drugs, and precisely documents all patient care.

B.W. is to have a CT scan of the abdomen. His abdomen has become distended and rigid.

5. What are the possible reasons for the abdominal distention and rigidity? **[E/an/PI/ct]**
   - Blood, or blood plus air in the abdomen with peritoneal irritation.
   - Air in the stomach causing distention.

6. List 5 nursing diagnoses for this patient. **[PD/ap/S,PI/ct]**
   - Impaired gas exchange r/t actual injury.
   - Ineffective breathing pattern r/t tissue injury.
   - Fluid volume deficit r/t hemorrhage.
   - Pain r/t disrupted nerves and tissue.
   - High risk for altered tissue perfusion r/t hypovolemia and/or decreased cardiac output.
   - Anxiety r/t critical and possibly fatal illness.

The CT scan shows a large liver laceration. B.W. will be taken directly to the OR for an exploratory laparotomy with repair of liver laceration, then to the ICU. When you return from transporting the patient to the OR, B.W.'s wife is in the ED very upset and frightened. The social worker has been called to another emergency.

7. How would you interact with B.W.'s wife? **[I/an/PI/ni,tc]**
   - Take her to a quiet private place.
   - Explain what has happened to her husband and that he is in very serious condition.
   - See if there is anyone you can call to come and be with her.
   - Give her tissues, make her comfortable, offer her liquids, provide a phone for her use, and tell her to let you know if she needs any assistance.
   - Make sure she appears to be stable before directing her to the OR waiting room, and make sure the OR staff know she is on her way.

BIBLIOGRAPHY

Ackerman, L. (1992). Interventions related to neurologic care. *Nursing Clinics of North America, 27*(2), 325-346.

Acute Pain Management Guidline Panel. (1992). *Acute pain management: Operative or medical procedures & trauma. Clinical Practice Guideline*. Rockwell, MD: Agency for Health Care Policy & Research, Public Health Service, U. S. Department of Health and Human Services (AHCPR Pub. No. 92-0032).

American Diabetes Association. (1994). Nutrition recommendations and principles for people with diabetes mellitus (Position Statement). *Diabetes Care, 17*, 519-22.

American Heart Association. (1993). *Human blood pressure determination by sphygmometry.* Dallas, TX: Author.

American Thoracic Society/Center for Disease Control. (1990). Diagnostic standards and classification of tuberculosis. *American Review of Respiratory Disease, 142,* 725-735.

American Thoracic Society/Center for Disease Control. (1994). Treatment of tuberculosis and tuberculosis infections in adults and children. *American Journal of Respiratory Critical Care Medicine: 149,* 1359-1374.

Bachman, D. (1992). The diagnosis and management of common neurologic sequelae of closed head injury. *Journal of Head Trauma Rehabilitation, 7*(2), 50-59.

Baldwin, K., Seftchick, C., Martin, R., Sheriff, S., & Hanssen, G. (1995). *Davis's manual of critical care therapeutics.* Philadelphia: Davis.

Bartlett, J. (1995-1996). *Pocketbook of infectious disease therapy.* Baltimore: Williams & Wilkins.

Bates, B. (1991). *A pocket guide to physical examination and history taking.* Philadelphia: J. B. Lippincott.

Barton Burke, M., Wilkes, G., Berg, D., Bean, C., & Ingwersen, K. (1991). *Cancer chemotherapy: A nursing process approach.* Boston: Jones & Bartlett.

Beare, P. G., & Myers, J. L. (1994). *Adult health nursing.* St. Louis: Mosby.

Berkow, R. (Ed.). (1992). *The Merck manual of diagnosis and therapy* (16th ed.). Rahway, NJ: Merck.

Berne, R., & Levy, M. (1992). *Cardiovascular physiology* (6th Ed.). St. Louis: Mosby.

Brown, W. V. (1994). Lipoprotein disorders in diabetes mellitus. *Medical Clinics of North America, 78,* 143-161.

Brooks, S., Gochfeld, M., Herzstein, J., Schenker, M., & Jackson, R. (1995). *Environmental medicine.* St. Louis: Mosby.

Bryant, R. A. (Ed.), (1992) *Acute and chronic wounds, nursing management.* St. Louis: Mosby.

Burden, N. (1993). *Ambulatory surgical nursing.* Philadelphia: Saunders.

Burrell, L. O. (1992). *Adult nursing in hospital and community setting.* Norwalk, CT: Appleton & Lange.

Carlson, K. J., Eisenstat, S. A., Frigoletto, F. D., & Schiff, I. (Eds). (1995). *Primary care of women.* St. Louis: Mosby.

Carpenito, L. J. (1995). *Nursing diagnosis: Application to clinical practice* (6th ed.). Philadelphia: Lippincott.

Clark, J., & McGee, R. (1993). *Core curiculum for oncology nursing* (2nd ed.). Philadelphia: Saunders.

Clark, J. B. F., Queener, S. F., & Karb, V. B. (1993). *Pharmacologic basis of nursing practice.* St. Louis: Mosby.

Copstead, L. (1995). *Perspectives on pathophysiology.* Philadelphia: Saunders.

Cubbin, J. (1992). Managing resources in the community. *Nursing Standard, 7*(10), 31-34.

Cuzzell, J. Z. (1993) The right way to culture a wound. *AJN, 93*(5) 48-50.

Deglin, J., & Vallerand, A. (1993). *Davis's drug guide for nurses* (4th ed.). Philadelphia: Davis.

Devinsky, O. (1994). Seizure disorders. *Clinical Symposia, 46*(1), 2-34.

Devita, V., Hellman, S., & Rosenberg, S. (1993). *Cancer: Principles and practice of oncology* (4th ed.). Philadelphia: Lippincott.

Dodd, M. (1991). *Managing the side effects of chemotherapy and radiation.* New York: Prentice Hall.

Doughty, D., & Jackson, D. (1993) *Gastrointestinal disorders.* St. Louis: Mosby.

Driscoll, C., Bope, E., Smith, C., & Carter, B. (1996). *The family practice desk reference.* St. Louis: Mosby.

Expert Panel Report (1991). *Executive summary: Guidelines for the diagnosis and management of asthma.* National Heart, Lung, and Blood Institute, National Institutes of Health. U. S. Department of Health and Human Services. Bethesda, MD: U. S. Government Printing Services.

Fischbach, F. (1995) *Quick reference to common laboratory and diagnostic tests.* Philadelphia: Lippincott.

Folden, S. (1994). Managing the effects of a stroke: The first months. *Rehabilitation Nursing Research, 3*(3), 79-85.

Frederick, C., & Hotter, A. (1991). Discharge planning for the head-injured patient. *Critical Care Nurse, 11*(6), 42-45.

Goldberg, L., & Elliot, D. (1994). *Exercise for prevention and treatment of illness.* Philadelphia: Davis.

Groenwald, S., Frogge, M., Goodman, M., & Yarbro, C. (1993). *Cancer nursing: Principles and practice* (3rd ed.). Boston: Jones & Bartlett.

Haire-Joshu, D. (1992). *Management of diabetes mellitus: Perspectives of care across the life span.* St. Louis: Mosby.

Halstead, L. S., & Grimby, G. (1995). *Post-polio syndrome.* Philadelphia: Hanley & Belfus, Inc.

Hollander, P., Castle, G., Joynes, J. O., & Nelson, J. (1990). *Intensified insulin management for you: A personal program for advanced diabetes self-care.* Minneapolis, MN: Chronimed Publishing. [The authors are part of the International Diabetes Center in Minneapolis, MN, one of the centers involved in the Diabetes Complications and Control Trial.]

Holloway, B. (1996). *Stat facts: The clinical pocket reference for nurses.* Philadelphia: Davis.

Hudak, C., & Gallo, B. (1994). *Critical care nursing: A holistic approach.* Philadelphia: Lippincott.

International Diabetes Center. (1994). *Nutrition and diabetes: Implementing the 1994 American Diabetes Association nutrition recommendations.* Minnesota: International Diabetes Center.

Jardins, T., & Burton, G. (1995). *Clinical manifestations and assessment of respiratory disease.* St. Louis: Mosby.

Kim, M., McFarland, G., & McLane, A. (1995). *Pocket guide to nursing diagnoses* (6th ed.). St. Louis: Mosby.

Kinney, M., & Packa, D. (1996). *Andreoli's comprehensive cardiac care* (8th ed.). St. Louis: Mosby.

Kersten, L. (1989). *Comprehensive respiratory nursing.* Philadelphia: Saunders.

Lanros, N. E. (1988). *Assessment and intervention in emergency nursing.* Norwalk, CT: Appleton & Lange.

Lewis, J. (1994). *A pharmacologic approach to gastrointestinal disorders.* Baltimore, MD: Williams & Wilkins.

Lewis, S. M., & Collier, I. C. (1992). Renal and urological problems. In S. M. Lewis & I. C. Collier (Eds.), *Medical-surgical nursing: Assessment and management of clinical problems* (4th ed.). St. Louis: Mosby.

Lipman, M. M. (1993, June). Kidney stones: Painfully common, but preventable. *Consumer Report on Health,* 67.

Marrelli, T. (1994). *Handbook of home health standards and documentation guidelines for reimbursement* (2nd ed). St. Louis: Mosby.

McCance, K. L., & Huether, S. E. (1994). *Pathophysiology: The biological basis for disease in adults and children.* St. Louis: Mosby.

McCloskey, J. C., & Bulechek, G. M. (Eds.). (1992). *Iowa intervention project: Nursing interventions classification (NIC).* St. Louis: Mosby.

Metheny, N., Reed, L., Wiersema, L., McSweeney, M., Wehrle, M., & Clark, J. (1993). Effectiveness of pH measurements in predicting feeding tube placement: An update. *Nursing Research, 42*(6), 324-331.

Miller, C., & Hens, M. (1993). Multiple sclerosis: A literature review. *Journal of Neuroscience Nursing, 25*(3), 174-179.

Murphy, G., Lawrence, W., & Lenhard, R. (1995). *American Cancer Society textbook of clinical oncology* (2nd ed.). Georgia: The American Cancer Society.

National Asthma Education Program: Expert Panel Report. (1991). *Executive summary: Guidelines for the diagnosis and management of asthma.* National Heart, Lung, and Blood Institute (Publ. No. 91-3042A). Bethesda, MD: U. S. Government Printing Services.

National Cholesterol Education Program. (1993). *Second report of the National Cholesterol Education Program on detection, evaluation and treatment of high blood cholesterol in adults (adult treatment panel II).* National Heart, Lung, Blood Institute (USDHHS Publ. No. 93-3095). Bethesda, MD: U. S. Government Printing Services.

Neufeld, R. (1993). Human determination: A cherished ally in rehabilitation. *Rehabilitation Nursing, 18*(5), 326-237.

Office of Disease Prevention and Health Promotion, NIH, DHHS. (1994). *Clinician's handbook of preventive services.* Bethesda, MD: U. S. Government Printing Services.

Otto, S. (1994). *Oncology nursing* (2nd ed.). St. Louis: Mosby.

Pagana, K., & Pagana, T. (1995). *Mosby's diagnostic and laboratory test infobase.* St. Louis: Mosby.

Paul, R. (1993). *Paper prepared for the National Council for Excellence in Critical Thinking.* Sonoma State University, Rohnert Park, CA.

Phipps, W., Cassmeyer, V., Sands, J., & Lehman, M. (1995). *Medical surgical nursing-concepts and clinical practice* (5th ed.). St. Louis: Mosby

Physician's drug handbook (6th ed.). (1995). Springhouse, PA: Springhouse.

Price, S. A., & Wilson, M. W., (1992). *Pathophysiology: Clinical concepts of disease processes.* St. Louis: Mosby.

Report of the U. S. Preventive Services Task Force. (1989). *Guide to clinical preventive services: An assessment of the effectiveness of 169 interventions.* Baltimore: William & Wilkins.

Rubenstein, E., & Federman, D. (1995). *Scientific American medicine.* New York: Scientific American, Inc.

Schroeder, S., Tierney, L., McPhee, S., Papadakis, M., & Krupp, M., (1992). *Current medical diagnosis and treatment.* Norwalk, CT: Appleton & Lange

Shannon, M. T., & Wilson, B. A. (1992). *Drugs and nursing implications.* Norwalk, CT: Appleton & Lange.

Sheehy, S., & Jimmerson, C. (1994). *Manual of clinical trauma care.* St. Louis: Mosby.

Siconolfi, L. (1995) Clarifying the complexity of liver function tests. *Nursing 95, 25*(5), 39-43.

Skidmore-Roth, L. (1995). *Mosby's nursing drug infobase.* St. Louis: Mosby.

Sloane, E. (1993). *Biology of women* (3rd ed.). Department of Biological Sciences, University of Wisconsin. Milwaukee: Delmar.

Stein, J. (1994). *Internal Medicine* (4th ed.). St. Louis: Mosby.

Su, S. A. (1992). Nursing management of the larynx and tracheobronchial tree. In L. O. Burrell (Ed), *Adult nursing in hospital and community settings* (p. 755). Norwalk, CT: Appleton & Lange.

Thelan, L. A., Davie, J. K., Urden, L. D., & Lough, M. E. (1994). *Critical care nursing: Diagnosis and management.* St. Louis: Mosby.

Thompson, J. M., McFarland, G. K., Hirsh, J. E., & Tucker, S.M . (1993) Nosocomial infections. In *Mosby's clinical nursing series* (3rd ed.). St. Louis: Mosby.

Urban, N. A., Greenlee, K. K., Krumberger, J. M., & Winkelman, C. (1995). *Guidelines for critical care nursing.* St. Louis: Mosby.

Vogt, G., Miller, M., & Esluer, M. (1985). Mosby's manual of neurological care. St. Louis: Mosby.

Wachtel, T., & Stein, M. (1995). *Practical guide to the care of the ambulatory patient.* St. Louis: Mosby.

Wilson, B., Shannon, M., & Stang, C. (1995). *Nurses drug guide.* Norwalk, CT: Appleton & Lange.

Wright, J., & Shelton, B. (1993).*Desk reference for critical care nursing.* Boston: Jones & Bartlett.

Wyngaarden, J., Smith, L., & Bennett, J. (1992). *Cecil textbook of medicine* (19th ed., vol. I & II). Philadelphia: Saunders.

Zollo, A. (1995). *The portable internist.* St. Louis: Mosby.

INDEX

CASE STUDY PREPSHEET

Name: ______________________ Date: __________ Case: ________

Symbols/terms abbreviations	Meaning/definition

Diagnoses (+current and -past)	Description of diagnosis

Laboratory tests and diagnostic procedures	What is it and why is it done?

Drugs	Generic name, class, indications, contraindications, significant side effects, food and drug interactions

Notes, observations, comments.

CRITICAL THINKING IN MEDICAL/SURGICAL SETTINGS: EVALUATION/PROBLEM REPORT

Your comments are essential to the further development of this and similar books. Please share your thoughts—both positive and negative—about the material in this book.

Date: ______________________________

Name: ______________________________

Title: ______________________________

Institution: ______________________________

Address: ______________________________

City: ______________________________ State: ______ Zip: ____________

Telephone: ____________________ FAX: ____________________

E-MAIL: ______________________________

Class/Level Taught: ______________________________

Area of clinical practice/specialty/research expertise: ______________________________

____

____

What did you find useful about this book?

☐ Variety of cases ☐ Layout of this book ☐ Clinical relevance

☐ Instructor comments ☐ Other ______________________________

Please clarify the above responses: ______________________________

____

____

Did you find any errors in this book? If so, which chapter, case, page, and question. Please provide a reference for the correct answer. ______________________________

____

____

____

What aspects of this book would you like to see changed and why? ______________________________

____

____

What could we do to make this book more useful to you? ______________________________

____

____

What other books/topics would you like added to this series? ______________________________

____

____

Thank you for your comments! If you ever are at a meeting where either of us (Winningham or Preusser) are present, please introduce yourself and share your experiences with us.

M.L.W. & B.A.P.